Sociality is what it means to be human; it underpins love, solidarity and social rights. Through this engaging exposition Hartley Dean beautifully finesses his long-standing commitment to social rights. He takes the reader to an alternative humanistic framing of the practical, philosophical and post-national realisation of the meeting of human needs.

Fiona Williams, *Emeritus Professor of Social Policy, University of Leeds*

In his new and fascinating book, Hartley Dean augments his earlier work on needs and social rights with an analysis of sociality which refers to the inherent aptitude of human beings for cooperation, care and interdependence. Encapsulating complex ideas in an all-embracing and novel narrative, the book makes a major contribution to welfare theory.

James Midgley, *Professor of Public Services, University of California*

While the world is searching for non-exploitative models of co-living, this book comes as a stimulating breeze, instilling confidence in our search for innovative solutions in a world of inequality. The book is a comprehensive examination of the idea of sociality, whose philosophical foundations are re-examined to provide a new lens.

Sony Pelissery, *Professor, National Law School of India University*

SOCIALITY

This book develops a very particular concept of sociality: a holistic way of understanding how human beings have come to care about and collectively provide for their welfare as a species and to recognise each other's needs in terms of shared social rights. It tells not so much a success story as a hopeful story. It provides a new way of looking at how our rights to life's essentials have been in the past, are now and can in the future be understood. It is, potentially, a book for anyone interested in the human condition but will be especially interesting for those engaged in human service provision, community action, social development, welfare law and political debate, and particularly useful to students of social policy and human rights.

It is a radically revised edition of *Social Rights and Human Welfare*, first published in 2015. It provides modified, re-organised and updated versions of chapters from that book while offering a wholly new underlying narrative through which further to develop and apply the author's alternative theory of social rights. It is a book about the connections between social rights and human welfare; between theory and practice; between debate and reality in the spheres of human service provision and human livelihoods.

Hartley Dean is an Emeritus Professor of Social Policy at the London School of Economics. He had for 12 years been a welfare rights worker in Brixton, South London, before moving on to a 40-year academic career researching, teaching and writing about social justice issues.

SOCIALITY

Social Rights and Human Welfare

Revised Edition

Hartley Dean

Routledge
Taylor & Francis Group
LONDON AND NEW YORK

Designed cover image: PeterPencil / Getty Images 1290118946

Revised edition published 2025
by Routledge
4 Park Square, Milton Park, Abingdon, Oxon, OX14 4RN

and by Routledge
605 Third Avenue, New York, NY 10158

Routledge is an imprint of the Taylor & Francis Group, an informa business

First Edition Published 2015 by Routledge

British Library Cataloguing-in-Publication Data
A catalogue record for this book is available from the British Library

Library of Congress Cataloging-in-Publication Data
Names: Dean, Hartley, 1949- author.
Title: Sociality : social rights and human welfare / Hartley Dean.
Other titles: Social rights and human welfare
Description: Revised edition. | Abingdon, Oxon ; New York, NY : Routledge, 2025. | Earlier edition published in 2015 as: Social rights and human welfare. | Includes bibliographical references and index. |
Identifiers: LCCN 2024031129 (print) | LCCN 2024031130 (ebook) | ISBN 9781032587912 (hardback) | ISBN 9781032587905 (paperback) | ISBN 9781003451518 (ebook)
Subjects: LCSH: Social rights. | Social policy. | Public welfare. | Social rights--Great Britain. | Great Britain--Social policy. | Public welfare--Great Britain.
Classification: LCC HM671 .D384 2025 (print) | LCC HM671 (ebook) | DDC 361.6/14--dc23/eng/20240816
LC record available at https://lccn.loc.gov/2024031129
LC ebook record available at https://lccn.loc.gov/2024031130

ISBN: 978-1-032-58791-2 (hbk)
ISBN: 978-1-032-58790-5 (pbk)
ISBN: 978-1-003-45151-8 (ebk)

DOI: 10.4324/9781003451518

Typeset in Sabon
by KnowledgeWorks Global Ltd.

To Brendan and Nicola,
to whom I dedicated my very first book
over 30 years ago

CONTENTS

ILLUSTRATIONS

Figures

Tables

Boxes

BY THE SAME AUTHOR

SOCIAL SECURITY AND SOCIAL CONTROL, 1991

DEPENDENCY CULTURE: THE EXPLOSION OF A MYTH, *with Peter Taylor-Gooby*, 1992

PARENTS' DUTIES, CHILDREN'S DEBTS: THE LIMITS OF POLICY INTERVENTION, *Editor*, 1995

WELFARE, LAW AND CITIZENSHIP, 1996

POVERTY, RICHES AND SOCIAL CITIZENSHIP, *with Margaret Melrose*, 1999

BEGGING QUESTIONS: STREET LEVEL ECONOMIC ACTIVITY AND SOCIAL POLICY FAILURE, *Editor*, 1999

WELFARE RIGHTS AND SOCIAL POLICY, 2002

THE ETHICS OF WELFARE: HUMAN RIGHTS, DEPENDENCY AND RESPONSIBILITY, *Editor*, 2004

SOCIAL POLICY, 2006, 2009 and 2012 (also in Chinese language editions)

SOCIAL RIGHTS AND HUMAN WELFARE, 2015

SOCIAL ADVANTAGE AND DISADVANTAGE, Editor *with Lucinda Platt*, 2016

UNDERSTANDING HUMAN NEED, 2010 and 2020

ACRONYMS

ALA	Alliance for Legal Aid
BNA	Basic Needs Approach
CESCR	Committee on Economic, Social and Cultural Rights
CESCR	Committee on Economic, Social and Cultural Rights
CPAG	Child Poverty Action Group
CRAE	Child Rights Alliance for England
CROP	Comparative Research on Poverty
DRtD	Declaration of the Right to Development
ECHR	European Court of Human Rights
ECOSOC	Economic and Social Council (of the United Nations)
HRC	Human Rights Council (of the United Nations)
ICCPR	International Covenant on Civil and Political Rights
ICESCR	International Covenant on Economic, Social and Cultural Rights
ILO	International Labour Organisation
IMF	International Monetary Fund
MDGs	Millennium Development Goals
NCC	National Consumer Council
NEF	New Economics Foundation
NGO	Non-Governmental Organisation
NHS	National Health Service
OECD	Organisation for Economic Co-operation and Development
OHCHR	Office of the High Commissioner for Human Rights
SDGs	Sustainable Development Goals
SSHRL	Spanish Society for Human Rights Law
UDHR	Universal Declaration of Human Rights

UK	United Kingdom (of Great Britain and Northern Ireland)
UN	United Nations
UNCRC	United Nations Convention on the Rights of the Child
UNDP	United Nations Development Programme
UNESCO	United Nations Educational, Science and Cultural Organisation
UN-HABITAT	United Nations Human Settlements Programme
UNODC	United Nations Office on Drugs and Crime
US	United States (of America)
WBG	Women's Budget Group
WHO	World Health Organisation
WTO	World Trade Organisation

PREFACE

This book develops a very particular concept of **sociality**: a holistic way of understanding how human beings have come to care about and collectively provide for their welfare as a species and to recognise each other's needs in terms of shared social rights. It tells not so much a success story as a hopeful story. It provides a new way of looking at how our rights to life's essentials have been in the past, are now and can in the future be understood.

It is, potentially, a book for anyone interested in the human condition but will be especially interesting for those engaged in human service provision, community action, social development, welfare law and political debate, and particularly useful to students of social policy and human rights.

Background

This particular book has evolved over a period of nearly 30 years, having appeared in different guises as *Welfare, Law and Citizenship* (1996), *Welfare Rights and Social Policy* (2002) and – tentatively offering a new theory of social rights – as *Social Rights and Human Welfare* (2015). The volume you now hold is a 10th-anniversary revision of the immediately preceding edition, newly entitled *Sociality*, while retaining *Social Rights and Human Welfare* as its sub-title. It provides modified, re-organised and updated versions of substantive chapters from past editions, but it offers a wholly new underlying narrative through which to expand the conception of 'sociality' as a foundation on which further to develop and apply the author's alternative theory of social rights, a theory grounded in the realities of the human condition and of human sociality. Sociality is a term drawn from anthropological philosophy, which captures an essential characteristic of the human species and relates to the expectations and practices by which human communities engage with Nature and with one another. It captures a perspective that can reach across disciplinary boundaries and perceptions and provoke new debates. This is explained in an entirely new introductory chapter, and the argument culminates in a substantially recrafted concluding chapter.

For any reader who may be familiar with the book's past versions and/or in any event with the theoretical and practical topics they covered, the chapters that top and tail this edition might be read on their own. Indeed, for anyone with a general or specific interest in humanist thinking, these chapters might serve as stand-alone essays. The intermediate Chapters (2-10) may perhaps be more selectively accessed by readers according to their specialised interests. It should be stressed, however, that these chapters have not merely been updated but freshly inflected so as to incorporate the significance of sociality within the guiding narrative: they serve as accessible but specialised examinations of theory and practice in relation to key areas of social policy and welfare law, and extensive referencing is provided to enable readers to pursue specific topics in greater detail.

Concluding his review of the 2015 edition of *Social Rights and Human Welfare*, Mike Adler concluded, with some justice, that:

> The test of good theory is not whether or not just whether it puts forward an alternative conceptualisation of reality, however attractive that alternative may be, but, rather, whether it can help us to explain or change some aspect of the real world. Although there is much that can be learned from *Social Rights and Human Welfare*, when judged in these terms, it falls somewhat short.
>
> *(European Journal of Social Security, 2017, Vol. 19(1) – p. 85)*

The same may be said by some, perhaps, about this revised and expanded edition, though I would contend that developing the concept of sociality does help us to explain the relationship between social rights and human welfare in a 'real world' context. Whether it will help to change that world remains to be seen. In arguing for a fundamental switch in perception, this book offers not a solution but a challenge. Sociality, I would contend, is a concept that could and should be central to social policy.

Acknowledgements

I am grateful to Mike Adler for the review mentioned above, but also, having regard for the generous encouragement, support, reflection, criticism and advice that they have severally in different moments and in various ways provided to Tania Burchardt, the late Vic George, Ian Gough, Suyoung Kim, James Midgely, David Piachaud, Hakan Seckinelgin, Peter Taylor-Gooby and Fiona Williams. There are many others whom I have to thank, including

Pam for her unfailing love (and proofreading). And I should particularly mention the diverse cohorts of interested and interesting students who took the *Social Rights and Human Welfare* MSc option course that I taught for 14 years at the London School of Economics (through which I learnt as much as I taught) and, by no means least, erstwhile colleagues at the Brixton Advice Centre (where, long ago, I first engaged with social rights and human welfare issues).

1

HUMAN SOCIALITY

This book offers a new way of thinking about social rights and human welfare. Its premise is that rights – in particular, 'social rights' – are human constructs; conceptual inventions that specify essential requirements for individual well-being and relate more widely to collective social welfare provision. Social rights – as distinct from civil and political rights – may be understood as an articulation of human needs. However, properly to understand this, we should first reflect upon what it is that human beings definitively need in order to *be* human and how it is that, unlike any other species, human beings have come to conceptualise and articulate *rights* as a basis for the way in which they relate to and look after one another. The answer, it will be argued, lies in the interpretation of our essential 'sociality'. Sociality is concerned with the ways in which humans attend to each other's welfare and includes the construction and recognition of social rights.

Sociality as a word has lately been loosely used as a synonym for 'sociability', but its origin is traced by Axel Honneth (2017, p. 6) to the mid-seventeenth century, when, in the context of disputes as to the foundations of natural law, Hugo Grotius (b.1583–d.1645) contended that legal order in human society is rightly to be founded not on divine revelation but on human 'sociality'. Grotius' contention was that human nature is constituted through an interaction between competing drives, on the one hand for self-preservation, but on the other hand for sociality – that is, to say social connectedness and interdependency. These competing drives entail both rational desires and emotive impulses, which, in the interests of freedom, according to Grotius, may be mediated by law (see Miller, 2021). Honneth suggests that Grotius' notion of sociality was largely subsumed in the eighteenth and nineteenth centuries by the emergence of new strands of thinking within socialist

DOI: 10.4324/9781003451518-1

movements, which demanded more than just formal, legally defined individual freedoms but substantive, effectively supported social freedoms.

In the twentieth century, emergent notions of 'inter-subjectivity', for example in philosophy (Levinas, 1969) and developmental psychology (Vygotsky, 1978), captured other elements of Grotius' juxtaposition between the historical materiality of the human struggle for existence and the intersubjective sensibility by which humans can, uniquely in Nature, *consciously* transcend narrow or utilitarian self-interest. Most recently, Michael Tomasello (2021) has advanced the concept of 'ontogenetic sociality', by which he interrogates the link between the species-specific development of the individual human organism and the process of socialisation. Biological evolution, Tomasello contends, has prepared humans for unique forms of socio-cultural activity that must then be developed in each human individual as they socially mature, as they begin to relate to others and as they become co-operative, group-minded and morally responsible. Sociality is a distinctive characteristic of the human species: a premise at odds with claims (e.g. by Dawkins, 1976) that human beings are genetically predisposed to selfishness. There are other ostensibly social animals that live in herds or packs, but as Aristotle asserted, the human being is uniquely a *zöon politikon*, a term for which sociality has also been regarded as a synonym (Klein, 2011). *Zöon politikon* may be translated from classical Greek as 'social animal' as much as 'political animal', and Karl Marx contended this to be so in a most literal sense since human beings can only individuate themselves 'in the midst of society' (1857, p. 84).

This chapter will briefly consider:

- Just how humans emerged in Nature as a distinctively *un*natural species.
- An historically contextualised explanation of human sociality that may be distilled and developed from Marx's philosophical writings and, following from this, a discussion of the dynamics and dimensions of sociality in human beings' struggle for mutual recognition.
- The processes by which sociality may be mediated and obscured.

The chapter will conclude with an outline of the rest of this book, showing how the analysis set out here can be applied in relation to the theoretical and practical aspects of social rights and human welfare provision.

Homo sapiens: the unnatural species

Aristotle (c. 350 BCE) had sought to draw a categorical distinction between humans and other animals, regarding humans as a species apart from Nature, albeit one that exists *within* Nature. Charles Darwin (1871) observed that human beings, though descended from primates, possessed characteristics including 'moral sense' or 'conscience' that, he contended, distinguished them from the 'lower' animals. He noted that while there are other animals that exhibit 'sympathy' towards and take pleasure in society with other members of their own species, only humans can, with certainty, be ranked as 'moral beings'. Darwin observed in the human species characteristics attributable not necessarily to natural selection but to 'social instincts' and 'habits' developed and sustained by transmission from generation to generation. Modern biologists widely accept that the transmission of human behaviours is, in part at least, social or cultural rather than biological. Even Richard Dawkins (mentioned above) acknowledges this, invoking the term 'memes' to describe units of cultural transmission, akin to genes as units of biological transmission, that provide a means of copying behavioural characteristics from generation to generation.

From foraging

It is generally accepted that anatomically 'modern' humans (*homo sapiens*) had first appeared around 130–150,000 years ago in Africa, although various earlier hominin species in various parts of the world had existed for perhaps 2 million years and had already begun, for example, to develop tools and make controlled use of fire. Archaeologists, anthropologists and prehistorians consider that it was the development by *homo sapiens* of fictive language around perhaps 70,000 years ago that precipitated a 'Cognitive Revolution' (Harari, 2011) by enabling humans to communicate to one another not only about the material things they could see, hear or smell but also about what they were thinking and feeling. In relatively small foraging bands, it is assumed, they colonised different pockets of the world, hunting efficiently with bows and arrows, fishing and travelling in boats and developing ever more elaborate forms of language, communication and storytelling. However, the beginnings of the species were characterised as much by its unique social characteristics as its intelligence. The nomadic hunter-gatherer communities in which they lived were able to adapt and develop methods of social co-operation in advance of those of earlier species, taking advantage of brains with a proportionately larger neocortex (Dunbar & Shultz, 2007).

Established accounts of how human society developed from such beginnings have lately been questioned – especially, for example, by Graeber and Wengrow (2022), who contend that human beings never lived in a 'State of Nature'. There had never been an original form of human society which, according to opposing views, has been either corrupted or enhanced as a result of 'civilisation' and/or by the sheer scale and complexity achieved in later forms of human society. It is clear that early human societies were creative and collaborative, but they were far from uniform, and it is important not to generalise when telling the story of humankind. Human beings developed and manifested a range of different ways in which to organise themselves.

The paragraphs that follow contain a highly selective thumbnail sketch that demonstrates early humans' essential propensities for what we shall call 'sociality', albeit that such propensities were not necessarily fully or beneficially realised.

It has been suggested that early foraging communities were relatively egalitarian in the way they distributed food and conducted exchanges of gifts and goods amongst themselves (Sahlins, 1974). Inferences drawn from ethnographic studies of surviving indigenous kinship groups indicate they were or had tended in the past to be matrilineal, and that day-to-day social relations equated to a form of what might be termed 'primitive' communism (Engels, 1884; Morgan, 1887). Social relations appear to have been characteristically or in part matriarchal and by and large non-hierarchical. Some early human societies are thought to have adopted social strategies by which to constrain the tendencies to disruptive hierarchical dominance that typify some of our biological forebears (Boehm, 1993). While some groups or tribes may have appointed 'chiefs', their functions did not necessarily accord great privilege or enduring power since they would be restricted to particular seasons of the year or to particular roles as pacifiers or mediators (Graeber & Wengrow, 2022). While hunter-gatherers may have struggled for survival at particular times and during particular seasons, at others, they could clearly enjoy an abundance of food and did not seek to generate or accumulate a surplus of provision.

Thus, *homo sapiens* could also be a playful species (Huizinga, 1949), with time for curiosity, experimentation and learning; for feasting, assemblies, games, rituals and the construction of monuments; quite literally, for re-creation. Some commentators point to a flowering capacity for the representation of abstract and symbolic thought – a 'Dawn of Culture' (Klein & Edgars, 2002) – that occurred perhaps 40–50,000 years ago. It is not necessarily clear whether particular developments at this time resulted from relatively sudden (in evolutionary terms) genetic mutations or whether it had been changing circumstances that unleashed aspects of *homo sapiens'* latent cognitive capacity. It was as recently as 13,000 years ago, however, that *homo sapiens* finally outcompeted other hominin species and became the only humans on Earth. The Neanderthals, with whom *homo sapiens* had hitherto coexisted and (to a limited extent interbred), were in many aspects at least as sophisticated in their behaviour as *homo sapiens*. In fact, they had slightly bigger brains and were arguably more creative, albeit less socially efficient (Slimak, 2023). Rutger Bregman (2020) speculates that it was *homo sapiens'* unique capacity for social co-operation that enabled them to out-survive the Neanderthals. He draws on Belyaev's (1979) celebrated experiments by which, through an intensive programme of selective breeding, wild foxes were transformed into domesticated pets. The characteristic for which the foxes were selected was 'friendliness'. The resulting animals were not only more 'friendly' (to humans as well as each other) but more playful, retaining certain puppy-like characteristics and amenability to social adaptation. Selective breeding can 'artificially' achieve – or at least illustrate – changes that might take millennia to occur through 'natural' selection, and citing the work of Belyaev and others, Bregman (2020, p. 65) argues that dogs are to wolves what we are to Neanderthals. The idea that human beings are distinguished by the way they can creatively play together – and *therefore* more effectively work together – is a partial key to the concept of sociality that we are here developing.

To farming

Around perhaps 12,000 years ago – to differing extents and in disparate parts of the world – *homo sapiens* initiated the beginnings of a second revolution, the so-called 'Agricultural Revolution',[1] which entailed a change in the means by which human beings engaged with the natural world but also some fundamental changes to the ways in which human societies were therefore organised. This transition was neither instant nor universal. It took a further 3,000 years for farming fully to develop. Some foragers became farmers, cultivating crops, domesticating animals and establishing permanent settlements. The transition enabled the feeding of ever larger groups of humans and the production of surpluses that could be exchanged or traded with other groups of humans. Paradoxically, the transition from foraging to farming could sometimes make life less rather than more secure. It tied humans to their chosen lands, making them dependent on a narrower range of food sources and vulnerable to seasonal famines. The laying of claims to land as exclusive property opened the door to disputes regarding ownership and to territorial conflicts. As the scale and process of food production became far more labour-intensive, societies became increasingly hierarchical in their organisation and in the way they were regulated. Forms of slavery emerged as rulers and elites took control.

With the beginnings of written language around 4–5,000 years ago came the dawn of *recorded* history and our historical account of human 'civilisation', from which we may now draw evidence for the development of cities and states; of kingdoms, conquests and empires; of a variety of formal belief systems through which to explain, maintain and justify the particular social orders into which successive generations of human beings were born. Discrete and diverse centres of civilisation emerged in Mesopotamia, ancient Egypt and parts of what are now known as India, China and Latin America, as well as, of course, Europe. In the 'Classical' civilisations of Athens and Rome, the concept of private ownership and the written laws by which it could be governed were expanded so as to encompass a transition from matrilineality to patrilineality and the creation of the patriarchal family or household form in which the patriarchal head was the owner not only of family land and chattels but also the family's female members and its slaves, with the 'freedom' to dispose of them as he pleased. Human societies are increasingly interconnected not only through languages but also through trade, with the development in place of gift exchange and/or barter of money as a medium of exchange and as a means for conceptualising and defining relative value. Throughout much of the world, in the 11½,000 years covered by the period of the so-called 'Agricultural Revolution', humanity changed, but not to the benefit of the greater part of the human population. Wealth and power became vested in small (male dominated) minorities, while the majority were subject to forms of serfdom or slavery. The dynamics of human sociality changed. Day-to-day social interdependency remained focused in much of the world around an immediate family, with less emphasis on wider kinship groupings or tribes. Wider social provision for human needs was restricted, depending by and large on notions of charitable relief informed by diverse religious enjoinders and by notions of *noblesse oblige* (that is to say, often capricious interpretations of the obligations owed by the rich and powerful to the poor and powerless).

To enlightenment?

What is acclaimed as the next great step for human civilisation came with a 'Scientific Revolution' which began around 500 years ago from what in the Common Era (CE) we now call the sixteenth century. This was the era of (an essentially) European 'Enlightenment', when philosophers stepped beyond the bounds of the Classical era and embraced the cause of scientific inquiry, discovery and the rule of reason. The resulting advances in knowledge and scientific understanding would lead over the next 300 years to the burgeoning of new technologies and increased control over Nature, while the quest for knowledge justified global exploration leading to European conquests of the Americas and extensive tracts of the southern hemisphere, the development of global trade and the rise of capitalist imperialism. Yet even within the era of the 'Enlightenment', the philosopher Blaise Pascal observed that the human being had become a chimaera: 'a novelty, a monstrosity, chaotic, contradictory, prodigious, judge of all things, feeble earthworm, bearer of truth, mine of uncertainty and error, glory and refuse of the universe!' (1670).

Amongst the discoveries made by European colonisers were the ways of life once led by the indigenous peoples who, in the name of progress, they subdued and/or displaced. Those indigenous peoples could for their part question whether the way of life offered by 'enlightened' European society represented social progress in relation to that which they already or had once enjoyed, see examples in Box 1.1.

BOX 1.1 INDIGENOUS PEOPLES' PERSPECTIVES ON EUROPEAN 'CIVILISATION'

Characteristic statements attributed to the indigenous Mi'kmaq of Nova Scotia by Father Pierre Briard, an early French missionary (circa. 1608)

> *You [the French colonisers] are always fighting and quarrelling among yourselves; we live peaceably. You are envious and all the time slandering each other; you are thieves and deceivers; you are covetous, and are neither generous nor kind; as for us, if we have a morsel of bread we share it with our neighbour.*

Response during a dialogue between Baron de la Huton, a liberal-minded French aristocrat (and one-time Canadian Deputy Governor) and Kandiaronk, a 'statesman' representative of the indigenous Wendat of Quebec who had visited and observed European society for himself (published 1704)

> *You honestly think you are going to sway me by appealing to the needs of nobles, merchants and priests? If you abandoned conceptions of mine and thine, yes, such distinctions between men would dissolve; a levelling equality would then take its place among you as it now does among the Wendat. And yes, for the first thirty years after the banishing of self-interest, no doubt you would indeed see a certain desolation as those who are already qualified to eat, drink, sleep and take pleasure would languish and die. But their progeny would be fit for our way of living. Over and over I have set forth the qualities that we Wendat believe ought to define humanity – wisdom, reason, equity, etc. – and demonstrated that the existence of separate material interests knocks all those on the head. A man motivated by interest cannot be a man of reason.*
>
> [Cited in Graeber & Wengrow, 2022, pp. 38, 56]

What shortly followed – from the late eighteenth century onwards – was the Industrial Revolution, with the rise of manufacturing and an exponential acceleration of 'economic development', based on the mass extraction and consumption of fossil fuels and other natural resources. Processes of mechanisation transformed labour processes and precipitated rapid urbanisation in the countries most affected. Economic development led to social change: rising living standards for some and increasing exploitation and impoverishment for others. Since the late twentieth century, the development of electronics and information technologies has led to what has been described as 'cognitive capitalism' (e.g. Gorz, 2010), which, together with processes of globalisation and financialisaton, has led to new forms of economic inequality and social insecurity, while the accumulated consequences of intensive human activity upon the planet have ushered in what has been characterised as the Anthropocene era (Ellis, 2018), in which our species is now threatened by the impacts of its own activities on Nature such that currently the Earth is 'well outside the safe operating space for humanity' (Richardson et al., 2023).

It is upon the industrial and post-industrial eras that academic studies in the field of social policy and social development have largely focused, as will the chapters that follow in this book, which will examine in some detail the impact and significance for human expressions of sociality. Broadly speaking, the unfolding of the Industrial Revolution entailed a transition away from social distribution and provision for human welfare within families and kinship groups, and/or through forms of charity administered or promoted by religious institutions, and towards market provision and/or provision administered or co-ordinated through welfare states.

Sociality in context

The preceding section has sought to outline the way in which the human species differs from others in the way it is able to interact with Nature. The species is a social rather than a natural phenomenon, albeit that its sociality has emerged in contradictory ways, given the species' demonstrable propensity for mutual exploitation, conflict and violent combat. A particular meaning to the concept 'sociality' may be attributed not necessarily directly to Marx but to a distillation from his philosophical writings made initially by the Hungarian theorists, Agnes Heller (1974) and György Márkus (1978) and its recent elaboration by Dean (2020; and see Boltvinik, forthcoming).

Radical needs and human essence

Heller draws from Marx a theory of radical human need. 'Radical' here is a term she applies not to the revolutionary nature of Marxist theory, but to the distinctiveness of human beings and what is needed for them to be human. Marxist theory, she contends, offers an understanding of human need as the radical essence present in the human species itself: in Marx's own words, 'To be radical is to grasp things by the root, but for Man the root is Man himself' (1843, p. 137). Human needs are not defined by the laws of economics; they are the 'Ought in collective being'; the necessity 'of subjective action, of collective activity, of practice' (Heller, 1974, p. 90).

Márkus carries the interpretation of Marx's anthropological insights further by drawing out four fundamental yet interconnected and universally constitutive characteristics of the 'human essence'. Of these, sociality is the one to which this book pays particular attention. However, sociality cannot be understood except in relation to the other three characteristics, namely consciousness, 'work' and what is perhaps best captured by the expression 'history making'. These four characteristics define the human species in relation to other species and in relation to the natural world. Márkus's contention is that the human essence lies in the 'inner unity of the total social development of humanity' (1978, p. 63). Together, these characteristics prescribe the universal parameters within which each member of the species is generically human. We have already captured something of what is meant by 'sociality', but let us outline what is entailed by the other characteristics:

- *Consciousness* is the dynamic relationship between thinking and being, and for Marx, while thinking and being may appear distinct, for human beings 'they also form a unity': individual consciousness is shared, ratified or confirmed through 'species consciousness' (1844, p. 351). Thinking by individuals depends on neurological processes, which may in part be similar to those occurring in the brains of other animals and which can be artificially replicated or even extended by sophisticated machines designed by humans. Consciousness is not to be conflated with intelligence (see Box 1.2), and human consciousness is distinct in that it is constructed through human processes (Malik, 2001). Consciousness is the means by which human beings have a personal and an inter-subjective awareness of their selfhood and identity in relation to the natural world and to each other as vulnerable and interdependent social beings. It is also the means by which they seek meaning in the world around them and in their relationships to others, and by which they can reflexively engage with that world as autonomous beings while remaining interdependent with others. A person may be recognised as human by their unique potential amongst other persons as a thinking being, though their freedom to think and therefore their humanity may be compromised by oppressive social and economic conditions.
- *Work*, for Marx, meant consciously conducted human activity that is purposeful and/or creative. He regarded work in terms of the human species' 'social-ecological metabolism' (see Foster, 1999); its potentially symbiotic but more lately parasitic and/or destructive appropriation of natural resources and its manipulation of natural forces. It is through necessary labour that humans secure the material means for survival. But there is also work entailed in processes of social caring and reproduction in order that such labour may be undertaken and developed. And once sufficient means have been obtained, human beings can (when free to do so) creatively interact with Nature and with one another in other forms of work, which may include, for example, artistic endeavour or forms of cultural

BOX 1.2 HUMAN CONSCIOUSNESS: A CONTROLLED HALLUCINATION?

A recent contribution to the philosophical and scientific debate regarding the 'mystery' of consciousness (Seth, 2021) has suggested that consciousness should be conceived quite simply in terms of the subjective experiences of living organisms. Artificially intelligent machines may exceed human beings in their intelligence, but they are not living organisms and cannot experience subjective consciousness. On the other hand, even primitive living organisms can experience external stimuli and respond reflexively. They may be minimally conscious, though they are not intelligent. More complex living organisms – including octopuses, whales, dolphins, elephants, domesticated dogs and especially primates – are capable in their various ways of 'predictive perception'. They display responsive awareness to their environment (and each other) and forms of cognitive capacity or intelligence. Their intelligence – and even, in some instances, the moods and emotions they exhibit – may in some respects be similar to, but are not necessarily the same as, those of human beings.

Human beings are embodied living organisms. We are 'beast machines' engaged in a process of biological survival. Yet we have subjected ourselves to religious and philosophical perceptions of the soul, the mind or the 'self'. The self-conscious human being looks out on the world from within itself and experiences a kind of hallucination – an external phenomenon which it interprets and to which it accommodates itself. Anil Seth contends that as human beings, 'we perceive ourselves in order to control ourselves' (p. 170). There remains, perhaps, a teleological element to this argument, but it represents a neuroscientist's way of expressing the distinctive unity of thinking and being that characterises the human species.

expression where the boundary between work and constructive play may dissolve. At certain stages of human history, however, necessary labour has been undertaken for the most part by slaves, serfs or waged labourers, while the work of ruling them is undertaken by others, and freedoms for 'playful' modes of creative activity are unevenly shaped. The distribution of work – whether it be manual or mental, productive or reproductive – has in practice been neither voluntary nor cooperative but externally imposed in ways that can alienate people from their work and from their essential humanity (see Gorz, 1999).

- *History making*. Human beings, unlike any other species, make their own history. Marx's interpretation of the dialectical unfolding of human history was drawn in part from Hegelian philosophy, but while borrowing Hegel's term *gattungswesen* (meaning 'species essence' or 'species-being'), he asserts that this is not, as Hegel would have it, a spiritual essence, but an essence borne out by the materiality of history, by the reality of social action and by the substantive consequences of human development. Eric Fromm interprets this succinctly (albeit in gendered terms) when he says, 'History is the history of man's self-realization; it is nothing but the self-creation of man' (1961, p. 26). When Marx asserted that 'Philosophers have hitherto only interpreted the world; the point is to change it' (1845, p. 199), his appeal was to the everyday reality of human beings' continuing and ever-evolving struggle for a better life, for self-fulfilment, for 'moral progress' (Gilbert, 1992). As species beings, humans are defined and constrained not merely by Nature but by their historical context. The world may be shaped around them by the state, laws, religion, ideology, culture and customs, but these things have been created by humans and can and most certainly will be changed by humans, whose actions have meaning not only for themselves and for those around them and potentially for the processes by which the species might or might not survive or flourish. It may be noted that Marx was already appraised of the potential 'metabolic rift' between human activity and Nature (Foster, 1999), though he could not have foreseen the extent of the currently unfolding environmental crisis: a beneficial outcome of human history is not assured!

Despite the chimeric propensities attributed to them by Pascal (see above), human beings are radically conscious, creative, historically self-determining and social. However chaotic, human history has been a continuing tale characterised by practical and social struggles not only to fulfil the need for material survival as a species but also to realise the dynamic essence of humanity – not to fulfil some naturally ordained purpose but essentially human purposes. These have been, on the one hand, socially co-operative struggles with or against Nature, but on the other, competitive and sometimes damaging or counterproductive struggles amongst social beings. Key, therefore, to human species' realisation of its essential sociality is a struggle for mutual recognition.

The struggle for recognition

To be human, we each must recognise and identify ourselves by recognising and engaging with others (see Box 1.3). Humans are essentially communal creatures: though individually vulnerable (Turner, 2006), they are inherently interdependent. We have seen that it is not intelligence alone, but sociality – socially organised caring, sharing and collaboration – that have allowed human beings to survive and adapt in spite of their limited size and strength relative to other larger, more physically powerful species and often in the face of challenging natural circumstances and climatic conditions. Human survival

BOX 1.3 RECOGNITION AND IDENTITY: A BUNYIP'S TALE

The *Bunyip of Berkley's Creek* is a children's story by Jenny Wagner (illustrated by Ron Brooks) published by Puffin Books in Australia in the 1970s. It tells of a strange, large creature who emerges from a muddy creek in the dead of night in a state of perplexity, repeatedly murmuring, 'What am I? What am I?'. But nobody answers. In the morning, he asks a succession of passing creatures, 'What am I?'. A platypus dismissively tells him he's a bunyip. When asked 'What do bunyips look like?', a wallaby and then an emu tell him that bunyips look horrible and have horrible features. Wandering along the creek, he meets a man – a scientist – who tells him that bunyips don't look like anything, because in fact bunyips don't exist. The bewildered creature sets out and walks alone all day before settling for the night beside a quiet billabong, where he examines himself in a mirror (which implausibly he has in his bag), unable to interpret or evaluate what he sees. In the middle of the night, something stirs in the bottom of the billabong, and another strange, large creature emerges from the depths, repeatedly murmuring, 'What am I? What am I?'. The Bunyip cries in delight, 'You are a bunyip!'. The other bunyip asked, 'What do I look like?', to which the first bunyip happily replied, 'You look just like me'. The story ends, 'And he lent her his mirror to prove it'.

This simple, ostensibly banal story perhaps illustrates fundamental existential questions: how can we know we are more than a self-hallucination without recognising and engaging with other members of our own species?

has depended on humans' capacity for loyalty to one another; upon their 'clinging together against the dark' (Rorty, 1982, p. 166). As we have seen, that 'clinging together' is made possible through, on the one hand, shared language, customs, institutions, knowledge and beliefs – all of which are dynamically socio-historically constructed and contested – and, on the other, by social and inter-psychological processes which shape the personal development of every human being. As Anil Seth puts it, 'our perceptions of our selves are refracted through the perceptions of others' (2021, p. 167). Clinging together entails a struggle for mutual recognition between the members of our unnatural species, and it is in this that the meaning of sociality may be found.

The idea that humanity may be characterised in terms of its continuing quest for mutual recognition dates back at least as far as Hegel (1807), who, departing from the individualism of the Romantic philosophers emphasised, that none of us can resign from society. We are defined by and through the recognition accorded or denied to us by other human beings. Hegel identified the family, civil society and the state as three 'spheres of recognition' (1821), a point to which we shall return below. Honneth (1995), however, has drawn on Hegel's philosophy – and upon social-psychological influences from Mead (1934) – to formulate a claim that the three requirements for a fully human or 'ethical' life are to be found in three phases, or modes of mutual recognition: love, solidarity and rights. These, we may argue, represent three constitutive dimensions of human sociality (Dean, 2020):

- *Love* entails discovering and being oneself in and through another. It is through intimate relationships that we discover ourselves, by which we establish who we are and affirm our self-identity.
- *Solidarity* entails participation and engagement with others in communities or social groups. It is through solidarity with neighbours, peers and colleagues that we can achieve self-esteem and establish ourselves as actors with shared collective identities and shared goals and responsibilities.
- *Rights* entail shared responsibilities in relation to strangers as well as neighbours and intimates. They provide a basis on which to recognise, accommodate and respect each other as beings defined by difference. Rights provide the basis on which we can come to recognise, accommodate and respect each other as bearers of a universal capacity that characterises us as humans. It is through exercising our own and respecting others' rights that we are able mutually to engage with relative strangers and more distant members of our species and to acknowledge the legitimacy of the claims that can mutually be made upon one another.

It is with rights to make claims upon one another that this book is concerned. However, such rights are dependent upon mutual recognition and, thereby, a shared awareness and understanding of human sociality.

Misrecognition and the denial of sociality

We therefore now turn to the issue of 'misrecognition' and its *de*humanising effects and also to consider how, in the course of human history, perceptions of sociality have been distorted or obscured.

Though we have considered human beings as 'unnatural' creatures, we must nonetheless remind ourselves that they are defined in part by their biology. While human beings share essential biological features, they also differ from one another biologically, and biological differences can and do take on social meanings. It is socially constructed conceptions of biological difference that have significance for the extent to which people and groups within human societies are recognised, accepted and respected as fully human in terms of their status and inclusion within society. By reason of the social significance attached to biological variations, large numbers of people within the human population are or have been in key respects misrecognised and/or dehumanised by reason of their 'otherness' (Fraser, 2008; Lister, 2004, ch. 5). This applies in relation to:

- *Gender and sexuality*. We have already commented on how, in the course of human history, women came to be systematically disempowered and discounted as less than fully human, more so in some societies than others. Similarly, dominant norms relating to gender and different expressions and experiences of sexuality have meant that the humanity of gay, lesbian, bisexual and transsexual people has been misrecognised or denied.
- *Race and ethnicity*. Though phenotypical differences between humans (e.g. skin colour) may have resulted from incidental or minor adaptive biological variations between different groups of human beings in different parts of the world, they have assumed social significance in the course of historical processes of migration and settlement, invasion and conquest, subjugation and slavery. A mistaken belief that phenotypical differences between humans signify that they belong to different 'races' results in racialised misrecognition. Where it is believed that some races are superior to others, this has resulted in dehumanising practices. Additionally, when genetic characteristics that human beings share with their immediate forbearers differentiate them from other members of the human species, such characteristics will invariably be accompanied by distinctive cultural, linguistic and often religious differences that together go to make up a person's ethnicity. Ethnic minorities, whether they be indigenous or diasporic, have perennially been victims of misrecognition, especially if different ethnic groups may be perceived or misrepresented as competitors for scarce resources.
- *Disability and ageing*. Some humans are born with genetic impairments. Others, in the course, of their lives experience illness, injury or degenerative conditions that impair their physical, mental or cognitive functioning. The lives of some people are therefore impaired by pain, discomfort and distress resulting from biological factors. But what constitutes impairment is also defined with reference to socially accepted or imposed standards of normality. The humanity of people who cannot walk, see or hear or who have difficulty learning or relating to others can be undermined as much as anything else by the norms of society around them. Chronological ageing is a biological process, and yet the meanings that attach to stages in the human life-course and the respect and care accorded to older people are shaped by social customs and practices. The biological basis of the relative strength and frailty that we can expect to experience and the recognition and support that we receive at any stage in the course of a human lifespan are overlaid with socially and politically constructed expectations; in other words, by the extent to which sociality is realised.

Mutual recognition is integral to sociality. And sociality may be, and has been, realised and understood in ways which are limited or limiting, especially in relation to the nurturing of solidarities beyond immediate kinship groupings and the mutual negotiation of rights between more distant strangers. This book is concerned with social rights and the means by which to promote and sustain human welfare, something achieved to different extents in differing parts of the world through the development of social policy. It was noted towards the beginning of this chapter that in his account of the evolution of the human species, Charles Darwin alluded to the particular 'social instincts' that human beings possess, an observation that arguably prefigured a developed understanding of sociality. In a prescient passage, he says:

> As [humanity] advances in civilisation, and small tribes are united into larger communities, the simplest reason would tell each individual that [they] ought to extend [their] social instincts and sympathies to all the members of the same nation, though personally unknown to [them]. This point being once reached, there is only an artificial barrier to prevent [their] sympathies extending to the [persons] of all nations and races.
>
> *(1871, pp. 100–101) [non-gender specific nouns and pronouns substituted]*

For an answer to what that 'artificial barrier' might be – and to whether in the course of human history there have been other inhibitions that constrained the realisation and understanding of sociality – we may consider the role played by fetishisms (see Morris, 2017). The concept of the fetish has fallen in and out of fashion in anthropology, philosophy, political economy and psychoanalysis,[2] but the concept appears to have had its origins in a report of an anthropological study of fetish Gods in West Africa by Charles de Brosses (1765) and has been applied in various ways to describe how symbolic objects, cultural constructs or moral ideals may obscure or distort the perception of human relationships (Dean, 2023).

In a seminal attempt to portray the twentieth-century welfare state as a form of institutionalised altruism, Richard Titmuss (1970) alluded to anthropological studies recounted by Mauss (1925), who (while not explicitly endorsing de Brosses' interpretation of fetishism) aptly described certain pre-modern tribal societies as 'gift economies' in which gift exchange played a vital social function, albeit that gift-giving was not (as Titmuss perhaps unintentionally implied) a conscious act of altruism, but governed by fetishised beliefs in magic: gifts were invested in some contexts with magical powers which bound the recipient upon pain of illness or death eventually to return or pass on the gift according to customary dictates. The term 'altruism' should be noted alludes to selflessness, rather than sociality. The term was first coined by Augustus Comte (1851), the founding father of positivist sociology. Comte's sociology was a form of 'social physics' by which he meant to inform and develop a rational altruistic social order that would, he claimed, supersede not only the 'immature fetishism' of a paternalistic pre-Enlightenment social order governed by irrational theology but also the intrinsically selfish individualism of the new Enlightenment era informed by abstract metaphysics. In later work (1896), Comte went so far as to propose a new non-theistic 'Religion of Humanity', which he offered as his own supposedly mature '*Grande Fétische*': a non-governmental institution through which to proselytise and subjectivise an altruistic social order.

Comte recognised fetishism as a mechanism for the cultural transmission and maintenance of altruistic behaviours while apparently failing to acknowledge links previously made between religion and philosophy. Kant, for example, drawing upon de Brosses' conceptualisation of fetishism (see Morris, 2017, pp. 166–167), critiqued the exteriority of religion as a regulator of collective moral principles but recognised the pedagogic functions that may nevertheless be served by religious observance when this promotes the observance of *morally desirable* duties or altruistic behaviours as distinct from *logically imperative* obligations. In a somewhat different vein, Hegel argued that older forms of fetish worship and belief systems founded on magic were religions of 'unfreedom' since they denied human beings an awareness of their own essential spiritual being (*ibid.*, pp. 179–187). But, he claimed, such spiritual awareness can be achieved in an *objective* sense by the processes of mutual recognition enabled through the institutions of civil society and the liberal state and achieved in an *absolute* sense through the revealed religions (along with such pursuits as art and philosophy).

Marx, in his interpretation, appraised the constitutive human essence not as something abstract or spiritual but as something material and real. He accused Hegel of inverting reality by deriving empirical institutions from abstract ideals. For Hegel, Marx claimed, the subjective reality of human beings and human activity becomes objectified in the institution of a state, which, like the church, has a mysterious, or we might say fetishised, autonomy of its own. 'Reality is not deemed to be itself but another reality instead. The ordinary empirical world is not governed by its own mind, but by a mind alien to it' (1843, p. 62). Marx was aware of the concept of the fetish originated by de Brosse (Worrel & Krier, 2018) and deployed it further in his critique of the prevailing perceptions of value that are inherent to the capitalist mode of production and exchange. He famously demonstrated the fetish-character of commodities, in which the social character of the human beings who produced them appears as an objective characteristic of the products themselves. The commodity form inverts reality by constructing 'material relations between persons and social relations between things' (1887, p. 73). Marx's focus on the commodity form is especially significant for understanding how the commodification of labour power reduced 'work', as a constitutive human activity, to potentially exploitative and anti-social wage labour. He contended that within capitalist societies, human beings can be 'alienated' not only from their work but also from their essential sociality by the objectifying forces of both market and state.

The invention of social rights through the creation of the capitalist welfare state was at best an ambiguous expression of human sociality. Titmuss claimed it represented a form of institutionalised altruism, but altruism is concerned with individual motivation, not our species being. It will emerge in the course of this book that though welfare states in liberal democracies may sustain limited social solidarities by affecting some redistribution of resources and ensuring the provision of certain human services, they can also undermine as much as give effect to human sociality. The rights they create are hedged around with conditionalities and are premised on a fetishised conception of the sovereign individual that obscures the social interdependence that is essential to our humanity. The account to be given in this book will nevertheless be critically supportive of a role for social rights in the promotion of human welfare but will contend that they should be more clearly perceived and founded upon an understanding of sociality.

Outline of the book

The remainder of this book is as follows:

PART ONE is concerned with *Established Theories of Social Rights* and begins in Chapter 2 by considering social rights as rights of national citizenship and the way they have been theorised in relation to capitalist welfare states. The chapter will bring the concept of sociality to bear in order to reframe T.H. Marshall's (1950) classic theory of social citizenship. Chapter 3 will move on to consider theories of human need and the extent to which understandings of human need are reflected in the framing of international human rights and specifically, 'social, economic and cultural rights'. The chapter will specifically revisit Marx's notion of radical human need and critically discuss the extent to which the human rights agenda might guarantee the fulfilment of the human species' constitutive characteristics, including and particularly sociality. Chapter 4 will address just how the social rights agenda has impacted within conflicting approaches to human development in the global South. Chapter 5 provides a discussion of ethics, ideologies and social rights and will elaborate upon the role of religious, philosophical and political influences on provision for human welfare and the emergence of social rights. Finally, Chapter 6 will consider a range of theoretical challenges to the validity of rights-based approaches to human welfare.

PART TWO will consider *Social Rights in Practice* and systematically address the extent to which existing forms of provision for human welfare are fulfilling humanity's needs and whether they amount to expressions of human sociality. It begins in Chapter 7 with a discussion of rights to human services, specifically to health, education, housing and social care. Health is axiomatically necessary for human activity. Education is critically relevant in relation to the development of human consciousness. The organisation of housing is an essential element to human beings' survival within their environment and to the functioning of human communities. Social care is key to the ways in which human beings look after vulnerable members of society. Chapter 8 is concerned with rights to livelihood and, as such, bears directly on social security, the protection of living standards and the human need for creative, self-sustaining activity or 'work' (in its widest meaning). Chapter 9 is concerned with social rights in a global context and will consider in broad outline the current stage and direction of the historical development of social rights across different regions of the world. Chapter 10 on rights of redress is practically addressed to the tactical concerns of welfare rights lawyers, community activists and others involved when social rights are violated or denied.

The book concludes in Chapter 11 with an evaluative summary. It will offer some speculative remarks regarding the future for rights-based approaches to human welfare provision. It will argue for a shift in perception: a shift by which to humanise the social rights agenda and alter dominant understandings of human sociality, its realisation and expression.

Notes

1 The following passages draw upon several of the sources already cited, albeit that the manner of their synthesis is attributable to this author's attempt to provide a succinct preface to arguments to be developed later in this book.
2 The use of the term that survives in popular discourse is unfortunately premised on, and tainted by, a crude interpretation of Freud's (1905) development of the concept of the fetish in his study of sexuality.

PART I

Established Theories of Social Rights

2

THE SOCIAL RIGHTS OF CITIZENSHIP

Chapter 1 has already introduced the reader to an encompassing concept of social rights as the articulation of human needs and as an expression of human sociality. Conventional understandings, however, treat social rights primarily as an invention of the twentieth-century capitalist welfare state. In this context, they are rights relating to education, health and social care, housing, social security and employment protection. These are rights that originated in industrialised capitalist countries but which have since been emerging in various forms and to varying degrees in the global South. Social rights are construed as the creatures of social policy, as specialised individual entitlements specifically created and legally framed in social legislation. We shall see in later chapters how the term social rights may also be used in a normative sense to refer more generally to societal objectives and international norms as to the levels of social protection that are, or ought to be, mutually guaranteed within all human societies. Terms such as 'social' or 'welfare' rights may be used within the arena of vocational or professional practice in which activists, development workers, advice workers and welfare lawyers engage. Such rights can be more than technical phenomena or abstract principles, but practical tools and discursive resources for campaigning, negotiation and advocacy – particularly by or on behalf of vulnerable, poor or disadvantaged people. But as matters stand, it is primarily as rights of citizenship of a nation-state that social rights may be substantively established and enforced.

The implication is that as a medium for the expression of human sociality, social citizenship rights have a constrained horizon. In this chapter, we shall start, nevertheless, with a conceptual discussion of the social rights of citizenship. We shall discuss the way in which the concept of social rights emerged explicitly as a defining feature of welfare state capitalism, before reflecting

DOI: 10.4324/9781003451518-3

on the prior origins of citizenship rights and finally analysing recent developments affecting the nature of social rights in the welfare states of the global North. We shall broaden the discussion in later chapters to consider the place of social rights within the international human rights agenda and further reflect on the deeper origins of social rights.

The coming of welfare capitalism

Social rights, according to the sociologist T.H. Marshall (1950), were the unique achievement of the twentieth-century capitalist welfare state. His exemplar was the British case. In Britain, the struggle to achieve civil rights (i.e. civil liberties, property and legal rights) had by and large succeeded by the eighteenth century, and the struggle to achieve political rights (i.e. voting and democratic rights) took major strides in the nineteenth century. The establishment of social rights – that is, entitlement to basic standards of education, healthcare, housing, income maintenance and employment protection – was completed with the formation of the 'modern' welfare state after the end of the Second World War. Marshall may be accused of overgeneralisation, particularly in his characterisation of different historical periods, but this ought not to obscure the importance of his argument and the idea that the coming of the capitalist welfare state – in Britain and elsewhere – had ushered in a new form of rights for a new economic and social order. His contentions were first that social conflicts and inequalities based on class divisions had been or could be 'ameliorated' through the development of citizenship, and secondly, that full citizenship required three components – not just civil and political rights but social rights as well.

Beyond class society?

The first of these points finds support among many commentators and supporters of the welfare state, including those on the social democratic left (George & Wilding, 1994, ch. 4). However, Marshall was a social liberal rather than a social democrat. His use of the term amelioration had been directly drawn from the works of the nineteenth-century economist, Alfred Marshall. It was in a series of lectures in memory of Alfred Marshall that T.H. Marshall advanced the proposition that the post-Second World War welfare state as founded in Britain represented the 'latest phase in an evolution of citizenship which has been in continuous progress for some 250 years' (1950, p. 7). In so doing, he claimed he was addressing a question raised by his erstwhile namesake some seven decades before, namely 'whether the amelioration of the working classes has limits beyond which it cannot pass [or] whether progress may not go on steadily, if slowly, till by occupation at least, every man is a gentleman' (Alfred Marshall, 1873 – cited in T.H. Marshall, 1950, pp. 4–5).

The equality foreseen by Marshall, the nineteenth-century economist, was an equality of opportunities and status rather than a material equality of incomes or wealth. Technological advances he believed would ameliorate the arduous nature of manual labour, while compulsory elementary education would civilise the manners of the working classes. Marshall, the twentieth-century sociologist, similarly believed that 'equality of status is more important than equality of income' (1950, p. 33). The development of a range of social services and cash benefits financed through taxation clearly did involve an equalisation of incomes, but this was not its only or even its primary achievement:

> What matters is that there is a general enrichment of the concrete substance of civilised life, a general reduction of risk and insecurity, an equalisation between the more and the less fortunate at all levels - between the healthy and the sick, the employed and the unemployed, the old and the active, the bachelor and the father of a large family. Equalisation is not so much between classes as between individuals within a population which is now treated for this purpose as though it were one class.
>
> *(ibid.)*

The argument then is that social rights could abolish inequality based on class differences. Social policy scholars, such as Titmuss (1958, 1968), agreed that the development and maintenance of state welfare provision constituted a moral imperative insofar as it represented the peaceful means of mitigating the unacceptable consequences of class inequality; social rights were a civilising force which compensated for the diswelfares of the industrialised capitalist system.

One British Labour politician, Tony Crosland (1956), went so far as to argue that the development of social legislation and the rise of labour and trade union power could together shift the balance so far against the old capitalist class system as to promise the imminent realisation of a democratic form of socialism. In reality, however, Marshall's concept of citizenship was not at all consistent with socialist aims. Marshall saw citizenship, particularly through the effects of a meritocratic state education system, as an alternative instrument of social stratification (1950, p. 39). Certainly, he believed the emergence of social rights signalled the extent to which *laissez faire* capitalism had been superseded. But the result would be a society based on status and dessert rather than contract and mere good fortune: 'Social rights in their modern form imply an invasion of contract by status, the subordination of market price to social justice, the replacement of the free bargain by the declaration of rights' (1950, p. 40). Paradoxically, as we shall later see, shorn of any commitment to economic equality, this liberal view of social rights can be rendered consistent or at least cohabit with a form of one-nation conservatism and its ideal of a non-conflictual or stable social order.

Unstable citizenship?

Capitalism, of course, never did achieve a non-conflictual social order. David Lockwood has argued that the structuring of life chances in capitalist welfare states was 'the direct result of the institutionalisation of citizenship under conditions of social and economic inequality' and that the tension between state and market was managed by 'the fine-tuning of social rights' (1996, pp. 532–553). The result he called a process of 'civic stratification', which depends, on the one hand, on the extent to which citizenship rights are allowed to develop and, on the other hand, on the nature of the relative gains and deficits citizens might experience depending on their social status. We shall see in Chapter 4 that the administrative power of the capitalist welfare state can be implicated in the perpetuation or shaping of social divisions. Class structures have been changing, but despite the welfare state, socio-economic class status still strongly correlates with an unequal distribution of life chances (Crompton, 2008). Social inequalities remain endemic throughout much of the developed world (OECD, 2019).

Elements of the instability of post-industrial capitalist societies could, from the end of the twentieth century, be said to stem from consequences of individual risks rather than active class conflict (Beck, 1992). The predominant fault line in the occupational structures of post-industrial capitalist societies was by then more passive in nature and lay not between 'workers' and 'bosses' or even between manual and non-manual workers, but between securely employed, highly trained and well-paid 'core' workers on the one hand and precariously employed, low skilled and poorly paid 'peripheral' workers on the other (Standing, 2009, 2011). Changes in class structure had been driven by changes in the nature of capitalism itself rather than by any direct influence of the welfare state (Esping-Andersen, 1999).

For the moment, however, let us return to the second limb of Marshall's argument, which was that civil, political and social rights are all necessary to a mature form of citizenship. Marshall recognised the sense in which citizenship based on a broad equality of rights might potentially conflict with the workings of a capitalist market economy. Nevertheless, he stressed that full citizenship need not inhibit a market economy, provided a state of equilibrium can be sustained between political, social and civil rights in what he characterised as a 'hyphenated' society: 'democratic-welfare-capitalism'. The hyphens in this formulation symbolise the interconnectedness of a democratic polity, a welfare state and a mixed economy, all functioning in harmony (1981). The maintenance of a flourishing 'hyphenated' society is therefore a matter of achieving the right balance between the constituent components of citizenship. Upon this premise, if too much emphasis is being placed in capitalist societies on our rights as producers and consumers and not enough upon our rights to participate in democratic decision-making and enjoy guaranteed living standards and social provision, this may create an imbalance between the civil, political and social aspects of citizenship. It poses a potential threat to stability. Similarly, social upheavals in post-communist regimes, such as the former Soviet Union, were regarded as a consequence of violent shifts in the equilibrium of citizenship. Under former Stalinist regimes, social rights had been guaranteed, while civil and political rights were either suppressed or neglected, albeit that subsequently political rights were promoted at the expense of social rights and without an adequate framework of civil rights (Deacon, 1993).

Marshall's sociological model of citizenship, though highly influential, has attracted criticism on a number of counts. First, feminists complained that his analysis failed to address social divisions other than class and the extent to which his 'image of an ideal citizenship' (1950, p. 29) might not include women, disabled people or migrants on equal terms as indigenous, able-bodied male citizens (e.g. Lister, 2003). These are issues to which we shall return in Chapter 6. Second, though Marshall theorises the functional role of social citizenship in relation to the amelioration of social class, he failed to account for the impact which social classes have had on the development of citizenship (Bottomore, 1992). The development of civil rights and the beginnings of political rights resulted from the struggles of an emerging capitalist class to wrest power from the feudal aristocracy. The more recent development of political rights and aspects of the beginnings of social rights owed much to the struggles of working-class organisations: the Chartists, the trade unions and socialist and social democratic parties. Marshall expresses the conflicts from which citizenship has emerged in terms of clashes between opposing principles rather than between opposing classes. The development and maintenance of capitalist welfare states were analysed, from differing perspectives, by other commentators (e.g. Esping-Andersen, 1990; Korpi, 1983; Offe, 1984) with reference on the one hand to political pressures applied directly through the democratic process and on the other to the influence of corporatism. Corporatism, in this context, is the process of tri-partite negotiation between the representatives of capital, labour and the state (customarily referred to in this context as 'social partners'). What is often involved in the development of social rights is not an impersonally established equilibrium between formal principles but a directly negotiated compromise between substantive class interests.

A third objection is that Marshall's account of state and market is, at best, reductionist. It may be observed that the antagonism between state and market to which social citizenship can supposedly bring equilibrium is not a simple opposition, since in some circumstances responsive market systems can and do fulfil social needs, while in others authoritarian state welfare systems can frustrate them (Hindess, 1987). What is more, there are parts of the world where effective markets and legitimate state apparatuses upon which Marshall's citizenship ideal depends simply do not exist (Gough et al., 2004).

Finally, Marshall, at the time he presented his theory of social rights, was strangely silent with regard to the contemporaneous emergence of an international human rights regime (Davy, 2013) and the idea of rights that are universal. Seven decades later, in a globalised world, his nation-based approach to social rights has been superseded (Dean, 2013). Notions of what constitutes citizenship have been changing. It is increasingly recognised that the basis for shared identities and community memberships extends beyond or regardless of national or other spatial boundaries. 'Citizenship' has become a fluid term, applied in a variety of contexts to the loyalties that people experience or feel they owe within a range of intersecting social groupings and institutions (e.g. Isin et al., 2008; Clarke et al., 2014). Human sociality may find expression but can also be constrained through forms of citizenship. These are arguments, which we shall revisit in later chapters. But for the moment we shall consider where conceptions of, and assumptions about, 'citizenship' and 'rights' first came from and how they have evolved and changed in the capitalist welfare states where they originated.

The origins and categories of rights

Rights and citizenship are intimately linked, and the orthodox assumption is that their common origins lie in antiquity and the creation in the fifth century BCE of the Athenian city state, where rights of citizenship were implied through rules of self-governance adopted by a patrician male elite (Held, 1987, ch. 1). Such rights did not extend beyond the city. Nor – as was discussed in Chapter 1 of this volume – did they extend to women and slaves within the city. Citizenship entailed membership in a distinctly exclusive political community but also a practice based on principles and procedures. Later forms of citizenship similarly invoke principles or *doctrines* on the one hand and provide procedures for the making and resolution of *claims* on the other. Through the dialectical engagement between doctrines and claims emerge competing understandings of rights, both *formal* and *substantive*. Our rights may be determined 'from above' by abstract or constitutional *doctrines*, or they may be driven 'from below' through *claims* or political demands. They may be framed in terms of *formal* freedoms premised on minimalist (or 'thin') expressions of sociality or in terms of *substantive* entitlements premised on fuller (or 'thicker') expressions of sociality. (The 'thin' vs. 'thick' distinction will be mentioned again below and discussed further in Chapter 3 in relation to human needs).

Doctrines and claims

It is important to recognise that what might once have been successfully demanded from below as claims-based rights may through processes of compromise and acceptance assume the character of doctrinal orthodoxies handed down from above, while conversely, rights that are conferred by doctrinal decree may establish themselves or be adapted as a basis for formulating or articulating new claims-based demands. Historically speaking, the form of rights in 'hyphenated' democratic-welfare-capitalist societies is inescapably traceable to 'Enlightenment' attempts in the seventeenth and eighteenth centuries to achieve a formal separation between market (the economy) and state (politics), but just as fundamentally to establish the inalienability (or 'freedom') of property.

Prior to this, in pre-Enlightenment feudal Europe, classical Greco-Roman conceptions of citizenship had lapsed into obscurity, and there had been no rights other than the right to govern, a natural right supposedly bestowed by God upon the sovereign and the nobility. To the extent that there were paternalistic duties attaching to such rights, then privileges and gratuities might be conferred from time to time upon the common people (Kamenka & Tay, 1975), but they enjoyed no rights in the modern legal sense. Though lauded for having prefigured the modern concept of rights, England's *Magna Carta* of 1215 was no more than a concession of restricted liberties by the Crown to the nobility, and it was not until the English *Petition of Rights* in 1628 that the process that would lead to the modern concept would unfold (Perry, 1964). A necessary precondition was the invention throughout Europe of the sovereign nation state (partially attributable to the Treaty of Westphalia of 1648) and conceptions of citizenship that now applied beyond the narrow sphere of the city state.

The doctrines of 'natural' law upon which feudal beliefs and practices had been founded afforded absolute power to a potentially capricious crown and aristocracy while imposing constraints upon property ownership. Natural law frustrated the market freedoms necessary to the economic foundation of capitalist society. Belief in natural law had therefore to be replaced over time by liberal beliefs in 'man-made' laws (women continued at that time to have no legal status). Bob Fine (1984) has contended that the doctrines which laid the foundations for man-made laws were inseparable from the doctrines of political economy. In the philosophical writings of Locke (1690) and the political writings of Paine (1791), we see reflected a moral discourse by which 'natural' rights were first recast as inalienable individual rights to 'life, liberty and estate [i.e. property]' and then exchanged, as it were, to become civil rights under doctrines of liberal governance (Raphael, 1989). This in essence was the discourse of rights that informed the English *Bill of Rights* of 1689 and, a century later, the American *Declaration of Independence* of 1776, the USA *Constitution* of 1787 and the French *Declaration of Rights* of 1789. By these constitutional instruments, it was not the claims of ordinary people that were ascendant over governments, so much as the interests of incipient property-owning middle classes over those of old aristocracies.

Nevertheless, the subsequent interpretation and influence of these various instruments would differ significantly. The celebrated French Revolutionary slogan, *Liberté*, *Egalité*, *Fraternité*, embodied a set of potential contradictions:

the objectives of freedom, equality and solidarity are not easy companions (Hobsbawm, 1962). Equality is capable of competing interpretations – a point to which we shall shortly return – while, at root, freedom and solidarity are conflicting principles. Hegel (1821) clearly understood this. He asserted that the ultimate freedom is the right of personal as opposed to common ownership, but he also acknowledged that citizens are mutually interdependent, such that public provision should be made for poor relief, health, education and public works. This he recognised to be controversial. The notion of property was as contestable as it was essential. For heuristic purposes, we can draw a broad distinction between the liberal citizenship tradition that came to characterise the Anglophone world and the civic-republican tradition that came to characterise the Western continental European world. The former prioritised individual freedom; the latter acknowledged solidarity. The liberal tradition reflected Locke's view of property rights as individual prepositive rights (1690); the civic-republican tradition reflected Rousseau's (1762) view of property rights as possessive claims upon common assets, legitimised only through the collective will (Davy, 2012).

The origin of rights in ownership leads to competing understandings of social rights. Rights and equality before the law are universal only in the formal and abstract sense that in an ordered (capitalist) society everybody has to relate to and respect everybody else as proprietors. Even people without land or goods at their disposal may 'own' (and therefore sell) their labour power. It has been suggested that social rights are, or ought to be, directly analogous to property rights and that 'government largesse' (such as welfare benefits, subsidies, grants, education, etc.) constitutes a kind of property which may be subject to the same legal rules and categories as other property forms (Reich, 1964). This is one way of looking at social rights: as an expression in legal form of the logic of individual ownership. Such benefits – provided all the conditions of eligibility are met – are available as an entitlement rather than as a gift, and the principles which give rise to that entitlement are supposed to operate with indifference to the personality and status of the recipient. They can be rights within the liberal definition of the rule of law. In contrast, the rhetoric of social rights campaigners and activists is more usually cast in terms of a very different doctrinal understanding of property. For example, opposition by nineteenth-century Owenites and Chartists to the tightening of the English Poor Laws was founded upon solidaristically conceived 'birth rights', that is to say:

> the right to have a living out of the land of our birth in exchange for labour duly and honestly performed; the right in case we fell into distress, to have our wants sufficiently relieved out of the produce of the land, whether that distress arose from sickness, from decrepitude, from old age, or from inability to find employment.
>
> *(William Cobbett, cited in E. P. Thompson, 1968, p. 836)*

The claim here – the right to work, the right to a living wage, the right to an adequate income in the event of incapacity, unemployment or retirement – is premised on the idea of common ownership through birth, yet it speaks none the less to the significance of property for social rights.

The doctrines that informed the coming of the twentieth-century human rights agenda, which we shall discuss in Chapter 3, centred neither upon the ordinances of God (Klug, 2000) nor necessarily upon principles of property ownership (Jacobs, 2013), but on the potentially problematic idea of humanity's inherent 'dignity'. Nevertheless, as Barry Clarke (1996) has argued, it was citizen rights that provided the model for human rights and not the other way round. The history of the rights-bearing subject, as 'citizen', as 'proprietor' and (more recently) as a 'client' or a 'customer', or indeed most fundamentally, as a 'human', is a narrative of social construction. It is a continuing story of shifting doctrinal orthodoxies and innovative claim-making.

The formal and the substantive

The language or 'discourse' of rights, as should be evident, is shot through with ambiguities. Not only is there a distinction to be drawn between the kinds of rights that are prescribed from above by established doctrine and the kinds of rights that are framed and claimed from below. There are also competing understandings of what it means for citizens, proprietors or humans to have *equal* rights. The liberal citizenship tradition has tended towards a formal or procedural approach to equality; the civic-republican tradition has tended towards a more substantive approach. The liberal tradition embraces the ideal of equality under the law. At its meanest, this is captured by Anatol France's celebrated aphorism: 'The law, in its majestic equality, forbids the rich as well as the poor to sleep under bridges, to beg in the streets, and to steal bread' (1894). More inclusive understandings of liberalism recognise that free markets can perpetuate social disadvantage and so favour equality of opportunity and the idea that every citizen should be allowed to succeed on the basis of their ability. Communitarian versions of the civic-republican tradition emphasise equality of belonging, inclusion and respect rather than strict material equality, though social democratic derivations of the tradition support broad equality of material outcomes.

These are issues to which we shall repeatedly return. But for the moment, we shall remain focused on the rights of citizenship. Lawyers make a distinction between 'black letter' rights that are written down and enforceable as opposed to 'moral' rights that are extolled and debated but have no necessary effect. The utilitarian philosopher Jeremy Bentham (1789) dismissed as 'nonsense on stilts' the very idea that there can be basic moral rights that naturally belong to every individual citizen. What matters, he believed, are the laws we might make to ensure the greatest good for the greatest number of citizens.

This represents a legal positivist tradition which refers to any right which is legally defined as a 'positive' right as distinct from a mere 'moral' right which is unspecified and unenforceable.

Other legal scholars, however, have debated a quite different distinction between 'negative' rights, which formally protect the individual from external interference, and 'positive' rights, which substantively guarantee state intervention. Here the term positive is being used with a different meaning. The distinction between negative and positive 'liberties' was drawn by Isiah Berlin to mark the difference between a 'right' to forbearance by others as opposed to 'the freedom which consists in being one's own master' (1967, p. 149). The words 'liberty' and 'right' are not necessarily synonymous, but they can refer to different categories of rights. Hohfeld (1946) identified four kinds of rights: liberties, claims, immunities and powers. Liberties and immunities are what might be called a category of negative right, because they signal a *freedom from* something, whereas claims and powers are positive rights because they signal an *entitlement to* something. In practice, if one takes, for example, what might be regarded as the most elemental of social rights, the right to be free from hunger, this would imply a right to food or, at least, to the means of subsistence. To be positive in this sense, the right must have substance; it requires someone or somebody not merely to refrain from action but to act.

The distinction between formal and substantive can be expressed not only in terms of negative and positive rights but in terms of different theories of rights: the *will* or *choice* theory on the one hand and the *interest* or *benefit* theory on the other (e.g. Campbell, 1988, 2006; Jones, 1994). The former is premised on the idea that every human individual with free will must necessarily have the right to exercise choice in relation to their dealings with others. The latter is premised on the idea that rights are created by rules which benefit the human individual by imposing obligations on other individuals to protect or further their interests. The theories resonate, respectively, with liberal and civic-republican citizenship traditions, and neither alone can account for the ways in which social rights necessarily have both procedural form (through the way they are established) and material substance (in terms of what they actually deliver). An attempt to do this has been made by Ronald Dworkin (1977), who draws a different kind of distinction between *background* rights and *institutional* rights. Background rights embody the fundamental formal principles that justify political and judicial decision-making, while institutional rights are policy or goal-directed and impose substantive duties on people or the government. The background rights that inform institutional rights imply not an empty morality of the kind dismissed by Bentham but a notion of social justice, such as that espoused by Rawls (1972). It may be seen, however, that background rights may be translated into more or less substantively generous institutional rights, depending on just how they are framed. Dworkin's background rights would seem to equate to what Michael Walzer (1994) has described as 'thin' or minimalist moralities: they represent, as it were, the lowest common denominator in terms of the principles upon which policy actors might agree, rather than a 'thick' or maximalist moral understanding of the substantive rights of citizenship.

We may conclude: firstly, that rights are ideological constructions, albeit that they have real consequences; secondly, that their character and meaning are inevitably fluid and change over time.

Post-industrial capitalism and the privatisation of social rights

The final set of preliminary debates that this chapter must address relates to the distinctive nature of social rights as demands upon resources and the extent to which, having been supposedly invented as creatures of capitalism, they will survive in the capitalist world as capitalism itself evolves. We shall be concerned firstly with the way in which social rights entailed or enabled a partial de-commodification of both labour power and human services; secondly, with the crisis of the modern welfare state and the resulting processes of re-commodification or 'privatisation'. We shall see that in the welfare states where they were first created, the nature of social rights has been changing.

Social rights and de-commodification

The development of twentieth-century capitalist welfare states was achieved through bodies of social legislation that extended the 'positive' or substantive rights of citizenship by expanding public services. While civil and political rights primarily entail 'negative' or formal rights (e.g. freedoms of movement and opinion), social rights entail substantive rights to the provision of goods and services necessary for human wellbeing. Social rights came onto the agenda when the state began to adopt a role in relation to such goods and services rather than leaving their provision entirely to the mechanisms of the market; in other words, when through social policy intervention certain goods and services were to some extent 'de-commodified'. It is a process that had actually begun in many countries before or during the early years of the twentieth century with partial reforms to nineteenth-century systems of poor relief. We have seen that according to Marshall, social rights developed only after certain 'negative' or formal rights had successfully secured the legal and economic infrastructure necessary for a free market economy – an economy in which not only land but goods and services, and even labour power, were instituted as alienable property that could be traded as commodities. However, Karl Polanyi (1944) has contended that labour power is in reality only a 'fictitious commodity'. Unlike ordinary commodities, labour power cannot be separated from its owners and is uniquely dependent for its existence upon the health and well-being of those owners. While it is possible for the owners of ordinary commodities to withhold them from sale until the price is right, the owners of labour power cannot do so unless they can secure an alternative means of subsistence. If labour power is to be traded as if it were a commodity, certain conditions must be met, including certain non-commodified support systems (Offe, 1984), including social security, healthcare and education. Marshall's analysis is arguably misleading since the development of substantive social rights was as necessary to the effective development of capitalism as the development of formal civil and political rights.

The development of social rights has been messier and more complex than Marshall suggested, and Esping-Andersen has elaborated the concept of de-commodification in order to explain the emergence of different kinds of welfare states in different capitalist regimes. He makes clear that:

> ... de-commodification should not be confused with the complete eradication of labour as a commodity; it is not an issue of all or nothing. Rather the concept refers to the degree to which individuals, or families, can uphold a socially acceptable standard of living independently of market participation.
>
> *(1990, p. 37)*

We shall return to Esping-Andersen's work in Chapter 5, which will examine how social rights can differ between countries, but this chapter will consider a particular element of his argument about the development of social rights. Esping-Andersen suggests that historically there were three kinds of responses to the commodification process, reflecting in effect three different ways of thinking about social rights. He defines these in terms of conventional paradigms of conservatism, liberalism and social democracy while seeking to demonstrate that all welfare state regimes are in fact compromises between these competing notions of what social rights should achieve.

- The *conservative* approach is suspicious of commodification because it undermines traditional authority. Characteristically, therefore, this approach favours 'rights' in a paternalistic sense: the kind of rights which come from imposing obligations on employers to look after their workers; from encouraging corporatist guilds and mutual self-help societies; or from state intervention in a paternal-authoritarian mode (e.g. compulsory national insurance schemes).
- The *liberal* approach embraces commodification and seeks to intervene only to the extent that intervention will assist the commodification process or correct 'market failures'. Characteristically, this approach favours 'rights' of a conditional nature (such as means-tested social assistance schemes).

- The *social democratic* approach is inclined to resist commodification because it is the basis of social alienation and class exploitation. Characteristically, this approach favours 'rights' which are emancipatory, which minimise stigmatising conditions and maximise equality.

Following the 1970s, a combination of forces – economic globalisation, the ascendancy of neo-liberal ideological orthodoxies and concerted social and demographic pressures – provoked continuing crises for the capitalist welfare states of the world (Pierson, 1998; Esping-Andersen, 2002; Taylor-Gooby, 2013). Writing in the 1980s, Claus Offe suggested that advanced capitalist societies were facing a paralysis of the commodity form, precisely because of the competing tendencies towards commodification and de-commodification. In the face of this, neither inaction, a return to economic *laissez faire*, nor further development of an extensive and fiscally unviable welfare state were tenable. The alternative, presciently identified by Offe as the underlying basis of emerging policies in welfare state societies, was 'administrative re-commodification' (1984, p. 125). What Offe anticipated is the use of the administrative power of government to sustain the commodity form. This may be achieved by regulating the self-destructive tendencies of market competition; by investing in the 'supply-side' of the economy (in education, training, research and development, transport and communications systems, etc.); and/or by introducing new forms of joint public/private decision-making and financing. The concept of re-commodification captures the sense in which the social rights of citizenship in capitalist welfare states have been transformed. It is not that social rights have been extinguished, but rather that they are being made less democratic and more akin to the property rights of classical jurisprudence. Social rights are now less about enabling people to exist independently of the market and rather more about requiring them to participate in markets, including 'quasi-markets' within the public sector. Paradoxically, however, social rights are no less administrative in nature; it is simply that administrative power has been made more technical than political in character (Barry et al., 1996; Foucault, 1991). This has been primarily manifested through two processes: a shift to welfare pluralism and the introduction of new public managerialism, processes that have played out in different ways and have varied in their significance in different welfare state regimes.

Re-commodification and privatisation

The capitalist welfare state can protect, promote or secure the fulfilment of social rights by a variety of means, not only by directly providing services but also by financing and/or regulating services delivered by non-state providers (Burchardt, 1997, 2013). Re-commodification or privatisation (which – as we shall see – are not necessarily the same thing) can be contrived through a restructuring of public spending and a transition to what is widely termed the 'mixed economy of welfare' or 'welfare pluralism' (e.g. Johnson, 1987; Powell, 2007). The concept of welfare pluralism rests on the idea that, instead of the public sector (the state) being the dominant or principal provider of welfare goods and services, an increasingly significant level of provision should also come from the 'informal' sector (families and communities), the 'voluntary' sector (independent, self-help or non-profit making organisations) and the 'commercial' or private sector. The suggestion is not that the state should cease to guarantee the social rights of the citizen, but that that guarantee need not necessarily be honoured through the direct provision of services by public sector organisations. The state might instead fund the provision of services by other agencies, or it might do no more than regulate the standards of provision made by such agencies.

- The very idea of an *informal sector* amounts in one sense to an oxymoron: it refers to the ostensibly 'unorganised' everyday care and support that people provide for one another within households and neighbourhoods (Rose, 1988); services expected and provided not by way of formally negotiated rights and responsibilities but in terms of common understandings (Finch & Mason, 1993). Nevertheless, households and communities are the original source of personal welfare and the elemental resource on which people the world over, to varying degrees, depend. Indeed, some developing countries with ineffectual state provision but strong kinship and community traditions have been defined as 'informal welfare regimes' (Gough et al. 2004; and see Chapter 9, this volume). In economically developed countries, however, social and demographic changes have diminished the scope for informal care, and some governments have been seeking to counter this trend by re-harnessing and supporting the kind of care that can be provided, for example, to disabled and frail elderly people in their own homes by family members, sometimes as an alternative to publicly provided or financed care (Balloch & Hill, 2007).
- The *voluntary sector* is also known as the Third Sector or the civil society sector (to distinguish it from the public and private sectors) or sometimes the NGO (non-governmental organisation) sector. It has been dubbed a 'loose and baggy monster' (Kendall & Knapp, 1995) on account of the number and diversity of the forms, functions and purposes of the local groups, mutual societies and national and international bodies by which it is constituted. Historically speaking, it is the sector from which all organised social welfare provision once stemmed and from which during the twentieth-century welfare states to a large extent took over. Provision for poor relief, education and healthcare were once primarily the preserve of charitable or religious organisations and were provided not as a right but out of calculated beneficence. Many welfare state governments, in seeking

to re-commodify a range of human services, have sought to revitalise the voluntary sector as a source of unpaid time and commitment in the service of the wider community or to engage voluntary sector organisations contractually as independent providers (Billis & Glennerster, 1998). Where voluntary sector provision represents a return to the feudal charitable principle of *noblesse oblige*, it amounts, according to Ruth Lister (1990), to a 'privatisation' of citizenship and a negation of social rights. Where it amounts to a direct substitution for public sector provision, the implications for social rights can be ambiguous and may depend on by whom and on what terms the provision may be accessed (Ishkanian & Szrerter, 2012).

- The *commercial sector* consists of organisations that sell social or human services as commodities. They differ from some public and voluntary sector providers primarily because they do so competitively and for profit. The commercial sector can trade in the open market in pension plans, employment services, unemployment and health insurance, healthcare, education, housing, residential and domiciliary care services and so on. Controversy surrounds the extent to which the World Trade Organisation's Global Agreement on Trade in Services (GATS) may ultimately open all forms of public services to worldwide competition from commercial providers (Deacon, 2007). There is a clear trend among welfare state governments on the one hand to admit such competition and to allow commercial organisations to provide a range of state-funded services and on the other to promote private alternatives or additions to public sector pensions, healthcare and educational provision (Drakeford, 2000; Papadakis & Taylor-Gooby, 1987). Once again, the implications for social rights are ambiguous and clearly depend on whether and on what terms citizens can access commercially provided services. And, as we shall see, even if no payment is required at the point of delivery of a privately provided public service, the rights of the service user are likely to be more akin to the civil rights of a customer than the social rights of a citizen.

Even where the provision of services remains within the public sector, provision can be made for services to function according to market principles and/or in a more 'business-like' way. This was the purpose of informing the doctrines of New Public Managerialism (Hood, 1991; Clarke & Newman, 1997). The application of such doctrines may entail the introduction of quasi-markets (Le Grand, 1990), whether by creating purchaser-provider splits within public sector organisations (such that some parts of the organisation commission services from others) or by generating funding mechanisms that require providers, such as schools or hospitals, to compete with one another for pupils or patients by improving the standards or the accessibility of their services. New managerialism also challenged the efficacy of the public service ethos by seeking to incentivise service providers through the imposition of performance targets and, for example, by instituting public service user or customer charters. Such charters amounted to symbolic contracts between social security claimants and administrators, pupils (or their parents) and schools, patients and healthcare professionals.

Perhaps the most iconic example was Britain's overarching *Citizen's Charter*, which aimed to make public services more open and accountable by offering 'more privatisation; wider competition; further contracting out; more performance related pay; published performance targets - local and national; comprehensive publication of information on standards achieved; more effective complaints procedures; tougher and more independent inspectorates; better redress for the citizen when things go badly wrong' (Prime Minister's Office, 1991, p. 5). Central to the idea of the *Citizen's Charter* is to link the payment for services (whether directly or through taxes) and the quality of those services. The competent citizen is therefore the successful consumer, able to get the best out of services. The users and providers of services are cast as opponents of each other's interests. What is more, the 'business' of service provision is uncoupled from the politics of welfare: policymakers may evade responsibility for policy failures (because customers are encouraged to blame the providers of services) and the collectivist ethos of the welfare state is diluted (because service provision is driven by individualised incentives rather than policy or vocational or professional commitment). In T.H. Marshall's terms, the *Citizen's Charter* strengthened civil rights (the kind of rights 'customers' enjoy in the marketplace) at the expense of political rights and social rights.

Re-commodification, therefore, involves more than simple privatisation; the selling off or transfer of public services from one sector to another (cf. Starr, 1988). It is also about the framing of the citizen and their rights. One aspect of privatisation relates to the way in which decisions are transferred from public agencies to private individuals (Burchardt, 2013). The key mantra of the new managerialism was the importance of choice: customers, however vulnerable or confused, must choose their service provider or have the opportunity to do so. Services provided by a private or third-sector supplier need not be financed by way of direct transactions between the state and the provider but by the medium of state-financed tax reliefs, allowances or vouchers provided to citizens to enable them to purchase services in the marketplace, compelling them to choose between providers and so drive competition. Service user charters may guarantee or even require service users to choose between schools, hospitals, pension funds, etc. Citizens are thereby accorded formal rights of choice above their substantive rights of benefit. Substantive benefits may be constrained or conditional, especially if resources are scarce and must be rationed. Re-commodification amounts to privatisation in the sense that the fulfilment of social rights must be individually sought through personal transactions. Marshall's conception of social rights – as the 'invasion of contract by status [and] the replacement of the free bargain by the declaration of rights' (see above) is displaced, or at best qualified, through the application of principles based on economic as opposed to social liberalism; principles primarily premised on the ownership and exchange of property, rather than considerations of social justice.

3

HUMAN NEED AND HUMAN RIGHTS

The last chapter discussed social rights as a component of citizenship within a democratic-welfare-capitalist state. Just as citizens of such a state are supposedly guaranteed rights to legal protection and political participation, so they are also entitled to have their needs for certain essential goods and services met. But which needs and to what extent? Understandings of need are not only a part of everyday life but are also central to social policy. And yet need is a deeply contested concept with an extraordinary array of meanings (Dean, 2020).

It has been contended that social rights may be understood as articulations of human needs. Citizenship, as we have seen, entails a more or less inclusive process by which needs can be named and claimed, claims may be recognised and rules for the distribution of resources can be made. Citizenship has been the principal arena in which rights have been formulated. And what have conventionally been identified as social rights were first specifically formulated at a particular point in the development of industrial capitalism, when a particular set of social ills warranted a particular kind of state intervention. We have considered Marshall's account of this process in Chapter 2. This was an account premised on the British example and on a welfare state whose foundations had been consolidated at the end of the Second World War. It was an era in which it was believed that the administrative power of the warfare state could be turned, like a sword into a plough shear, into a peacetime welfare state that would engage and defeat what were characterised in a report by Sir William Beveridge (1942) as five metaphorical 'giants': disease, idleness, ignorance, squalor and want. Each giant represented an unmet human need: the need for health, for work, for education, for decent housing and for a means of subsistence.

Meanwhile, on the other side of the Atlantic, the US President, Franklyn D. Roosevelt (1941), was propounding 'Four Freedoms': the freedoms *of*

DOI: 10.4324/9781003451518-4

speech and worship and the freedoms *from* fear and want. Roosevelt later elaborated explicitly on freedom from want when he declared that 'Necessitous men are not free men. People who are hungry and out of a job are the stuff of which dictatorships are made' (1944). When it came to developing its post-war welfare state, the United States would later be regarded as something of a 'laggard' compared to Western European countries (e.g. Offe, 1972), but the legacy of Roosevelt's Four Freedoms declaration (in part through the role played by his widow, Eleanor, as Chair of the UN Commission on Human Rights) is nonetheless to be found in the preamble to the Universal Declaration of Human Rights of 1948. This proclaimed that 'the advent of a world in which human beings shall enjoy freedom of speech and belief and freedom from fear and want [to be] the highest aspiration of the common people'. The rhetoric of mid-twentieth-century social liberalism was implicated not only in promoting rights of welfare state citizenship but also in the social rights component of the international human rights agenda. The idea of freedom from want – of needs as a basis for the construction of rights – though potentially ambiguous is conceptually compelling. It will lead us in this chapter to a broadening of the discussion, including an introduction to the international human rights agenda, but also to an evaluation of the extent to which the needs of humanity remain unequally or insufficiently satisfied. To begin, however, we shall turn to a discussion of human needs.

Concepts of need

The word 'need' in English is both a verb and a noun. The things we need, we call needs. Need may be defined in terms of that which we feel or experience, or in terms of things we must have or must do. Needs may be equated (though they are not necessarily synonymous) with wants, preferences, or desires. Insofar as people may suffer for 'want' or lack of that which they find necessary, Agnes Heller has argued that 'All needs considered by humans to be real must be considered as real' (cited in Soper, 1981, p. 215). We may say that we need to eat, we need to work, we need a home, we need to rest, we need to love and be loved, we need to understand the world in which we live, or that we need to lead a 'good' or fulfilling life. Picking up the discussion begun in Chapter 2 of the ways in which rights may be differently interpreted, we might now begin to unpack the different ways in which needs may be interpreted, according not only to whether they are being defined from the top-down or the bottom-up, but also – later in the chapter – whether they derive from a 'thin' or a 'thick' understanding of human wellbeing.

Top-down vs. bottom-up

Top-down definitions of human need can be described as 'inherent' conceptions in that they are needs that have been adjudged to be inherent to the human person. They therefore require an implicit or explicit theory of personhood, whether this is scientifically, philosophically, ideologically or theologically derived. They are top-down in the sense that they are needs that are prescribed for us on an *a priori* basis, which is not to say that we might not accept or embrace them as needs. Bottom-up definitions of human need can be described as 'interpreted' conceptions in that they are needs that we may name and claim for ourselves, albeit that our claims may be culturally shaped or else our claims may sometimes be named and claimed on our behalf by legitimate advocates or beneficent welfare professionals. They are pragmatically formulated and bottom-up in the sense that they are articulated through demands people make on other people or on social institutions. In practice, the distinction between top-down and bottom-up can be difficult to sustain (for the same sort of reason that it can be difficult to sustain the distinction made in Chapter 2 between doctrinal and claims-based rights): today's bottom-up definitions can become tomorrow's top-down definitions and *vice versa*. But the distinction is heuristically valuable. It helps us reflect upon and make sense of the dynamic way in which needs are defined.

Top-down definitions can be diversely informed: by utilitarian assumptions that regard the person as an independent rational actor with objective interests (Thomson, 1987); by economistic beliefs that regard the person as a market actor with subjective preferences (e.g. Menger, 1871); by psychological theories that regard the person as a sentient being with inner drives (e.g. Maslow, 1943). In the field of academic social policy, the most influential attempt to provide a theory of universal human need has been provided by Doyal and Gough (1991), who draw out a distinction between, on the one hand, basic or universal needs for physical health and personal autonomy; and, on the other, the intermediate needs that must be met if basic needs are to be optimally satisfied in any given socio-economic or cultural context. Doyal and Gough's list of intermediate needs or needs satisfiers (see Box 3.1) can be, and sometimes are, read as if they are a list of social rights.

BOX 3.1 DOYAL AND GOUGH'S 'INTERMEDIATE' NEED SATISFIERS

- Adequate nutritional food and water
- Adequate protective housing
- A non-hazardous work environment
- A non-hazardous physical environment
- Appropriate health care
- Security in childhood
- Significant primary relationships
- Physical security
- Economic security
- Safe birth control and childbearing
- Basic education

Bottom-up definitions of need can similarly be shaped through a diversity of processes: not only through active resistance to perceived injustices (Moore, 1978; Thompson, 1993), but also through passive acceptance of the local customs by which a shared understanding of 'necessaries' is established (Smith, 1776, p. 691), or through everyday expectations fuelled by consumer culture (Marcuse, 1964; Galbraith, 1992; Bauman, 1998). From an earlier social policy perspective, Jonathan Bradshaw (1972) suggested that need may be not only 'normative' (as when it is determined by welfare professionals and experts); but also 'felt' (and revealed, for example, by opinion polling); 'expressed' (and voiced through democratic participation); or 'comparative' (as when it is evaluated through social research). Nancy Fraser (1989) has since expressly advocated more active bottom-up processes of definition through a 'politics of needs interpretation', an idea to which we shall return in later chapters.

Both top-down and bottom-up understandings of need contribute to the construction of social rights. Social citizenship is a process that sets the parameters within which understandings of need are negotiated (Dean, 2013); within which the top-down and the bottom-up meet one another. The outcomes may vary. Bryan Turner (1990; 1991), when considering the emergence of different kinds of citizenship during the period of the European Enlightenment, draws a broadly framed historical distinction between a 'descending' and an 'ascending' view of citizenship: 'In the descending view, the king is all powerful and the subject is the recipient of privileges. In the ascending view a free man was a citizen, an active bearer of rights' (1990, p. 207). Turner suggests that the English outcome was a triumph for a descending constitutionalist view, whereby the rule of the sovereign-in-parliament was established over subjects as citizens. In contrast, the aspirations – but not necessarily the eventual outcome – of the French Revolution epitomised the ascending view. In the event, the post-absolutist settlement in France, as across much of continental Western Europe, represented a brokered rather than a constitutionalist outcome and the kind of power-sharing arrangements that prefigured modern corporatism (Mann, 1987).

But this is a retrospective analysis of power struggles at a macro-level. The social rights of citizenship are about human needs and human encounters that are experienced at a micro-level. Citizenship encompasses both the systems in which power operates and the living agents of that power. The distinction between top-down and bottom-up is also reflected in Jürgen Habermas' celebrated distinction between 'system' and 'lifeworld'. Habermas' (1987) characterisation of late Western 'modernity' is that it exhibits a separation and continuing tension between, on the one hand, the technical systems by which rights of citizenship are formulated and administered and, on the other, the lifeworld that gives meaning to social participation and in which the wellsprings of behaviour and aspiration are located. Perhaps, however, there has always been a tension between systemic top-down prescriptions for meeting human needs and bottom-up agency through which voice is given to lifeworld needs. The enduring question is whether – and in what circumstances – this can be a creative tension or a destructive one.

Thin vs. thick

In Chapter 2, passing mention was made of Walzer's notions of thin and thick moralities. A similar distinction can be made between thin needs and thick needs (Soper, 1993). Both kinds of needs are important, but whereas 'thin' needs relate to what is required for bare survival, 'thick' needs relate to what is required for true fulfilment (cf. Ignatieff, 1984). The distinction captures the relativity of need and different levels of necessity. Insofar as needs are articulated through rights, thin needs may in part be met through the protections offered by formal or procedural rights, which guarantee equality of access and opportunity. Thick needs may be met through substantive rights, which ensure universal protection or provision. But even when there is provision for substantive social rights, provision may be thin – a parsimonious safety net against total destitution. A universal minimum level of social rights may be sufficient for some citizens but provide too thinly for those with complex needs. Relatively generous levels of rights-based social provision may meet the thick needs of some citizens but not the needs of others.

Doyal and Gough's list of needs satisfiers in Box 3.1 was intended as an attainable standard to which even poorer countries might aspire, but arguably it implies a relatively thin definition of need. It refers only to 'adequate' food and housing, to 'appropriate' healthcare and to 'basic' education. Thicker definitions might insist on plentiful and palatable food, good standard housing, high-quality healthcare and secondary and even tertiary education. The terms thin and thick are, of course, metaphorical and though it is a banal analogy, it is often used in relation to soup. It may be seen, however, from Box 3.2 that deeper meaning can be read even into such an analogy. Human well-being necessarily depends on physical survival, but it has other – thicker – dimensions because human well-being depends on social context. This is plainly recognised by Doyal & Gough when they include such things as 'security in childhood' and 'significant primary relationships' as intermediate needs. We might quibble that it would be preferable to demand ontological security *throughout* the human life course and significant social relationships *beyond* the bounds of immediate family, but in fairness, Doyal & Gough's emphasis here is upon 'optimising' rather than maximising needs satisfaction (1991, ch. 7). Clearly, if one were to hold to a meanly Hobbesian view of human nature and assume that human society entails

BOX 3.2 THIN SOUP/THICK SOUP

All soup is made from ingredients taken from nature and gathered and prepared by human endeavour. But there is a distinction to be drawn – sometimes metaphorical but often literal – between 'thin' soup and 'thick' soup.

Thin soup may be perfectly nutritious, even wholesome, but it is characterised as thin because it is insipid, relatively flavourless and unappetising, if not unpleasant to taste. It is likely to have been prepared impersonally, in a factory or institutional kitchen, by anonymous people with little or no culinary skill. It relieves hunger or is minimally satisfying, and it keeps you alive. The consumption of a thin soup is an act performed solely to ensure personal survival.

Thick soup may be equally nutritious, but it is characterised as rich because it is richer in texture and flavour. It is likely to have been prepared with care by a skilled chef or a loving parent, partner or companion. It provides enjoyment and can make you feel not merely satiated but fulfilled – good to be alive. The appreciation of a thick soup cements respect for others' skills and/or gratitude for their love.

nothing more than 'a war of all against all' (1651), one's view of human need is likely to be minimalistically thin. But as soon as one acknowledges human society to be an association of vulnerable and fundamentally interdependent beings (e.g. Turner, 2006), one's view of human need will begin to take on thicker dimensions.

It should by now be evident that the term 'wellbeing', though widely used, is ambiguous and, like the term 'welfare' (Daly, 2011), conceals significant controversies with regard to the nature and meaning of human need. Competing understandings of human needs lead to radically different debates about the role of policy. A distinctly thin, if not explicitly hedonic, approach to human need has driven a recent global preoccupation with subjective wellbeing or 'happiness', which now widely figures as a measure of human progress and as a metric, potentially, to inform social policy (Helliwell et al., 2024; Stiglitz et al., 2009). It is a trend informed by the so-called Easterlin 'paradox' (2005), which observes that economic growth does not necessarily correlate with increased subjective wellbeing. The implication that it is time for humanity to rein in its destructive pursuit of wealth is one that finds favour with some (Marks, 2006; New Economics Foundation, 2012; Hickel, 2022), but the alternative implication – that the wellbeing of poor and disadvantaged people may be addressed other than by policies for wealth redistribution – would seem to be the more dominant assumption. By contrast, a thicker approach to wellbeing is evident, for example, in scholarly work around concepts such as 'social quality' (Beck et al., 1997) and 'social value' (Jordan, 2008), concepts that challenge the essentially individualist-utilitarian premises of the subjective wellbeing agenda and seek to re-establish a notion of wellbeing premised on the 'centrality of the *social* human being' (McGregor, 2007, p. 321).

Revisiting radical need and human essence

Emphasising the centrality of the *social* human being brings us back to the discussion begun in Chapter 1 and the concept of sociality as one of the essential and defining characteristics of the human species. The provenance of the distinction between thin/survival needs and thick/fulfilment needs might arguably be traced back to classical philosophy and, in particular, Aristotle's (c. 350 BCE) distinction between, on the one hand, *hedonic* well-being, which associates human welfare with the pursuit of pleasure and the avoidance of pain, and on the other *eudaimonic* wellbeing, which associates welfare with the living of a good or ethical life. Clearly, hedonic needs matter because their measured satisfaction ensures survival and will better enable a person effectively to achieve eudaimonic wellbeing and so achieve the characteristics that differentiate human beings from other species. We might here revisit Marx's analysis of radical needs and human essence. Marx, it might be said, implicitly reinterprets or translates Aristotle's notion of eudaimonic well-being by interpreting human 'essence' in terms of that which is materially essential rather than that which is spiritually essential. The radical needs of human beings are reflected in the realisation of all four of the essential species characteristics that may be inferred from Marx's philosophical writings (see Table 3.1). Insofar as those characteristics are interdependent, it may be argued that sociality – including the recognition of social rights as an expression of sociality – are indeed central to the realisation of our humanity and to human welfare as a whole.

TABLE 3.1 The eudaimonic character of our human species being

Essential *species characteristics*	*Which define ....*	*Are* realised *through ....*	*Are ethically fulfilled when ...*
Sociality	how we relate to one another	our mutual interdependence	we can sustain love, solidarity and rights
Consciousness	who we are	our search for meaning	we can exercise critical reason
Work	what we do	our substantive activities	we can express human creativity
history making	what we might accomplish	our part in human history	we can contribute to human 'betterment'

Source: Adapted from Dean (2016).

The international human rights agenda

There is no global consensus as to the definition of human need. In some languages, there is no single word that directly corresponds with the ambiguous and encompassing English word 'need' (Lederer, 1980). And yet we do have an internationally agreed Universal Declaration of Human Rights (UDHR), a declaration that defines certain substantive social rights and, by implication, accords recognition to certain agreed human needs (Freeman, 2011; Woodiwiss, 2005).

The United Nations Organisation, founded at the end of the Second World War in 1945, established a Human Rights Commission to draft a Universal Declaration, which was eventually adopted and proclaimed by the UN General Assembly in 1948. The Declaration explicitly included well-established 'first generation' civil and political rights (to life, liberty, property, equality before the law, privacy, fair trial, religious freedom, free speech and assembly, to participate in government, to political asylum and an absolute right not to be tortured), but also, more controversially, a 'second generation' of economic, social and cultural rights. Though distinctions can be and are drawn between 'economic', 'social' and 'cultural' rights, they may and shall, for our purposes, be encompassed within a single expanded concept of 'social' rights and they specifically included rights to work, education and even leisure. Most particularly, Article 25 states:

> Everyone has the right to a standard of living adequate for the health and wellbeing of himself[/herself] and his[/her] family, including food, clothing, housing and medical care and necessary social services, and the right to security in the event of unemployment, sickness, disability, widowhood, old age or other lack of livelihood in circumstances beyond his[/her] control.

First and second-generation rights were declared to be inalienable and indivisible, but for the purposes of preparing legally binding international covenants, they were in fact separated. The resulting covenants – the International Covenant on Civil and Political Rights (ICCPR) and the International Covenant on Economic, Social and Cultural Rights (ICESCR) – were presented to the UN General Assembly in 1954 and eventually adopted in 1966. Unlike the ICCPR, the ICESCR admits a principle of 'progressive realisation' (Article 2), requiring states parties unable immediately to fulfil rights prescribed by the covenant to 'take steps' towards achieving the full realisation of such rights. Monitoring and reporting arrangements under the ICCPR require states parties to report periodically on their progress to a committee – the Committee on Economic, Social and Cultural Rights (ECOSOC).

The discussion between state parties' representatives on the Commission on Human Rights as to the drafting of the UDHR and the ICESCR and their subsequent reports to, and discussions with, the ECOSOC reveal divergent interpretations of social rights, but perhaps a greater degree of convergence since the 1990s (Davy, 2013). What clearly emerges is the extent to which, initially, the social rights framed by the UDHR and the ICESCR represented an uneasy compromise between different understandings of social rights: between a social citizenship ideal espoused by the US and Western European nations; a developmental approach espoused especially by Latin American nations; and a state socialist approach espoused by Eastern European nations (who, in practice, abstained from much of the debate). The liberal social citizenship ideal was focused on individual freedom from want; the developmental approach on collective need for economic and thereby social development; and the state socialist approach on state duties for the meeting of needs. Social rights or social rights-related clauses were subsequently written into a variety of supra-national treaties and instruments (see Box 3.3) and, in various forms, into many national constitutions (Jung et al., 2013). While generally replicating or borrowing features of the UDHR, these clauses would appear

BOX 3.3 SUPRA-NATIONAL TREATIES CONTAINING SOCIAL RIGHTS OR SOCIAL RIGHTS RELATED CLAUSES BEARING UPON PARTICULAR GROUPS OR GLOBAL REGIONS

UN Conventions

- International Convention on the Elimination of All Forms of Racial Discrimination (1966)
- Convention on the Elimination of All Forms of Discrimination Against Women (1979)
- Convention on the Rights of the Child (1989)
- International Convention on the Protection of the Rights of All Migrant Workers and Members of Their Families (1990)
- Convention on the Rights of Persons with Disabilities (2006)

UN Declarations

- Declaration on the Right to Development (1986)
- United Nations Principles for Older Persons (1991)

Regional Charters

- European Social Charter (1961 – amended 1996)
- American Convention on Human Rights (1969) and the Additional Protocol of San Salvador (1988)
- African Charter of Human and People's Rights (1981)

to have had quite different and, in some instances, limited substantive effects. However, the apparent convergence mentioned above, following the collapse of communism in Eastern Europe and the development of new forms of social assistance provision in the emerging economies of the global South (Leisering & Barrientos, 2013), suggests elements of a global shift in favour of the liberal social citizenship ideal, with its focus on individual freedom from want.

By the turn of the Millennium, the United Nations Development Programme declared that the rhetoric of human rights, having been reduced during the Cold War years 'to a weapon in the propaganda for geopolitical interests' (UNDP, 2003, p. 3), should henceforth be harnessed to a common vision and a common purpose for the respective concepts of human rights and human development. The framing of this vision was significantly influenced by Nobel laureate, Amartya Sen, who argues that human rights guarantee the basic freedoms necessary for 'human development'. They are, therefore, primarily means to an end, namely the realisation of human *capabilities* (Sen, 1999, 2004; UNDP, 2000, ch. 1). By capabilities, Sen was alluding to the freedom of the human individual to be and do in their life that which they value and have reason to value. What has come widely to be known as the 'capabilities approach' (Deneulin, 2006; Nussbaum, 2011) had some direct impact in the framing of the Millennium Development Goals (UNDP, 2003; UN, 2000). It served in some respects to re-inflect the international human rights agenda and to re-frame the distinction that may be drawn between social rights development and human development. The capabilities approach was regarded as a palatable alternative: first, to the 'Basic Needs Approach' (BNA) that had informed the broadly social democratic conception of social development that was initially promoted by the ILO in the 1970s and fleetingly adopted within the World Bank (Reader, 2006; Streeten et al., 1981); and more immediately, to the widely discredited neo-liberal Washington Consensus that had displaced the BNA in the 1980s and '90s (see Chapter 9 in this volume).

In essence, the capabilities approach is fundamentally liberal individualist in the sense that individual fulfilment is constituted through the capacity to exercise choice (Dean, 2009). The implication for human rights is that they may be seen (contrary to the protestations of Jeremy Bentham mentioned in Chapter 2, this volume) to be consistent with a utilitarian ethic (Sen, 2004). Human development is about maximising individual freedom and so:

> Human rights can include significant and influenceable economic and social freedoms. If they cannot be realized because of inadequate institutionalization, then, to work for institutional expansion or reform can be a part of the obligations generated by the recognition of these rights. The current unrealizability of any accepted human right, which can be promoted through institutional or political change, does not, by itself, convert that claim into a *non*-right.
>
> *(ibid., p. 320)*

According to this view, the social rights component of human rights may for the time being (and perhaps unavoidably) be violated for want of individual freedom. But freedom, which does not need satisfaction, is the paramount consideration.

This draws us back to the question of the relationship between social rights and human needs. The UDHR came into existence in the aftermath of the horrors of two world wars, at a time of deep concern about the consequences of totalitarianism and 'rightlessness' and a conviction that human rights offer us the 'right to have rights', independently of any nation-state or government (Arendt, 1951). There is a sense in which 'social rights' is a term that might be used to refer to all rights created by sovereign nation-states, whereas human rights are the innate or imprescriptible rights of human beings (Turner, 2006, p. 2). This is not a terminology adopted in this volume (since there are important distinctions to be drawn between different species of citizenship rights), but the argument points us to a different vein of reasoning wherein the most fundamental of rights relate at least as much to human *sociality* as to individual *autonomy*; as much to solidarity as to freedom. Contemporary claims to cosmopolitanism of a human rights approach are suspect: 'because [human rights discourse] very clearly privileges autonomy over reciprocity, it also allows some individuals to be more autonomous than others' (Woodiwiss, 2005, p. 123). In fact, long before the current era, Hannah Arendt, mindful of the ontological essence of human existence, had warned that:

> The concept of human rights can again be meaningful only if they are redefined as the right to the human condition itself, which depends on belonging to some human community, the right never to be dependent on some inborn human dignity which de facto, aside from its guarantee by fellow men, not only does not exist but is the last and possibly most arrogant myth we have invented in our long history.
>
> *(1951, p. 439)*

Social rights – whether they are considered as citizenship rights or human rights – are social. While writing about social rights of citizenship rather than human rights, Fred Twine (1994) located social rights in relation to the 'interdependence of self and society'. Similarly, in pursuit of a theory of human rights, Bryan Turner has argued that 'it is from a collectively held recognition of individual frailty that rights as a system of mutual protection gain their emotive force' (1993, p. 507). Social rights are located in relation to the shared vulnerability that characterises the human condition. Such approaches at present stand, at best, as a 'minor tradition' within human rights discourse (Woodiwiss 2005, p. 134). While the major hegemonic tradition attributes violations of human rights to the lack of *freedom*, the minor tradition attributes violations to failures of *solidarity*. But it is to the deficits and failures in *equality* and equality of needs satisfaction to which we now turn. The 'myth' against which Arendt railed was the premise contained in Article 1 of the UDHR, that 'All human beings are born free and *equal* in dignity and *rights*' [emphasis added]. Leaving aside the hollowness of the concept of dignity in this context, this begs the question – what is the relationship between equality and rights?

The failures of social rights

The survival of social inequality and poverty, even within developed welfare state nations, suggests that their approach to social rights has failed. At best, it would seem citizens' needs are unequally satisfied. At worst, their needs remain unsatisfied. The problems of inequality and poverty in the richer countries of the world imply a failure of the social liberal citizenship ideal (Lister,, 2010). It has already been noted in Chapter 2 of this volume that in OECD countries, socio-economic inequality remains persistent. Thomas Picketty (2014) has demonstrated that in the twentieth century, the effects of two world wars followed by the extensive development of welfare states may have moderated a previously ineluctable growth in inequality of income and wealth, but that such inequality has since been rapidly accelerating. Across the world as a whole, in the decades immediately preceding the 2008 global financial crisis, global per capita income was rising, but it was that of the richest which rose, while that of the poorest fell (Milanovic, 2007). Even in one of the richest countries, the United Kingdom, it has been shown that in 2021–2022, 30 per cent of the population in practice experienced what a majority of Britons would consider to be an unacceptably low standard of living (Padley, et al., 2024). In Chapter 9, this volume, we shall see in greater detail how inequality and poverty in the rich and poor countries compare and how social development interventions by the UN and other agencies and social rights provision by poorer nation states have yet fully alleviated inequality and poverty.

Inequality

It was noted in Chapter 2, this volume, that equality is a fiercely contested concept when it comes to the distinction between formal equality under the law and substantive equalities of entitlement to social protection or provision. There are related contests between arguments for equality of outcome as opposed to equality of income; equality of opportunity as opposed to equality of reward; equality of dignity as opposed to equality of power; equality of status as opposed to equality of condition. As we might expect, when Amartya Sen contentiously posed the question 'Equality of What?' (1982a), he concluded that his preferred concept – equality of capabilities – could effectively settle such arguments. The concept of capabilities entails both formal and substantive freedom: freedom of choice as to the life one leads. But this doesn't necessarily deal with the question of just how free human beings can 'really' be when in the course of their lives they are so necessarily interdependent with and upon one another; when they live in a world so dominated by an economic system (capitalism) founded on the exploitation of human labour power; when they may be systemically subordinated by relations of power that oppress, control or simply exclude them (Dean, 2009).

Inequality, as the negation of equality, provides tangible evidence of when and where needs are not fully met. It is in attempts to identify inequality that connections between needs and rights are often made. In Britain, for example, an independent review, set up in preparation for the creation of an Equality and Human Rights Commission (EHRC), made recommendations for a measurement tool by which to evaluate dimensions of inequality across Britain. The review identified and operationalised a framework of ten 'domains of valuable capabilities' (see Table 3.2) quite explicitly distilled from the international human rights framework (Equalities Review, 2007; Vizard & Burchardt, 2007). A rather different approach has been taken by Baker et al. (2004), who, in an attempt to forge a substantive multidimensional egalitarianism reaching beyond that implied by Article 1 of the UDHR, have proposed five 'dimensions of equality'. Their dimensions, they claim, establish a framework 'that helps to map the differences between liberal egalitarians and equality of condition' (2004, p. 25). What may be seen in Table 3.1 are two contrasting ways of reflecting on equality and human need. Using the notions of 'thin' and thick' we might say that Baker et al.'s dimensions are thicker than Vizard and Burchardt's domains. But important connections can be made between the two lists. What is clear is that discussions about equality and equal rights lead back to definitions of need.

TABLE 3.2 Equality and need

Vizard and Burchardt's 'domains of valuable capabilities'	*Baker et al.'s 'dimensions of equality'*
• life; • physical security; • health; • education; • standard of living; • productive and valued activities; • individual, family and social life; • participation, influence and voice; • identity, expression and self-respect; • legal security	• respect and recognition; • resources • love, care and solidarity • power • working and learning

We saw in Chapter 2 that Marshall's theory of social rights explicitly claimed that social rights would and should ameliorate class inequality, which they have not. What has happened is that the structural dynamics of class and inequality have changed. Marx and Engels had claimed that 'the history of all hitherto existing society is the history of class struggles' (1848, p. 16) and under capitalism, inequality of needs satisfaction stems from the fact that workers are unequally and inequitably rewarded for their labour. Under classic industrial capitalism, the boundaries between bosses and workers and between relatively privileged non-manual and manual workers were reasonably clear. But fundamental changes in the nature of labour processes associated with shifts towards post-industrial service and information economies have resulted in, on the one hand, increasing labour diversification and associated income inequalities and, on the other, the fragmentation of traditional classes. Paradoxically, while socio-economic and occupational status continued to be a key determinant of life chances across the capitalist world (e.g. Goldthorpe et al., 1982; Marshall, 1997; Meiksins-Wood, 1995), the transparency of class relations evaporated. The phenomenon has conventionally been captured by dual labour market theory (e.g. Watson, 1995, ch. 5) and the idea that labour markets are now polarised between a securely employed, highly skilled and well-paid 'core' and a chronically precariously employed, lower-skilled and badly paid 'periphery'. Guy Standing (2009, 2011) has attempted an alternative global class analysis focusing on seven groups of actors in the globalised economy and hypothesising the emergence within this fluid structure of a new class, the 'precariat', situated beneath a 'global elite', the 'salariat', a class of highly expert 'proficians' and the diminishing 'traditional working class' on the one hand, but above the officially 'unemployed' and what he would seem to regard as an underclass, which he describes as 'the detached'. The precariat is a class ill-served by social rights, as will be further discussed in Chapter 6.

Classic Weberian class analysis (Scaff, 1998; Weber, 1978) has focused more on the interrelationship between socioeconomic and sociocultural differences in society; it considers lifestyles as much as living standards. Sociologists have presented us with insights into how it is not only a person's standing in relation to the means of production but their engagement with relations of consumption that characterise and give meaning to inequalities in needs satisfaction. Social divisions came to depend not so much on people's occupational status as upon whether they are able to meet their needs for housing, healthcare and education independently in the marketplace, as opposed to having to depend on inferior or stigmatised forms of state provision (Saunders, 1984). In consumer societies, people's sense of subjective sufficiency and social inclusion depends on their capacity to comply with a prevailing 'aesthetic of consumption' (Bauman, 1998); to follow fashions and be able, for example, to afford to have one's children wear 'the right trainers' to school (Ridge, 2002).

More recent analyses of inequality have moved beyond class analysis to consider how the substantive differences in human experience and life chances may result from other dimensions of human diversity. This has resulted, in part at least, from the 'cultural turn' that occurred in the global North with the advent of the post-industrial era (Clarke, 1999), the significance of which can, paradoxically, be linked as much to the maturity of capitalist welfare states as to the crisis that apparently befell them in the 1970s (Mishra, 1984, 1999). The welfare states of the post-Second World War era had developed to the point that they provided a degree of material security for a comfortable majority; indeed, there is evidence that it was the comfortable middle classes rather than the poorest in society who benefited most (Le Grand, 1982). This made way for more individualistic or introspective cultural concerns as issues of personal identity took precedence over issues of material survival (Inglehart, 1990). At the same time, new social movements – the second wave feminist movement in particular – and new forms of community activism began to challenge monolithic, inflexible and sometimes oppressive state welfare institutions (Lewis et al., 2000; and see Chapter 6, this volume). There was a shift from a politics of class to a politics of identity: a new awareness of social diversity and difference and, in particular in the 1970s, the inequalities associated with gender, ethnicity and disability. Increasingly now, the focus is on multiple and intersecting inequalities (in the plural) and on a range of systemic manifestations of social advantage and disadvantage (Dean & Platt, 2016).

Inequalities in human society are perhaps inevitable. Some would even say that inequality can be functional (Davis & Moore, 1945); others say that, within limits, it may be socially just (Rawls, 1972). What is clear, however, from a body of international evidence (Wilkinson, 2005; Wilkinson & Pickett, 2009; WHO, 2008) is that inequality has consequences for human well-being. Those countries in which material needs are more equally satisfied tend by and large to exhibit not only higher levels of subjective well-being but less variation in health outcomes and life expectancy.

Poverty

Poverty is perhaps the most ancient and encompassing concept associated with systemic social disadvantage. It has been defined as the 'unacceptable face of inequality' (Tawney, 1913), which begs the question, how do we define acceptability and unacceptability and the point at which something should be done about inequality or poverty; the point at which, perhaps, a right to poverty relief might kick in? Elements of this question will be addressed in Chapter 8 of this volume, but here we shall seek a link between definitions of need and definitions of poverty.

There is an enduring debate as to whether poverty should be defined in absolute or relative terms. But beneath this distinction lies a question of the standard, which should be applied in relation to some level of absolute need as opposed to a broader conception of relative need. In practice therefore, what are generally identified as absolute definitions may apply a spectrum of different standards: a person may be adjudged poor only if they have insufficient resources to avoid *starvation*, or, more generously, if they have insufficient resources to achieve a sometimes arbitrarily defined minimum level of *subsistence*. What are generally identified as relative definitions may similarly apply different standards: a person may be adjudged to be poor if, though they have enough resources for bare subsistence, they are unable to *cope* in the context of prevailing social standards; or, more generously still, if they are unable fully to *participate* in the society of which they are a part (George & Howards, 1991). Associated with debates about definition is a host of underlying controversies:

- Technical controversies with regard to where to draw the 'poverty line'; how to set a 'budget standard' that defines an adequate standard of living; whether there can be a social consensus as to what is minimally necessary; is there a resource threshold below which people cannot socially participate? (e.g. Alcock, 2006, ch. 6);
- Explanatory controversies with regard to whether poverty is attributable to individual pathology, cultural malaise, policy failure or the structural consequences of capitalism (Alcock, 2006, ch. 3; Jordan, 1996; Novak, 1988);
- Political controversies with regard to whether governments should be responsible for minimally relieving poverty if and when it occurs, or whether they should attempt to prevent poverty from happening in the first place (Alcock, 2006, ch. 3; Townsend & Gordon, 2002);
- Sociological controversies with regard to whether, on the one hand, poverty is an objective phenomenon or social fact or whether, on the other, it is a symbolic process of subjection and a social construct (Dean with Melrose, 1999).

Just as Sen considers that his concept of human capabilities answers his own question, 'Equality of What?', he has also argued that it resolves the controversy about absolute and relative definitions of poverty. Poverty, Sen claims (1985), may be relative in the space of the commodities that human beings need, but it is absolute in the space of human capabilities. By this, he means we all need different things in order to fulfil our personal life projects and achieve acceptable kinds of human functioning, but we each absolutely need the freedom to choose how we live. This claim was challenged by Peter Townsend (1993, ch. 6), who feared that Sen's insistence on an 'absolutist core' of poverty could too easily perpetuate a narrow subsistence-standard conception of poverty. Sen, for his part, was alleging that Townsend's concept of relative deprivation was merely conflating poverty with inequality.

Sen and Townsend each recognised that human needs have a social context, but they had different conceptions of social justice. Townsend (1979) had been seeking to define an objective material threshold beneath which relative deprivation leads to a person's exclusion from social participation. He was not conflating poverty and inequality; his quest was to determine a definitive relationship between them. It has been suggested from a very different quarter that such a quest could nevertheless miss the point. The sheer diversity of human beings' lifestyles and behaviours makes it difficult to pin down a threshold by which to define where poverty starts and ends. Drawing on Titmuss' notion of 'diswelfare' (1955), we might suggest that, in its many forms and guises, poverty may be universally defined in terms of 'human diswelfare'. The term 'poverty', Piachaud points out, 'carries with it an implication and a moral imperative that something should be done about it' (1981, p. 119).

When, as we shall see in the next chapter, the UN Copenhagen Summit (UN, 1995) appeared to declare poverty to be a violation of human rights, it pronounced a call to action. Sceptics may claim that when the problem is hunger and malnutrition, the victims don't need rights, just action; they need farmers and doctors, not lawyers or philosophers (O'Neill, 1986). Here we may return to the contention that social rights are to be understood as the articulation of human needs. Debates about the distinction between absolute and relative poverty or absolute and relative need can most certainly miss the point. Embodied and 'needy' human beings and the societies they have created are diverse and complex, and specific needs differ in their framing (they may be prescribed from the top down or demanded from the bottom up) and in their immediate extent (they may be thin or thick). Human sociality entails the continual construction and renewal of what we may describe as social rights, which, however suboptimally or unevenly and however immanently or explicitly, express the outcome of a struggle for the mutual recognition and satisfaction of human needs.

4

SOCIAL RIGHTS AND SOCIAL DEVELOPMENT

We have seen that social rights were initially framed as rights of citizenship through substantive social legislation by capitalist welfare states, but also formulated as general principles within the Universal Declaration of Human Rights. Chapter 3 has focused on the relationship between needs and rights and concluded with a discussion of 'poverty' and the extent to which social rights – as currently framed and understood – have succeeded or failed to counter poverty and failures of universal human development. We shall be returning in Chapter 9 to consider the various ways in which social rights have in practice emerged in different parts of the world and debates as to the relevance of prevailing social rights discourse across all societies and cultures. But in this chapter, we shall first consider contested understandings of human development before addressing conceptual links between development, rights and poverty.

Economic development *vs.* social development

Human development, it might be supposed, is the process through which the human species organises to meet its needs. Marx, however, regarded human development not as a planned or unilinear process but as an immanent and dialectical historical struggle (see Chapter 1, this volume). In the capitalist era, explanations of relative wealth and poverty at the international level were first framed in terms of 'development' and 'underdevelopment' (George, 1988, ch. 10). Development was then considered to be synonymous with industrialisation. The dominant conception of development imported a hegemonically Western theory of 'modernisation', which assumed there is an

DOI: 10.4324/9781003451518-5

optimum, it not virtuous, path to democratic-welfare-capitalism (e.g. Lipset, 1963; Rostow, 1971). Insofar as some countries remained chronically poorer than others, it was supposed that this reflected a failure to 'modernise', occasioned by technological, political or cultural deficiencies. Poor countries were to be encouraged or assisted to 'catch up' with their richer capitalist neighbours. Structuralist critics of this view (e.g. Frank, 1971; Hayter, 1971) began to suggest that the continued disadvantage of the world's poorer countries should be attributed not to internal failings but to external factors, in particular the historical and structural economic dependency of poor and economically weak nations upon rich and powerful ones. Later commentators drew attention to the ways in which poor nations are more vulnerable than rich ones to the power of mighty transnational corporations and in which they could, in practice, be impeded rather than assisted by the regulatory interventions of supranational bodies, such as the International Monetary Fund (IMF) and the World Bank (Deacon et al., 1997). Pressure, largely from countries of the global South, led in 1986 to the UN's adoption of a Declaration to a Right to Development, expressing demands from poorer countries for self-determination and the right to develop on their own terms. Nevertheless, it may be argued that there are limits to economic growth, both social (Hirsch, 1977) and ecological (e.g. Jackson, 2009; Meadows et al., 1972). And so-called 'post-development' critics (e.g. Escobar, 2012; Sachs, 2010) now claim that the global race for capitalist economic development, in which there must be winners and losers, can be inherently damaging to human well-being. It results, according to James Midgley, in 'distorted development' (Midgley, 1995).

Insofar as development may be regarded not as an immanent process but as an explicit goal, it remains contested: is that goal the creation of wealth, or is it the provision through social rights of food security, clean water, sanitation, shelter, healthcare and education? Amartya Sen's contention is that the goal is the wider realisation of human capabilities or freedom, but this still leaves open the question of the relationship between economic development and social development. Are social rights a prize to be earned through economic growth or a pre-condition for economic success? What has been referred to as the Washington consensus, which once informed the thinking of key international agencies (see Chapters 3 and 5, this volume), was premised on the neo-liberal 'trickle-down' thesis: in a free-market world, it was believed, wealth will eventually trickle down from rich to poor nations, just as it should trickle down from rich to poor people within each nation. What matters from this perspective is that the engine of economic growth and development should be fired up and kept running – most certainly, that wealth creation must precede the development and funding of social rights. It was a thesis supported by economists such as Kuznets (1955), whose proposed 'Kuznets curve' suggested that as per capita income in a country grows, inequality will initially increase before plateauing and then falling as general living standards rise and as the economy can support the costs of redistributive social rights. Just as influentially, the US sociologist, Harold Wilensky (1975), specifically demonstrated a direct correlation between economic development and social security spending, from which he inferred a causal relationship: the former, he claimed, facilitates the latter.

Contrary evidence was provided, for example, by Newman and Thompson (1989), who assembled alternative data to suggest that provision for basic needs (measured by indices of basic literacy, perinatal mortality and life expectancy) tended to precede, rather than result from, economic development. We shall see in Chapter 9 that the internationally adopted metric for measuring different levels of 'human development' seeks to combine indicators of economic activity on the one hand and social provision on the other and that the relationship between such indicators is complex. A recognisable three-way tension exists around firstly, the enduring spectre of 'poverty' (or, as suggested in Chapter 3, 'human diswelfare'); secondly, the disputed conceptions of 'development' (as discussed above); and third, 'rights' (most pertinently social rights).

The poverty-rights-development triad incorporates a combination of links (see Figure 4.1), and these we shall explore. The link between development and rights is associated with a particular discourse concerning rights to self-determination or 'freedom'. The link between poverty and development is associated with an essentially technocratic discourse as to how a rights-based or 'rights standards' approach can alleviate poverty. The link between rights and poverty is associated with a normative or humanistic discourse

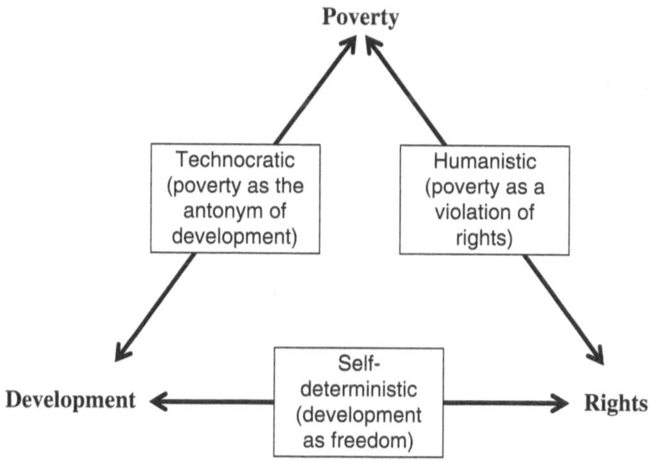

FIGURE 4.1 The links between poverty, development and rights: Contrasting understandings

that regards poverty as an unnecessary and unacceptable violation of rights. There are connections and intersections between these discourses, but for the purposes of discussion, we shall consider each in turn.

Self-determination and the right to development

We have seen that civil and political rights have together been characterised as 'first generation' rights, and social rights as 'second generation' rights. In 1986, the UN General Assembly's Declaration on the Right to Development (DRtD) gave expression to a central plank within a 'third generation' of human rights. Third-generation rights are widely represented as collective, group or solidarity rights: as rights to peace, to a healthy environment and to 'development'. Central to the concept of development was the principle of 'self-determination' (Rosas, 2001).

Agitation for a more holistic understanding of human rights had begun in the 1960s with the Peace Movement, the Green Movement and the Anti-racist/Anti-apartheid Movement. The instigation of the demand for a right to development is widely attributed to a call articulated by the Senegalese delegate to the UN, Justice Keba M'Baye, when he called not only for the right to live but for 'the right to live better' (1972). The agenda for the DRtD was driven largely from the global South, with some resistance from parts of the global North, most especially the United States (Marks, 2004). The Declaration did not give rise to legally binding covenants and remains aspirational in nature. Nevertheless, it had considerable symbolic significance. Its advocates contend that it transcended the unfortunate schism between civil and political rights on the one hand and the social rights agenda on the other (Sengupta, 2000, 2010) and set them in a broader context. The principal provisions of the Declaration are outlined in Box 4.1.

The Declaration reiterated rights proclaimed in existing treaties and instruments, including the right to self-determination. In seeking to reframe them in terms of an overarching right to development, there were some elements of ambiguity. The DRtD proclaimed the rights of people (in the plural) but stressed that the human person (in the singular) is the central subject. It proclaimed the duty of nation-states to formulate national policies but required all states to co-operate in the formulation of international policies. The question this begs is whether the right to development is the right of individual subjects, exercisable against nation-states, or a right of nation-states to international co-operation? The Declaration adds nothing to the exposition of social rights already contained in the UDHR and ICESCR, other than perhaps to call for international assistance in realising them.

The implicit premise is that self-determination cannot be achieved without international co-operation. If first-generation rights were about freedom and democracy and second-generation rights were about substantive equality

BOX 4.1 THE UN GENERAL ASSEMBLY'S DECLARATION ON THE RIGHT TO DEVELOPMENT, 1986

- Expresses the right of 'every human person and all peoples ... to participate in, contribute to, and enjoy economic, social, cultural and political development', which implies 'the full realization of the right of peoples to self-determination', including 'the exercise of their inalienable right to full sovereignty over all their natural wealth and resources' (Article 1).
- Asserts that 'The human person is the central subject of development'; but also that 'All human beings have a responsibility for development, individually and collectively' and should 'promote and protect an appropriate political, social and economic order for development' (Article 2 [1] and [2])
- Holds that states have:
    - ◊ 'the right and the duty to formulate appropriate national development policies that aim at the constant improvement of the well-being of the entire population and of all individuals' (Article 2 [3]);
    - ◊ 'the primary responsibility for the creation of national and international conditions favourable to the realization of the right to development' (Article 3 [1]);
    - ◊ 'the duty to co-operate with each other in ensuring development and eliminating obstacles to development' (Article 3[3]);
    - ◊ 'the duty to take steps, individually and collectively, to formulate international development policies' (Article 4);
    - ◊ and must ensure 'equality of opportunity for all in their access to basic resources, education, health services, food, housing, employment and the fair distribution of income' (Article 8).

and well-being, then third-generation rights were supposed to be about international solidarity and co-operation. The battle lines drawn between the interests of the 'non-aligned' nations of the global South who championed the right to development and those of the global North (especially the United States) revolved substantially around the challenges it posed to the structural economic and political imbalances of the status quo (Marks, 2004) and the prevalence of the neo-liberal pro-market ideological assumptions represented by the so-called Washington consensus (see Chapters 3 and 6, this volume). The right to self-determination expressed in the DRtD may be thought of as the combination of first-generation rights to freedom and democracy scaled up to the international level. Aristotle's famous reservation concerning democratic governance was that 'in democracies the poor have more sovereign power than the rich; for they are more numerous' (1981, p. 363). In the current context of extreme global inequalities, democracy between nations premised on an effective right to national self-determination would require a revolutionary upheaval to the global capitalist world order. Unsurprisingly, that hasn't happened. The editors of a collection of papers first presented in 2003 at a Nobel Symposium on the Right to Development and Human Rights in Development lamented that 'the operationalization of the right [to development] has not kept up with theory' (Andreassen & Marks, 2010, p. xxix).

The impetus for the elusive idea of a right to development has been sustained – paradoxically perhaps – by Amartya Sen's (1999) liberal-individualist framing of 'development' as *freedom*. This has been important, not least because it explicitly connects with the issue of poverty. Sen, though no supporter of solidarity rights, can be credited with inflecting UN agencies away from strict adherence to the Washington consensus and for shaping certain elements of the work of the United Nations Development Programme (UNDP). There is an implicit resonance, it may be argued, between Sen's framing of human development and certain underlying purposes of the DRtD. For Sen, human rights provide the means to guarantee basic human freedoms. But it is human development that enhances human capabilities so as to give full expression to freedom. Freedom is constituted through human development, not rights; rights are but a means to an end, not an end in themselves. The capabilities approach prioritises 'individual freedom as a social commitment' (1999, ch. 12). It fits with what has been characterised for the purposes of this chapter as a 'self-determinist' approach in that: it is more of an approach *to* than a theory *of* development; it expressly *challenges* top-down theories based on welfare utilitarianism and Rawlsian social justice; it attempts simultaneously to embrace potentially contradictory notions of freedom (freedom of individual opportunity and freedom of systemic process); and yet it supports a role for competitive markets (Prendergast, 2005). It is an elusive approach which (as we shall see in Chapter 5) pragmatically – albeit contrarily – synthesises elements of competitive individualism with elements of radical communitarianism and demands for personal freedom with expectations of collective support. It does not necessarily or expressly lay claim to do so, but it does lend some sense to the ambiguities inherent within the UN's generally somewhat neglected DRtD.

Development and the technical means to alleviate poverty

Though the DRtD itself may have slipped rather from prominence, the preoccupations of the UN with the monitoring of human development and global poverty have not. The initial debate around the DRtD had coincided with a realisation that attempts by the World Bank and the IMF to address poverty in the global South, through crude structural adjustment programmes, were failing (Deacon et al., 1997; Yeates, 2001). The conditions attached to aid and the loans provided to developing countries in the 1980s imposed free market solutions that, far from alleviating poverty, served to exacerbate it. The result in the 1990s was a partial shift towards a 'Post Washington Consensus': while still favouring free markets and restricted public spending, this espoused a social safety net approach to poverty alleviation (Deacon, 2007; World Bank, 1991). The emphasis was on 'getting the institutions right' (Yeates, 2008, p. 287); on promoting both private sector reform and good governance; on social risk management; on partial re-regulation and the use of 'smart' conditionalities; on the tailored use of social funds to promote community-level initiatives (e.g. Braathen, 2005).

The highpoint, perhaps, of this technocratic turn was the publication in 2000 of the UN's Millennium Development Goals (MDGs), the details of which will – together with those of the Sustainable Development Goals (SDGs) by which they were succeeded in 2015 – we shall discuss in Chapter 9. Insofar as the MDG initiative had been partly inspired by Amartya Sen, it is important to stress that the apparent softening of the Washington consensus did not extend to an accurate understanding of his concept of human capabilities. The first chapter of the *Human Development Report 2000* (UNDP, 2000), which had been penned personally by Sen, included a careful discussion of the capabilities concept. But in the rest of the report, other authors picked up the pen, and the notion of human capabilities was deftly appropriated as a malleable concept akin to that of human capital, notwithstanding that Sen himself is quite clear that human capabilities and human capital are *not* the same thing (1999, pp. 292–297). Capabilities are concerned with substantive freedoms, not productive capacity. Development, the UNDP still assumed, self-evidently requires economic growth, while rights require liberal democracy. Both require a pluralistic and apolitical social context in which NGOs and civil society groups can play a role as much as government. Lip service is paid to the importance of social rights, but their enforcement, according to UNDP, requires regulatory mechanisms akin to those by which global trade is governed. As it identified the gaps that exist in the global order, the UNDP's 2000 report began to draw on language bearing all the hallmarks of new public managerialist doctrine (see Chapter 2, this volume, and e.g. Porter & Craig, 2004). It spoke of the need for incentive structures, self-assessment techniques, benchmarking and culture change, and for poorer countries to avail themselves of the *opportunities* that globalisation offers (UNDP, 2000, p. 9). While accepting that this report was written a few years before the global financial crisis of 2008–2011, it failed to acknowledge that though powerful people might interpret the risks of a globalised capitalist economy in terms of new opportunities, the world's vulnerable people might experience such risks in terms of chronic insecurity (Vail, 1999). The significance of the language of the UNDP in this era – and that in a parallel report from the World Bank (Braathen, 2000; World Bank, 2001) – was that it reflected the context in which the UN's MDGs had been framed: their purpose was to urge upon the members of the UN the meeting of *goals*, not the realisation of *rights*.

Nevertheless, there had been an attempt to formulate a human rights approach to poverty reduction. In 2001, the UN's Committee on Economic Social and Cultural Rights had asked the Office of the High Commissioner for Human Rights to develop draft guidelines on integrating human rights into poverty reduction strategies. The OHCHR appointed consultants – two lawyers (Paul Hunt and Manfred Nowak) and an economist (Siddiq Osmani) – who produced and consulted on a first draft in 2002 before presenting a revised draft and a conceptual framework document in 2004 (Hunt et al., 2004). The draft guidelines were finally adopted and published as a set of *Principles and Guidelines for a Human Rights Approach to Poverty Reduction Strategies* (OHCHR, 2006). The authors, in their conceptual framework document, suggest that Sen's capability approach provides a useful conceptual 'bridge' between poverty and human rights (Hunt et al. 2004, p. 6). It is argued that the non-fulfilment of human rights counts as poverty if the rights involved 'correspond to the capabilities that are considered basic by a given society' (*ibid.*, p. 10). This contention seems to suggest that capabilities (as substantive individual freedoms) can be equated with, or read across from, agreed and established understandings of rights. What is meant by this is not especially clear. For Sen, human rights can create the space in which human capabilities may be realised. Be that as it may, the principles on which the OHCHR guidelines are premised require:

- specific and prioritised norms and defined standards;
- accessible mechanisms of accountability (that may or may not entail justiciability);
- democratic participation of poor people in the development of strategy;
- that particular attention be paid to the well-being of especially vulnerable social groups;
- the identification of immediate, intermediate and long-term targets;
- the use of indicators and benchmarks to monitor progress.

(Hunt et al., 2004, p. 21)

The end result (see Box 4.2) is a set of 'rights standards' (cf. Mishra, 1999), with ordered targets. The approach embraces the principle of progressive realisation and the methods of public managerialism. The document was to all intents and purposes a sister document to the MDGs. It may be noted that social rights to work, food, housing, health and education are included and clearly outlined, but the right to social security is omitted. Apparently, it was felt that to include the right to social security would be counterproductive since in some parts of the world 'social security' is, at best, an unfamiliar or ambiguous term and, at worst, a disputed concept (Nowak, 2011).

BOX 4.2 THE OHCHR PRINCIPLES AND GUIDELINES FOR A HUMAN RIGHTS APPROACH TO POVERTY REDUCTION STRATEGIES

Integrating specific human rights standards

Right to work

Target 1: Full employment
Target 2: All workers to be able to earn a minimum necessary income
Target 3: All workers to receive reasonable financial support during spells of unemployment
Target 4: To eliminate gender inequality in access to work
Target 5: To eliminate gender inequality in remuneration for work
Target 6: To eliminate child labour
Target 7: To eliminate bonded labour
Target 8: All workers should be able to work in safe and healthy working conditions
Target 9: No worker should be subject to unfair dismissal

Right to adequate food

Target 1: All people to be free from chronic hunger
Target 2: Eliminate gender inequality in access to food
Target 3: All people to be free from food insecurity
Target 4: All people to have access to food of adequate nutritional value
Target 5: All people to have access to safe food

Right to adequate housing

Target 1: All people to have a home
Target 2: All people to enjoy security of tenure
Target 3: All people to enjoy habitable housing
Target 4: All people to enjoy housing situated in a safe and healthy location
Target 5: All people able to afford adequate housing
Target 6: Adequate housing physically accessible to all
Target 7: All people to enjoy housing with access to essential services, materials, facilities and infrastructure

Rights to health

Target 1: All people to have access to adequate and affordable primary health care
Target 2: To eliminate avoidable child mortality

Target 3: To eliminate avoidable maternal mortality
Target 4: All men and women of reproductive age to have access to safe and effective contraception
Target 5: To eliminate HIV/AIDS
Target 6: To eliminate the incidence of other communicable diseases
Target 7: To eliminate gender inequality in access to health care

Right to education

Target 1: To ensure universal primary education for boys and girls
Target 2: To make free primary education available to all children
Target 3: To implement compulsory primary education
Target 4: To eradicate illiteracy
Target 5: To ensure equal access for all to secondary education
Target 6: To make free secondary education available to all children
Target 7: To eliminate gender disparity in primary and secondary education
Target 8: To improve the quality of primary and secondary education

[i.e. in addition to civil and political rights, including the rights of equal access to justice]

The OHCHR document articulates the links between development and poverty, drawing in the language of rights, but the implied premise is that poverty and development are opposites. The document is a response to the UN agenda that assumes that economic development is the *sine qua non* of poverty alleviation. It offers a sophisticated, but primarily technical, answer to a human problem.

Poverty as a violation of rights?

The process that led to the formulation of the MDGs had begun with the Vienna Declaration of the United Nations (1993), followed by its Copenhagen Social Summit (1995). These events have been taken as landmarks; the first is credited with having declared that poverty was a violation of human rights (Lister, 2004, ch. 7); the second resulted in a commitment to social development. At both events, the universality and indivisibility of human rights and the principles of DRtD were ritually reaffirmed. What the Vienna Declaration specifically affirmed was that 'the existence of widespread extreme poverty *inhibits* the full and effective enjoyment of human rights' (Article 14 [emphasis added]) and that 'extreme poverty and social exclusion constitute a violation of human *dignity*' (Article 25 [emphasis added]), an affirmation expressly restated by the UN General Assembly (2012). In fact, neither affirmation states that poverty *of itself* is a direct violation of rights. The report from the Copenhagen Summit commits itself to creating an environment that 'will enable people to achieve social development' and to 'eradicating poverty in the world' (UN 1995, pp. 11, 13). The means to such ends include provision for a stable legal framework, an enabling economic environment, and dynamic, open and free markets. The report added that the parties to the Summit would 'reaffirm, promote and strive to ensure the realization of rights set out [in the UDHR, the ICESCR and the DRtD] ... particularly in order to assist people living in poverty' (*ibid.*, p. 12).

Upon a close reading, therefore, it is clear that the UN was in no way retreating from the principle that social rights are progressively, not immediately, realisable and, in this sense, cannot be wholly inviolable. Poverty 'inhibits' the realisation of rights, and it violates human 'dignity'. The Vienna Declaration and the Copenhagen Summit fall short of declaring a right not to be poor. It was accepted, certainly, that the scale of global poverty amounted to an injustice, giving rise to obligations on the part of the international community to prevent hindrance to and facilitate the promotion of the right to development (Salomon, 2007, 2010). However, in 2001 the UN's Committee on Economic, Social and Cultural Rights submitted unequivocally that:

> The rights to work, an adequate standard of living, housing, food, health and education, which lie at the heart of the Covenant [the ICESCR], have a direct and immediate bearing upon the eradication of poverty. Moreover, the issue of poverty frequently arises in the course of the Committee's constructive dialogue with States parties. In the light of experience gained over many years, including the examination of numerous States parties' reports, the Committee holds the firm view that poverty constitutes a denial of human rights.
>
> *(2001: para. 1)*

The idea that poverty represents a violation of rights is an important and powerful one (Lister, 2004). It brings the symbolic and mobilising potential of rights discourse directly to bear on the issue of poverty. It can do so, broadly speaking, in two ways: through formal institutional approaches to combat global injustices and rein in the destructive forces that fuel and perpetuate poverty; or through substantive interventions that give expression to our universal humanity and/or acknowledge that people experiencing poverty/diswelfare are not passive victims or mere statistics, but human beings with their own agency, albeit – it must be said – that such agency may be systemically suppressed.

Approaches inspired by institutional justice concerns

An author and activist who most clearly brings a human rights perspective to bear on global poverty issues is Thomas Pogge (2002; 2007, ch.1). Pogge holds to an institutionalist conception of social rights, regarding them as 'moral claims on the organization of one's society' (2002, p. 64). His concern is with moral, not legal, rights and here he draws on the authority of the UDHR, Article 28: 'Everyone is entitled to a social and international order in which the rights and freedoms set forth in this Declaration can be fully realized'. On that basis, he contends that a global institutional order that continues to permit a foreseeable and extensive incidence of extreme poverty is in violation of human rights. By that standard, the commitment under the MDGs merely to halve the proportion of people living in extreme poverty by 2015 was simply not enough. The alternative, according to Pogge, depends first on the entrenchment of democracy. Currently, he contends, the most affluent have shaped the world order to the disadvantage of the poorest, and we must hold the powerful to account. At the very least, it would be necessary to obtain an international agreement that no kind of financial aid should be provided to non-democratic regimes. Secondly, he proposed the introduction of some form of international fiscal mechanism with which to fund development aid. One such mechanism would be a Currency Transfer or 'Tobin' Tax (see Nissanke, 2003), which would entail a UN-administered tax (that might be set at anything between 0.005 and 1%) on the 2 or more trillions dollars' worth of speculative currency transfers that take place each day. Pogge's own preference would be for a Global Resources Dividend, a tax that would redistribute from those in the world who make the greatest demands on the world's resources to those who make the least. It would work by raising a levy ($US 2 per barrel of oil, for example) on those countries that use or sell limited natural resources extracted from their own territories.

The third of Pogge's proposals is for some form of cosmopolitan citizenship. There are similarities here with other proposals for cosmopolitan or global citizenship emanating from a spectrum of authors (Falk, 1994; Delanty, 2000; Dwyer, 2010, ch. 10; Held, 2010). The common core of these proposals is a form of institutional cosmopolitanism premised on generalised and universal equality between all individuals; forms of post-national inclusion at both sub- and supra-national level; but subject in the foreseeable future to an enduring role for the nation-state within a system of multilateral global governance. David Held, in particular, has suggested that the initial stages in a transition to cosmopolitan governance might centre on a further reshaping of the Washington consensus in the direction of a social democratic agenda (Held, 2004, 2010). It is striking, however, that none of these proposals contain much, if any, explicit detail as to the role of social rights. The assumption appears to be that the realisation of social rights is somehow assured on the basis of generic cosmopolitan principles that include a commitment to social justice. It is possible to envisage reforms to the apparatuses of the UN that might facilitate such an agenda. Proposals here include the idea of strengthening ECOSOC by giving it Charter powers and a proper infrastructure or creating a UN People's Assembly or even a World Parliament (Patomäki & Teivainen, 2004). While none of these ideas may seem immediately feasible, we shall nonetheless return to reflect upon such possibilities in Chapter 11.

Approaches inspired by concerns for humanity

An approach distinguishable from, though not necessarily unsympathetic to, that of Pogge is that of Tom Campbell (2007). Campbell, who once attempted to explore the idea of socialist rights (1983), regards poverty as a violation of rights, not so much because it is unjust as because it is an affront to the humanity of the people who experience it. He contends that all human rights derive from the existence of needs (2007, p. 59), though, puzzlingly, he associates needs with Sen's concept of capabilities rather than – as a socialist might – with Marx's concept of human essence. Nonetheless, he conceives of social rights as rights to the resources required for a truly human life. Poverty therefore violates human rights in the same sense as torture or slavery might. Poverty should be eradicated, or indeed abolished, out of humanity by enforcing the rights of the poor. Campbell himself is somewhat philosophically preoccupied with competing utilitarian and deontological justifications, but as we shall see in Chapter 5, the broad implication of his argument might be that a eudaimonic/humanitarian ethic should prevail over a hedonic/justice-based ethic.

On this basis, Campbell would prefer a Global Humanitarian Levy to Pogge's Global Resource Dividend. A Global Humanitarian Levy would replace existing bilateral and multilateral overseas aid arrangements with an international system under which all national governments would levy a hypothecated tax, Campbell suggests, of 2 per cent on all personal incomes in excess (at the time he was writing) of $US 50,000 (or the equivalent) and 2 per cent on all personal wealth above $US 500,000. Such a mechanism, according to Campbell, would ensure the fulfilment of subsistence rights that are 'grounded primarily in the universal humanitarian obligation to participate in the relief of extreme suffering' (2007, p. 67).

It is possible to conceive of mechanisms – whether based on the taxation of currency transactions, natural resource usage, corporate wealth holdings or personal income/wealth (Zedillo, 2001; Atkinson, 2004; Alstadsaeter et al., 2023) – by which to garner resources for poverty eradication, but this leaves aside the question of just how such resources should be distributed. Peter Townsend had argued that such funding should provide the basis for establishing an international welfare state (Townsend & Donkor, 1996; Townsend, 2002, 2007; 2009, chs. 1 and 2). Townsend's demand was founded on a lifetime of scholarship and campaigning around poverty and was deeply rooted in Fabian socialism. His argument was that provision for a broadly construed right to social security was already internationally enshrined through the UDHR and the ICESCR and should be realised by building on the experiences of the richer OECD countries in developing social security systems. Elements of his argument are (albeit posthumously) reflected in the ILO's Social Protection Floor initiative (Batchelet, 2011; ILO, 2012). This is an approach that contrasts notably with that of the OHCHR's guidelines for a rights-based approach (see above). A concrete and practicable first step in the construction of an international social security system, according to Townsend, would be the introduction of an international universal child benefit, funded by a Tobin Tax, and rolled out globally, merging with and/or succeeding existing schemes as appropriate (including, for example, the conditional cash transfer schemes developed in parts of the global South) (2009, ch. 7; and see Leisering & Barrientos, 2013).

It remains to be seen whether it will ever be possible to pursue such ideas through the established institutional machinery of the UN. In the meantime, however, agitation for rights-based action against poverty can be detected at other levels. Callinicos (2003), for example, has suggested that through global networks such as the World Social Forum, it might be possible to build campaigns drawing upon diverse constituencies for rights-based demands for basic incomes, reduced working hours, and better public services. Some of these demands are also expressed in proposals by Guy Standing for the extension, globally, of a new form of 'occupational citizenship' (Standing, 2009). These are issues to which we shall return in Chapter 11, but for now, it is worth mentioning approaches taken by a campaign organisation in which poor people themselves are directly involved.

ATD Fourth World is a human rights-based, anti-poverty organisation founded in 1957 in France by Joseph Wresinski, a Catholic priest. It now has a presence in over 30 countries around the world. Wresinski made himself famous both in France and at the United Nations by promoting the claim that extreme poverty is a form of violence and a violation of human rights. It is fundamentally a campaigning and educational organisation that aims to give a voice to people in poverty and to promote poor people's participation in policymaking. As a contribution to the debate about the UN's post-2015 development agenda, the organisation published a report, drawing on a cross-national participatory evaluation. The evaluation was based on a well-developed methodology by which ATD Fourth World has for some years been seeking to empower people living in poverty to communicate, 'to build a collective understanding of their situation as well as construct a sense of pride that counteracts their stigmatisation and isolation' (2014, p 14).

The principal thrust of the report and other publications of this era is that whatever happens, poor people should not be 'left behind'. The rights it asserts are not specific social rights but the rights to be heard, to equal participation and not to be discriminated against. The concern is to combat not only poverty but 'poverty-ism' (Davies, 2008). Povertyism is a form of discrimination that may be equated with sexism, racism, disablism and ageism.

Poverty is an assault on a person's humanity as much through stigma and discrimination as it is through material deprivation (Dean, 1992; Lister, 2004). When people fight for their rights on the basis of a common identity, they characteristically mobilise and take pride in their shared identity – their class, their gender, their sexuality or their ethnicity, for example. But it is not possible for a person to take pride in their poverty – at least not in the same way. ATD Fourth World attempts to organise at the national level, but few other national or local organisations effectively mobilise poor people to speak for themselves rather than speaking on their behalf. Such organisations tend to be transient. The 1960s welfare rights movement in the United States is a case in point (Piven & Cloward, 1977), though there was a more recent attempt to build a Poor People's Economic Human Rights Campaign in the US to oppose the introduction of harsh welfare reforms in the 1990s (Baptiste & Bricker-Jenkins, 2002). The latter was significant for the way in which it sought explicitly to equate the struggle against poverty with the historic struggle against slavery. Both struggles had confronted class interests that demanded 'a flexible, contingent – and terrified – workforce and the substitution of mandatory work activity for real jobs'. The organisers' objective was to produce:

> a populace that questions, that demands, that moves. In those circumstances concessions might be possible. But we believe that this is a new period of history in which ending poverty is eminently possible. If we educate and organize around the realities and possibilities of this moment, the [welfare reforms] could have the same galvanizing effect as the Dred Scott decision of 1857 [by which the US Supreme Court ruled that a slave by virtue of his African descent could not be a citizen and had no right to sue for his freedom]. It is worth remembering that the abolition movement did eventually prevail. Poverty is no more inevitable or permanent than slavery.
>
> *(ibid., p. 200)*

In a similar vein, Tom Campbell concluded that 'We need to work for the emergence of moral progress of a kind that led to a universal acknowledgement that the one time-honoured practice of slavery is morally heinous' (2007, p. 4). The idea that poverty is as much a rights violation as slavery is especially powerful, but its mobilising potential requires more than solidarity among those whom poverty afflicts, whose voices will not be heard without the recognition of their social rights. While social rights have been acknowledged to have a part to play in measures that promote social development and alleviate global poverty, they have tended sometimes to be marginalised within the social development process; to have been denied a meaningful let alone a leading role; to have been reduced to standards, not imperatives; to be deployed as primarily rhetorical devices in support of abstract demands for global justice. Poverty like slavery is quintessentially dehumanising – something to abolish, not ameliorate. The argument of this book is that such rights should be regarded as translations or expressions of human sociality, which, as an essential, albeit partially suppressed, species characteristic, is as relevant in a global context as in national contexts.

5

ETHICS, IDEOLOGIES AND SOCIALITY

We have considered social rights as creatures of welfare state citizenship, as articulations of human need and as a key element in processes of social development. We turn now to consider the ethical and ideological foundations of social rights and connections that might be made with conceptualisations of human sociality.

Amartya Sen has defined rights as 'primarily ethical demands' (2004, p. 319), and in Chapter 3 (this volume), we have already touched on ethics when discussing 'doctrinal' conceptions of rights. But the focus of the current chapter is on the relationship between rights and responsibilities, with whether and when social rights should be conditional on the individual acceptance of responsibilities, with whether and when there can be collective responsibility for meeting individual human needs. Such concerns appear to have been uppermost in the thinking of Grotius when he coined the term sociality (see Chapter 1, this volume). Discussions of ethics do not figure too prominently in academic social policy texts, other than in relation to 'applied' ethics (e.g. Bochel, 2005; Fitzpatrick, 2008), but issues relating to rights and responsibilities – to human welfare and interdependency – clearly have ethical connotations that bear fundamentally on our discussion of rights and needs (Dean, 2004). First of all, this chapter will briefly set the scene by explaining a distinction that may be made between ethics and morality and their relevance for notions of human 'values'. It then returns to the distinction made in Chapter 3 between hegemonic (or dominant) and minor (or 'subaltern') traditions in rights discourse in order to reflect on their ethical underpinnings and how these may be reflected in different religious or ideological values. Finally, the chapter will endeavour to bring together elements of this discussion by presenting an overarching conceptual taxonomy of the competing and overlapping perspectives that have hitherto dominated or in part influenced the social construction of social rights.

DOI: 10.4324/9781003451518-6

Ethics, morality and human 'values'

Arguments about the difference between ethics and morals may be dismissed as mere pedantry. There is a tendency sometimes, even amongst philosophers, to treat the terms as if they were synonymous. Nevertheless, there is some purpose in wishing to make a distinction between the two. It is a distinction directly analogous to that which has already been drawn between the doctrinal and claims-based foundations of rights and between top-down and bottom-up definitions of needs. Ethics, as a branch of philosophy, is quite simply the study or the 'science' of morals: ethics is to morality what methodology is to methods in social science or what theology is to religion. (As to theology and religion, they too can have consequences for perspectives on social rights, as we touched upon in Chapter 2 and to which we shall return.) Clearly, therefore, ethics and morality are intimately related, but that relationship is important. The two inform each other; they evolve in relation to each other over time; they have a dialectical relationship.

If one considers the etymological origins of the terms, ethics comes from the Greek *ethos*, meaning 'character', while morality comes from the Latin, *mores*, meaning 'behaviour'. Contemporary English usage of the term ethos is concerned with cognitive awareness of the human context and the societal context in which a person acts. We speak, for example, of a 'professional ethos', a 'public service ethos' or even a 'sporting ethos' when specifying the common understandings shared respectively between the members of accredited professions, appointed or elected public servants, or sporting competitors as to their vocation, purpose and principles. Contemporary English usage of the term mores is concerned with cultural expectations as to the nature of acceptable behaviour; for example:

> The men, women and children who compose a society at any time are the unconscious depositories and transmitters of the mores. They inherited them without knowing it; they are moulding them unconsciously; they will transmit them involuntarily. The people cannot make the mores. They are made by them.
>
> *(Sumner, 1906, p. 477)*

This, however, is a jaundiced, if not misanthropic, interpretation of popular mores. It chimes with Dawkins' conceptualisation of the cultural memes by which human behaviours are transmitted (1976; and see discussion Chapter 1, this volume). It is an essentially mechanistic analysis that, according to Malik (2001), implies human beings are 'zombies', governed by the tyranny of predetermined replicators. Dawkins glibly claims that 'we [human beings] have the power to defy the selfish genes of our birth and, *if necessary*, the selfish memes of our indoctrination' (p. 200) [emphasis added]. But Malik questions how such defiance can be achieved without a deeper understanding than that offered by Dawkins as to what it means to be human and to possess the interdependent capacities both for scientific knowledge and abstract understanding on the one hand and for practical political conduct and action on the other.

While ethics is concerned with that which should be regarded as 'right', morality is concerned with norms and that which is popularly accepted as 'good'. Ethics is concerned with abstract reasoning, principles and doctrines; morality with everyday codes and agreed-upon or even implicit rules of conduct. There is once again a connection to be made with Habermas' (1987, 1996) distinction between 'system' and 'lifeworld': systemic ethics on the one hand, the morality of the lifeworld on the other, together framing the structure of communicative action. Ethical arguments dreamed up by past or present philosophers may or may not have an influence on everyday thinking in the real world of policymaking, where social rights may be named and claimed, but they do tell us something about what had once been, or is now, thinkable.

The dynamic relationship between ethics and morality may be considered a feature of the human essence; it is a factor within the evolving interdependency between consciousness, purposeful activity, history and sociality; it is intrinsic to life that is human. This can be lost in recent discussions of human 'values' when these are defined not in the context of objective or constitutive human characteristics but with reference only to currently observable subjective attitudes or stated beliefs which are empirically identifiable and whose extent may be quantified through the use by political scientists and cross-cultural psychologists of social survey techniques. Ronald Inglehart (1990) has observed shifts in cultural values that have been associated with processes of industrial development across the world and observed patterns and trends in, on the one hand, the secularisation of beliefs and, on the other, shifts away from concerns with immediate material survival and towards concerns with individual freedoms on the other. Inglehart's methodology has been developed in a range of work, most notably through the annual World Values Survey (Inglehart & Welzel, 2005; World Values Survey, 2023) which now draws and regularly updates a World Cultural Map of human values. In Chapter 9 of this volume, we shall consider the relevance of cultural values for the framing of social rights in the global context, but for, now we turn for a moment to work by behavioural psychologists closely related to that of the WVS, which identifies the values by which individual behaviour may be specifically motivated, positing the existence of 'near-universal' values, reflecting a combination of overlapping and sometimes mutually antagonistic individual desires, priorities and ideals which can be shown to be widely shared, albeit to varying extents across different countries and demographic groupings (Schwartz, 1992; Schwartz et al., 2012).

The approach is reflected in notions of 'national' values and 'corporate' values employed instrumentally in both political and managerial discourse when aiming to target or appeal to particular audiences and/or to promote behavioural change (Atkin et al., 2014; and see Box 5.1). The number of human

BOX 5.1 'BASIC VALUES' AND INDIVIDUAL MOTIVATIONS

An illustrative summary of the eleven overarching human values identified in a report by BCW Movatory-*Age-of-Values*-(2023) [p. 14] *https://bcw-global.com/newsroom/global/bcws-age-of-values-2023-report-highlights-values-void-between-governments-and-citizens*

Value	**Related behaviour**
Self-direction:	independent thought and action; emphasis on freedom, exploration and creativity.
Stimulation:	the pursuit of excitement and challenge in life; emphasis on novelty, variety and adventure.
Hedonism:	personal pleasure and enjoyment; emphasis on self-indulgence and sensuous gratification.
Achievement:	personal success according to social standards; emphasis on ambition and the demonstration of competence.
Power:	social status and control over people and resources; emphasis on social power, wealth and authority.
Security:	personal and societal safety and stability; emphasis on safety, harmony and stability.
Tradition:	commitment to and acceptance of customs and ideas that culture and religion provide; emphasis on the maintenance of cultural, family or religious traditions.
Conformity:	restraint and compliance with social expectations to avoid upsetting others; emphasis on adherence to rules, laws and obligations.
Benevolence:	concern for the welfare of the people with whom we are in frequent contact; emphasis on caring and dependability.
Universalism (Societal):	understanding, appreciation, tolerance and protection of all people in society; emphasis on equality, justice and protection for all.
Universalism (Natural):	preservation of the natural environment; emphasis on the protection of nature and animals.

DISCUSSION: It may be argued that the connections between the values and their related behaviours listed above reflect – albeit indirectly – a distinction between ethics and morality, though the tendency in this report and similar work is by implication to elide that distinction. Some of these disassociated 'values' may – in whole or in part – be identified as individualistic or communitarian, liberal or conservative, and all are addressed to individual motivations rather than essential species characteristics. Nevertheless, it may be noted that several of the descriptions of associated behaviours speak potentially *to* (but not explicitly *of*) the immanence of critical consciousness, purposeful/creative activity and human sociality.

values posited in such analyses varies widely, and it is expressly acknowledged that values may exist in opposition to each other across or along two bipolar dimensions: 'openness to change *versus* conservation', and 'self-enhancement *versus* self-transcendence'. It will be seen that these dimensions of variability have a degree of resonance with the discussion to be found towards the end of this chapter. It may, however, be argued that the study of individually held preferences or ideas, while potentially revealing, cannot by itself capture the dynamics of the underlying ideological conflicts and compromises through which the connections between ethics and morality are in practice negotiated. And it is through such connections that human sociality may be substantively inflected.

In Chapter 1, we considered the ways in which fetishised understandings of our essential or intrinsic human characteristics may conceal or distort the perception of human relationships, and there is a sense in which it is through the social construction of 'values' relating to human conduct that this may occur. 'Values' in this context are fluid and ambiguous constructs forged at intersections between ethical conceptualisations and cultural mores. They are potentially implicated in fetishised, compromised or restricted perceptions, with consequences – as we shall see – for the understanding and construction of social rights.

Hegemonic and subaltern traditions of rights discourse

The last chapter contrasted the hegemonic or major liberal-individualist conception that sees social rights as a condition precedent for personal freedom with what Woodiwiss (2005) has dubbed the 'minor' tradition that conceives of social rights as an intrinsic expression of human solidarity. For our purposes, it may be argued that the hegemonic tradition tends to marginalise or obscure human sociality, whereas the minor or 'subaltern' tradition embraces it. These traditions entail competing ethical premises, drawn from a range of established schools of thought. The connections can be tenuous and are messy. The account that follows, therefore, is highly simplified, but it represents one way of telling an otherwise complicated story.

Consequentialist and utilitarian foundations

Consequentialism reasons that human beings should act in whichever way will have the best consequences. If the consequence of 'necessity' or 'Want' (i.e. unmet human need) is a limitation upon individual freedom, social rights that substantively provide for human need are, we might think, justified (see, for example, Sen, 1982b). However, this 'welfarist' and ostensibly beneficent interpretation of consequentialism can be heavily qualified by strictly utilitarian versions of the creed (e.g. Bentham, 1789), which would argue that the utility of freedom is surely the pursuit of self-contentment or happiness. And, since we can't all be equally happy, the job of government is to maximise the happiness not of all citizens but of the greatest number. The utilitarian ethic reflects a tradition that reaches back to a particular strand in classical philosophy beginning with Epicurus (Fitzpatrick, 2018; George, 2010, ch. 2), who appears to have first articulated a very particular contractarian view of the relationship between the individual and society: the idea that society exists not to provide for human need but to provide the security wherein individuals might peaceably provide for their own needs. The Epicurean view of the good life was distinctly hedonic, though not hedonistic: life's aim was to pursue pleasure – both physical and spiritual – and avoid pain, but nevertheless to abjure wasteful luxuries or excess. Though Epicurus valued personal friendship, he insisted that human beings were essentially individualistic, self-interested and disinclined to community spirit or civic participation. Epicurean thinking was reflected in Stoicism, a philosophical movement which began in ancient Athens and achieved later prominence in classical Rome. Stoicism established an intellectual foundation for the principle of formal equality of rich and poor before the law, since rich and poor were deemed equally capable of leading a good life (though not necessarily equally comfortable lives). Towards the end of Europe's feudal era, this principle would eventually be re-inflected in liberal Enlightenment thinking, most conspicuously in the work of Hobbes (1651), who clearly and influentially advocated a form of government based on a notional compact or contract, whereby the individual citizen would forgo or trade certain elements of their own freedom in return for the protection of the state against the predations and irresponsible tendencies of their fellow citizens. The initial object was to secure the minimum necessary level of social order.

The utilitarian ethic may be called upon in justification of policy interventions that permit or inflict suffering on a minority of people so long as it is thought to benefit the majority. This was indeed what occurred in the more punitive kinds of Poor Law regimes that preceded the modern capitalist welfare state – regimes that incarcerated paupers in the workhouse. A utilitarian ethic justifies interventions that encourage or compel people to act in particular ways to ensure the greatest benefit to the greatest number in society. Such justification is premised on the assumption that all human beings are motivated primarily by self-interest and can be relied upon to respond to material incentives; they will be deterred by penalties and attracted by rewards. Social rights therefore can legitimately be made conditional on behaviour that is judged to be desirable and in the interests of society at large; social assistance claimants can be required to seek low-paid or uncongenial employment; penalties can be imposed on parents who fail to send their children to school; public housing can be denied or withdrawn from families deemed guilty of anti-social behaviour.

The utilitarian tradition – though potentially authoritarian and therefore illiberal in many important respects (King, 1999) – has clearly been an important component in the hegemonic liberal-individualist ethic. Its first priority is to secure a social order for the benefit of the individual through the rule of law and, therefore, the maintenance of civil rights. Its second priority is to ensure some influence of the sovereign individual over the state and, therefore, the maintenance of political rights. Within this context, the development of social rights, if it is supported at all, is likely to be a lower priority. And the framing of social rights is likely to entail elements of conditionality, a trend whose significance in the twenty-first century has been re-emerging across the world (Dwyer, 2000, 2004; Gaia et al., 2011).

We have seen in previous chapters, however, that other strands of liberal thought were decisive to the development of social rights in the mid-twentieth century. There had been important precursors to the reluctant liberal collectivism of Beveridge and Roosevelt. Political liberals, such as Paine (1791) in the eighteenth century and early social liberals, such as T.H. Green in the nineteenth century (see Carter, 2003; George, 2010, ch. 11) had each in their writing prefigured ideas of social rights. Fundamentally, however, all strands of liberalism are rooted in a belief in the autonomous individual as the bearer of rights. It was the economic liberalism of Adam Smith that most clearly captured the need for moral rules in the context of an amoral capitalist market system: the idea that though the free market could harness the pursuit of economic self-interest, a sense of selfless civic duty was necessary to the 'harmony of sentiments and passions' (1759, p. 72) on which human wellbeing depends.

Deontological and ontological elements

Deontological reasoning is concerned not with the consequences that follow from human actions but with principles, rules and duties that apply prior to such actions. And it is reason itself that matters above feelings and emotions. Deontology was the product of Cartesian dualism and the idea that the mind is separate from the body and that thinking is more than being. The deontological thinking of Immanuel Kant holds a vital place within the broader spectrum of liberal thought insofar as it furnished the rational argument for exactly that which Adam Smith had in mind: it could temper the naked pursuit of self-interest and encourage selfless civic duty. Deontological thinking requires an understanding of the human subject, not only as a competitive self-seeking individual but as a socially situated being who must recognise and respect the rationality of other human beings. From this flows the Kantian categorical imperative:

> Act in such a way that you always treat humanity, whether in your own person or in the person of any other, never simply as a means, but always at the same time as an end.
>
> *(Kant, 1785, p. 91)*

This imperative ostensibly resonates with the so-called 'Golden Rule' – 'Do unto others as you would have them do unto you' – subscribed to in broadly similar terms by all established world religions, though Kant himself insisted that the Golden Rule cannot amount to a universal law since it is not founded on reason. His insistence is that we should only do what we could rationally want any other person to do in the same circumstances (Walker & Walker, 2018). Kant's deontology is based, according to Fitzpatrick, 'on the freedom of rational beings who observe the laws and duties of universal reason in a moral and social system of mutual respect '(2008, p. 47). This is an understanding that clearly supports 'first generation' rights, namely, the liberal Enlightenment conceptions of civil liberties and constitutional government. But its implications for 'second generation' social rights are less clear. It is an understanding that can be developed in different directions.

One such direction – that is explicitly liberal – has been championed through Rawls' (1972) theory of social justice. This is a theory that is described as 'contractualist', as distinct from 'contractarian' (the term applied above to the Hobbesian bargain between individual and state). It is contractualist in the sense that Rawls envisages a hypothetical negotiation between rational actors as to the rules that should apply not only in relation to the defence of liberty but also with regard to the distribution of rewards in society. The parties to this hypothetical negotiation would not know what their own station in society would be, so would rationally determine principles of distribution that would be in the interests of everybody. This metaphysical proposition is capable (though not without difficulty) of political interpretation in relation to the construction of social rights and taxation policies in the real world (e.g. White, 2003).

The other direction in which Kantian deontology leads arises from the manner in which Kant himself opens a door to thinking about the nature and limits of individual autonomy and the ontological implications of human dependency and interdependency; of needs for care and recognition. It should be mentioned that strictly speaking, 'ontology' is not etymologically the opposite of 'deontology', since they stem from different roots. In classical Greek, *ont* means 'being', whereas *deon* means 'duty'. Nevertheless, the terms 'ontology' and 'deontology' have contrasting meanings. Kant draws a firm distinction between 'perfect' duties that cannot rationally be ignored and 'imperfect' duties that have ontological importance but cannot, he claims, be universally demanded. Sen (2004) has alluded to this distinction between perfect and imperfect duties and their correlative rights and argues that certain rights do not cease to be rights if they have not or cannot yet be realised. This argument is especially relevant with regard to social rights and the principle of 'progressive realisation' (see Chapter 3, this volume). The idea – whether explicit or implicit – that there is a realm of imperfect duties and correlative social rights that may be inferred or may yet be developed lies arguably at the heart not only of certain social liberal and democratic socialist ideological aspirations but also of religious interpretations of the Golden Rule. We observed in Chapter 1 that though Kant considered religion to be a non-rational or fetishised medium of collective regulation, he acknowledged its potentially beneficent influence. For Kant, the existence of imperfect as opposed to universal duties required a doctrine of virtue (Fitzpatrick, 2008, pp. 48–51). Virtue had been a central feature of Aristotelian ethics, but Kant alludes to virtues not simply as characteristics of a good life but as rationally contestable (and in that sense imperfect) moral duties.

Virtue ethics is sometimes presented as a third branch of moral philosophy – after consequentialism and deontology – though Nussbaum (1999) suggests its intersections with the other branches (including Kant's work) render it insufficiently distinctive. It is important, nevertheless, since it addresses ontological issues – issues to do with the fundamental nature of human interdependency and well-being. Virtue ethics is concerned not so much with effects or rules of action as with moral character and moral rationalities. In a sense, it attenuates the distinction between ethics and morality. MacIntyre (2007), in particular, drawing from Aristotle, is profoundly critical of the values of the liberal Enlightenment and the construction of the 'liberal self'. Instead, he advocates what he calls the 'narrative self', rooted not in abstract reasoning but in the context of communal life and substantive social practices. The approach can be seen as essentially, even nostalgically, conservative, but it connects, for example, with important recent debates about ontological identity and the ethic of care.

Mention has been made in Chapter 3 of the recent shift towards a politics of identity, a shift that is consonant with liberal values of equality and tolerance. However, David Taylor (1998) has suggested that in addition to focusing on categorical identities and the importance of ensuring just treatment for women, ethnic minority groups, older, young, disabled and LGBT+ people and other systemically disadvantaged communities, social rights must surely also ensure the maintenance of ontological identity and wellbeing. Ontological identity, irrespective of the multiplicity of our particular categorical identities, relates to our frailty and embodied-ness; our uniqueness as human beings; our inner or noumenal sense of 'self'; and the integrity of our moral being. This is an aspect of human need ill-served by the prevailing hegemonic tradition, but which is captured in the subaltern human rights tradition that prioritises solidarity and care.

An ethic of care represents a clear counterbalance to the liberal ethic of justice (Slote, 2001). Caring for one another is a daily social practice and moral obligation (Finch & Mason, 1993). The motivation to care for others may be regarded as a moral virtue, but feminist theorists (Sevenhuijsen, 1998; Tronto, 1994, 2013) have argued for an ethical approach premised on a construction of the individual not as an abstract individual rights holder but as a self-in-relationship: an approach that recognises that 'vulnerability is part and parcel of ordinary human subjectivity' (Sevenhuijsen, 2000, p. 19). Caring, Tronto has argued, is to be viewed as a species activity' (1994, p. 103). And here we have a direct connection to Bryan Turner's conception of human rights (see Chapter 3, this volume) and to a subaltern tradition that best represents or potentiates the essential sociality of the human species. Fiona Williams (1999) captures the sense in which an ethic of care, embracing concerns for interdependence, bodily integrity, ontological identity and voice, may be translated into 'good enough' principles of welfare: 'good-enough' in the sense analogously portended by Winnicott's (1953) notion of good-enough parenting, since while collective welfare provision may not always be absolutely perfect, sustained by essential human commitment, it can be good enough. We shall return to this assertion in Chapter 11. A subaltern ethic of care and human solidarity offers a foundation for social rights concerned not only with the provision of quotidian intimate care but systematic health and social care; not only with the provision of asylum and relief in the face of disaster or exceptional distress, but sustained protection against all forms of systemic disadvantage and exploitation.

Dependency and responsibility

Whereas interdependency is an essential feature of the human life course and the human condition, the dominant ethic is implicitly premised on an assumption that dependency and responsibility are somehow inimical (Dean 2004, ch. 10). Autonomy is conflated with self-sufficiency: sustaining oneself through dependency on an employer and/or within one's family is regarded, perversely, as independence. We shall see in the next chapter that there has been a tendency to denigrate social rights on the grounds that rather than promoting citizens' autonomy or independence, they promote an undesirable and stigmatising form of dependency. It had been argued (Dean & Taylor-Gooby, 1992) that this amounts to a form of 'dependency fetishism', analogous to commodity fetishism (Marx, 1887, ch. 1). However, the wider understanding of the concept of fetishism suggested in Chapter 1 of this volume (and see Dean 2023, p. 263) would indicate that, strictly speaking, the fetish here is not welfare dependency but the objectified ideal of individual sovereignty and independence, which distorts and obscures the perception and understanding of human relationships and transactions. The hegemonic liberal-individualist conventions upon which the development of capitalist welfare states are in large part founded – whether they are defended in whole or in part by utilitarian or deontological ethical principles – have been implicated in sustaining this distorted understanding of dependency and in constraining welfare state citizens' sense of interdependency and solidarity (Dean & Rodgers, 2004).

Economic globalisation and the ascendancy of neo-liberalism (Amin, 1997; Stiglitz, 2003) have accentuated this. When in the late twentieth century capitalist welfare states were subject to economic pressures, this was accompanied and fuelled by a significant backlash against social rights (Roche, 1992). The extension of social rights, it was feared, could eclipse individual responsibilities and was literally 'de-moralising' (Himmelfarb, 1995). We shall consider such critiques in Chapter 6, but what is important for now is the extent to which a new preoccupation with 'responsibility' pervaded debates about social rights, not only in relation to established welfare states, but more globally. What Nikolas Rose (1996a) once identified as a new form of 'advanced liberalism' sought to promote not only social rights but prudentialism, self-provisioning and the 'responsibilisation' of everyday life. However, it follows from our discussion above that responsibility is not a simple concept. Does responsibility equate with obedience, duty or moral obligation, or can there be such a thing as collective responsibility – a form of responsibility to which social rights, far from negating, give expression?

Philosophers have offered a range of answers. James Griffin (2008), for example, argues that as human beings we each have an ethical responsibility for everybody else and, insofar as minimum material provision is as constitutive of personhood as individual autonomy, that we should all contribute to collective provision for social rights. This is consistent with, on the one hand, Richard Titmuss' (1970, ch. 16) idea that welfare states enable their citizens to care not just for their family and neighbours but for strangers; and, on the other, with Tom Campbell's case for a Global Humanitarian Levy whereby the citizens of richer countries might contribute to the relief of poverty in poorer countries (see Chapter 4, this volume). The logic of the argument is illustrated by the anecdote in Box 5.2. Karl Otto Apel (1980, 1991) has similarly developed a concept of 'co-responsibility': a form of responsibility that links individual duty and collective obligation. The seeds of co-responsibility or collective responsibility may lie in love and human friendship, but for human beings, it can expand into wider loyalties and shared commitments premised on an explicit appreciation of our essentially constitutive human sociality.

We have already in Chapter 1 introduced Axel Honneth's argument that the requirements of an ethical life are constituted through the three ways in which human beings achieve mutual recognition: love, solidarity and rights. It is through *love* that we can achieve the most intimate kind of recognition, care and respect for another needy being, and so we discover our own being and self-identity. It is through *solidarity* that we can achieve shared recognition, accommodation and respect for members of a social group defined by their differences in unity, and so we establish our own human self-esteem. And it is through *rights* that we can achieve cognitive recognition, empathy

BOX 5.2 THE RIGHTS OF STRANGERS: AN ANECDOTE

Philosophers will often employ vignettes – imaginary situations – in order to illustrate some important argument or conundrum. Though the anecdote that follows is redolent of one such widely used vignette, it is actually a true story. It concerns a longstanding friend of the author, with whom he had grown up in South London in the 1960s. We'll call him Adam (not his real name).

A few years ago, Adam was revisiting some of his childhood haunts and was strolling through a popular inner-city park, in the midst of which, he remembered, was a little visited and isolated ornamental pond. As he approached the pond, he saw to his horror that lying motionless and face down in the middle of the pond was a child – a little boy of perhaps 4 years of age. There was nobody else in sight. The pond was shallow, and Adam, at no risk to himself other than the discomfort of getting his feet wet, was in a position to wade into the water and rescue the child. And this he did. The child, fortunately, was still alive, and Adam was able to remove him from the water and resuscitate him. Some minutes later, the child's mother appeared, wholly unflustered. She had been unaware of her son's predicament and was angry with him for getting wet rather than concerned that he had nearly drowned. She offered no word of thanks to Adam.

We might ask: in the circumstances, did that child (or his mother) have a right to expect Adam to save his life? The child had behaved irresponsibly; there is a fence around the pond over which he must have climbed. The mother had irresponsibly allowed her child to wander unsupervised. It was none of Adam's business. But most reasonable people would probably agree that the child's right to life placed an *accidental* responsibility upon Adam.

If any of us individually incur accidental responsibility to help even irresponsible strangers, can we not share collective responsibility (even at the cost of some modest sacrifice) to relieve or prevent the foreseeable suffering of strangers in need? Do systematically disadvantaged members of our society or even other societies have a right to collectively organised assistance, even if this is provided or funded by people who are not directly to blame for their disadvantage?

and respect for distant strangers who may have legitimate claims for our assistance, as we may have claims for their assistance. We have been developing this argument to make the case for social rights in a context that is primarily focused: not on utilitarian concerns but on the necessity of mutual human recognition, and which assimilates ontological with deontological ethics. It re-situates rights in relation to human interdependency and notions of co- or collective responsibility.

Competing rights-based perspectives

The analysis provided so far seeks to link rights and responsibilities, each of which may be approached or understood in relation to a variety of ideological leanings and from a variety of perspectives. One way of achieving a synthesis or overview of the story so far is through a taxonomy or classification of these different perspectives, such as that diagrammatically illustrated in Figure 5.1. The taxonomy is intended to serve – optionally – as a heuristic device. The method may not be one that every reader will find helpful, and certainly, it is not meant to provide a knock-down, all-inclusive explanation of current reality. That is impossible in a world messily shaped through contradiction and compromise. Nevertheless, despite its apparent complexity, the diagram is intentionally parsimonious: deliberately, it vastly oversimplifies some things in an attempt to understand a big picture and explain the contradictory influences that have played out and continue to shape systems for the provision of human welfare and competing conceptualisations of social rights.

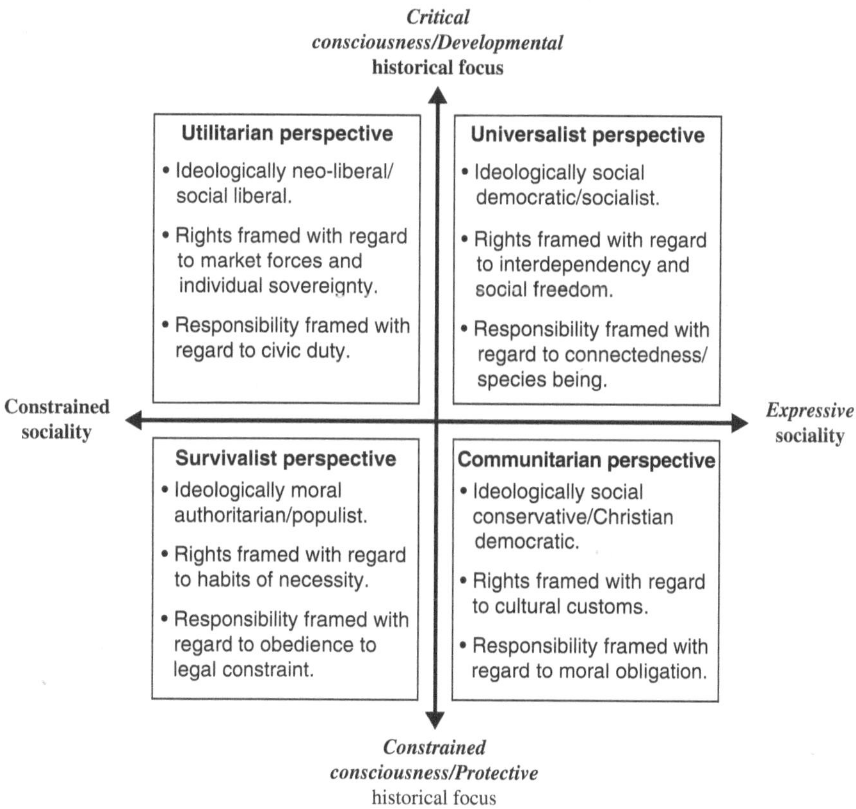

FIGURE 5.1 A taxonomy of perspectives contributing to the understanding of social rights

The taxonomy builds upon previous work by the author, the most salient of which was based on research that had used qualitative methods to explore not 'human values', but the extent to which discursive 'moral repertoires' identifiable in political discourse reflect and/or are reflected in popular discourses relating specifically to understandings of relative disadvantage and social citizenship (Dean with Melrose, 1999). The overarching analytical distinctions developed in that work – as will be seen – resonate to some extent with those drawn in the WSV surveys and the work of Schwarz (discussed earlier in this chapter), albeit the distinctions we shall make are differently informed by sociological and anthropological thinking. The analytical distinctions are represented by intersecting vertical and horizontal axes in the diagram, each of which represents a dimension or continuum bearing upon the dynamics entailed by the essential human characteristics identified and discussed in Chapter 1 of the volume. We shall consider each axis in turn.

The vertical axis – top-down and bottom-up dynamics of human consciousness and historical struggle

The vertical axis is concerned with relations of power in human society; relations that bear not only upon controls exercised over human activity – and resulting inequalities – but also on the formation of human consciousness and the direction of human development. In Chapter 2, we discussed a distinction between doctrinal and claims-based conceptions of social rights; in Chapter 3, we have already related this to a distinction between top-down and bottom-up definitions of need; and in this chapter we have discussed distinctions between ethical and moralistic understandings of responsibility and between hegemonic and subaltern understandings of rights. Readers may already have an intuitive sense that there are commonalities between these several distinctions. They are each and together associated with communicative relations of power: the hierarchical relations within which rights, needs and responsibilities are negotiated. The tensions between doctrinal and claims-based social rights, top-down and bottom-up need and ethical and moralistic responsibility are all dialectically mutually constitutive; they feed off each other.

Though not directly analogous, there is a resonance between the vertical axis and the 'grid' axis in Mary Douglas's (1977) highly influential cultural theory. Douglas's grid axis signified the extent to which individuals were either 'free' (or isolated) from or 'locked' (or included) into a culturally dominant view of the world. However, the horizontal axis in Figure 5.1 is premised on the idea that hegemonic relations of power can lock people in different ways; that powerful people can be as constrained by fetishised ideological beliefs as powerless people are constrained by customary mythologies and/or the mind-numbing effects of oppressive living conditions. And powerless people are not necessarily cultural dupes but may be capable of artful or counter-hegemonic forms of resistance as opposed to passive compliance (Scott, 1985). Power and communication flow up as well as down.

The principal advocates of doctrinal rights, top-down needs and ethical responsibilities are those in authority: rulers, sages or priests. The principal advocates of claims-based rights, bottom-up needs and moralistic responsibilities are subaltern members of society or their representatives: civil society organisations, trade unions and community activists. In practice, however, dissident politicians, radical scholars and liberation theologists may side with the subaltern, while civil society organisations, trade unions and community activists can be co-opted by the authorities (Piven & Cloward, 1977). And fundamentally, of course, systemic orthodoxies can 'colonise' the lifeworld (Habermas, 1987); they can shape and ossify the claims, the needs and the mores of the people. Conversely, yesterday's dissidents may sometimes become tomorrow's governors. It should be clear that rights, needs and responsibilities are dynamically negotiated and renegotiated at the point where competing perspectives engage with one another.

We have seen that psychologists, without detecting the underlying processes, may capture how this is reflected in individual human 'values' (see Box 5.1) when they observe a distinction between individuals who value 'openness to change' as opposed to those who value 'conservation'.

The horizontal axis – the thin and the thick of human sociality

The horizontal axis engages directly with sociality as an essential human characteristic. In Chapter 3, we discussed a distinction between thin and thick definitions of human needs. The notions of 'thin' and 'thick' chime well with the expressions 'constrained' and 'expansive' used here to describe different expressions or levels of realisation of human sociality. In Chapter 2, we discussed a distinction between formal and substantive conceptions of social rights; in this chapter we have been teasing out a distinction between individualistic and solidaristic understandings of responsibility. Once again, readers may already have an intuitive sense that these distinctions are associated. They are each and together associated with social relations and social connectedness: with the ways in which needs, rights and responsibilities are constituted and articulated. Thin and thick conceptions of need, formal and substantive social rights and individualistic and solidaristic understandings of responsibility stand respectively in relation to each other as opposing ends of a spectrum of theories, discourses and practices upon which social actors may draw in a variety of combinations.

Once again, there is a resonance in this instance with the 'group' axis in Mary Douglas' cultural theory. Douglas' group axis signified the extent to which individuals were free from, or protectively bound by, social group membership. There is a clear correspondence between the distinctions captured by the group axis and the distinction between the principles of liberty and solidarity. These are competing principles by which different people in different societies will in different ways live out their lives.

It may be inferred that the principal advocates of thin needs, formal rights, needs and individualistic responsibilities are likely to be found towards the 'right' of the ideological spectrum, and the principal advocates of substantive rights, thick needs and solidaristic responsibilities would be found towards the 'left'. The reality, however, is more complex than that. These are not always distinctions that fit neatly into conventional ideological categories. What is more, people are perfectly capable of embracing more than one principle at a time and combining them in inconsistent, complex and even ostensibly contradictory ways (Dean, 1998). We have also seen that psychologists may capture how this is reflected in individual human 'values' when they observe a distinction between individuals who value 'self-enhancement' and 'self-transcendence'.

We should, however, turn now to the four categories generated within the taxonomy, remembering that these are not perfect descriptions but heuristic constructs.

The synthesis

What we here identify as the utilitarian perspective (constructed at the intersection of the axes that delineate the top left quadrant in the top part of Figure 5.1) might currently be regarded, as we have seen, as a *dominant* perspective. The perspective:

- Is ideologically liberal, though the spectrum of liberal beliefs is wide. There is an important divide between economic and social liberalism. Economic liberalism is rooted in 'classical' liberal-individualist egalitarianism, but variants of what is dubbed 'neo-liberalism' may share *some* ground with far-right neo-conservative authoritarianism. Social liberalism, as we have seen, has been dubbed 'reluctant. collectivism' and can share *some* political centre ground with social democrats. All liberals, however, share a commitment to the autonomy of the individual.
- Adopts a selective approach to social rights. Rights are doctrinally conceived on the basis of a belief in the fundamental efficacy of a competitive market economy; an efficacy that depends, however, on formal equality of opportunity and on a 'level playing field' for all. A right to targeted social assistance is considered legitimate where – for example, through unemployment or infirmity – a citizen is excluded from economic participation. Or else there can be a right to provision at the basic minimum 'floor' necessary to ensure a person's readiness for economic participation. A right to education and/or healthcare is considered legitimate in circumstances where markets fail or are unable to maintain the skills and health of the labour force.

- Adopts an economistic approach to human need in the sense that the human subject is defined *a priori* as an economic actor who, as a producer of goods or services, should have freedom to compete and, as a consumer, should have freedom to choose. Needs reflect people's wants and preferences and are thin in the sense that they are particular to the individual.
- Conceives of responsibility as civic duty: an individual duty to be self-sufficient on the one hand, but respectful towards one's competitors and their freedoms on the other; to act and to contribute in such a way as is commensurate with the maintenance of a functional market economy. The performance of duties should, ideally, be a self-regulating process.

The survivalist perspective (constructed at the intersection of the axes that delineate the bottom left quadrant in the top part of Figure 5.1) might currently be regarded as a *resurgent* perspective. Though redolent of the principles of social assistance that preceded the capitalist welfare state, elements of the perspective have endured and are evident, as we shall see in later chapters, within current policy innovations. The perspective:

- Can be difficult to define in conventional ideological terms but is best captured by the terms 'moral authoritarian' and/or 'populist' (Rosanvallon, 2021). It has diverse elements: nineteenth-century Benthamite political utilitarianism on the one hand, twentieth-century neo-conservatism (Elliott & McCrone, 1987; Thompson & Brook, 2011) on the other. Its essence is individualist yet anti-libertarian.
- Adopts a conditional approach to social rights (when and insofar as it recognises social rights at all). Rights are properly the conditions on which bilateral exchange between competitive individuals is conducted, but they may, under certain circumstances, be transposed to a multilateral context. An individual right to any form of social assistance, if claimed, will necessarily be conditional on the deservingness of the supplicant and/or their compliance with behavioural constraints.
- Adopts a circumstantial understanding of human needs. Needs equate with that which is required for survival in a competitive and hazardous social environment.
- Conceives responsibility in terms of compliance with authority and conformity. The baseness of human nature must necessarily be constrained. Irresponsible behaviour should be suppressed by the inculcation of habitual obedience or through the imposition of rules or conditions by which all are equally bound.

The Communitarian perspective (constructed at the intersection of the axes that delineate the bottom right quadrant in the top part of Figure 5.1) might currently be regarded as a *declining* perspective. Its influence on social rights development, though by no means exhausted, is arguably waning. The perspective:

- Is ideologically communitarian, though this covers a spectrum of beliefs. There is an important divide between the communitarianism of traditional conservatives – such as Burke (see Lock, 1999) or Bismark (see Steinberg, 2011) – and that of radical democrats – such as Rousseau (1762) or, in recent times, Michael Walzer (1983). In essence, however, whether the emphasis is on the traditions of *noblesse oblige* or the general will of the people, its commitment is to some version of social solidarity.
- Approaches social rights as rights to social protection. Such rights arise because people share certain risks and vulnerabilities. Conceding the people's claims to protective rights serves to bind them together and to the social order (which will nevertheless be subject to certain inevitable inequalities); it guards against subversive influences and so protects the institutions of society.
- Adopts a paternalistic approach to human needs. Human needs are needs held in common. They are thick in the sense that they encompass the ontological need to belong. They are responsively defined in accordance with principles of subsidiarity, with priority accorded to support for families and communities.
- Conceives of responsibility in terms of mutual moral obligation. Responsibility is constructed with reference to collective loyalties and traditions, to moral norms and social values and to the expectations that arise from membership in a particular community. Failure to comply is seen as shameful.

The universalist perspective (constructed at the intersection of the axes that delineate the top right quadrant in the top part of Figure 5.1) might currently be regarded as a *potentiating* perspective. It may be noted that it is the only perspective that potentially combines an embrace of human sociality, critical consciousness and historical development.

- May be defined in ideological terms as social democratic or as democratic socialist. The ideological integrity of social democracy, some would argue, has arguably been compromised by an ever closer association through the so-called Third Way with neo-liberalism (Pierson, 2001) and through accommodation with the politics of austerity (Farnsworth & Irving, 2015), but the principles of democratic socialism still offer a vision that is both solidaristic and informed by what might be described as a social humanistic ethic (Fromm, 1965) or 'social humanism' (Fitzpatrick 2008, pp. 21–26 & 91–93).
- Has a preference for universal social rights; rights that should, as a matter of principle, attach to every citizen, or even to every human being;

that are comprehensive and should extend to substantive and appropriate support during every stage of the human life course; and that should be unconditional.

- Adopts a humanitarian approach to human need in the sense that the human individual is regarded as a social actor, defined inherently by her humanity. Its focus is on people's need not merely to survive but socially to participate and to be personally fulfilled.
- Conceives of responsibility as collective: a form of co-responsibility that is cosmopolitan in nature, in that it is as far as possible inclusive.

No actual existing social welfare/development regime conforms exactly to the perspectives caricatured within this taxonomy. But the perspectives outlined have all played a part and continue to have influence on policy development and, in the process, upon the multiple ways in which the human species conducts its metabolism with nature, its activity and its 'work'. The utilitarian perspective may be predominant, albeit that it may be constrained by residual or newly emerging survivalist influences, and it may in some instances sustain compromises with policy legacies premised upon pre-established communitarian or universalist perspectives. These, however, are matters to which we shall return in future chapters.

6

CRITIQUES OF SOCIAL RIGHTS

Challenges to the idea that citizens can, or should, enjoy social rights have been issued from several quarters, and this chapter will explore certain of these. It should by now already be clear that social rights, when conceived as rights of citizenship rather than as an element of human sociality, are an ambiguous phenomenon capable of dichotomous interpretations (see Box 6.1). Firstly, therefore, we shall briefly consider just how the fragile ideological

BOX 6.1 THE DICHOTOMOUS NATURE OF SOCIAL RIGHTS

Do social rights:

accord people **emancipation** and freedom from want	or	subject them to **control** and the regulation of need?
provide **entitlement** to social services	or	subject people to **discretion** and judgement?
ensure **substantive protection** across the life course	or	offer merely **procedural guarantees** of equal life chances?
promote **creative justice** amidst social diversity	or	ensure merely **proportional justice** as between individuals?

DOI: 10.4324/9781003451518-7

consensus that permitted the original development of the capitalist welfare state was possible. We shall then consider the critiques of the consensus that emerged from the extremities of the ideological spectrum before turning to a range of newer critiques that have emerged in the late or post-modern era.

An uneasy consensus

We have already seen that the social rights agenda, whether framed in terms of welfare state citizenship or the international human rights framework, was driven primarily by what may be regarded as a social-liberal consensus (broadly, within the **utilitarian** perspective portrayed in the last chapter in Figure 5.1). This of itself was an uneasy consensus between factions within liberalism: right-leaning economic liberals who broadly favoured 'negative' rights (which demand *freedoms from* things) had to concede to left-leaning social liberals who were prepared, reluctantly perhaps, to countenance 'positive' rights (which demand *entitlements to* things). However, the consensus had also somehow to embrace or accommodate both traditional conservative and moderate socialist opinion (elements of the **communitarian** and **solidaristic** perspectives in Figure 5.1) while, at the same time, tempering the authoritarian tendencies of populist politics (an element of the **survivalist** perspective in Figure 5.1).

Giving people rights is ostensibly one way of protecting their liberties – of safeguarding them from arbitrary power. This was fundamental to the historic strategy by which the property-owning bourgeoisie, in their bid to wrest power from the crown and the feudal aristocracy, had sought to displace conceptions of 'natural' rights with laws which were 'man-made' (Thompson, 1975). For precisely this reason, conservatives in the mould of Edmund Burke were mistrustful of any extension of rights, since the only common right that they would recognise was the 'right to adjudication'; that is, the right to be governed by the decisions of established authority with the power to translate imagined rights into realities (see Scruton, 1991, pp. 16–18). Rights are an explicit challenge to traditional paternalistic authority. There is a paradoxical resonance between this reservation about the consequences of a rights-based approach and that expressed by Richard Titmuss as a representative of the peculiarly British 'Fabian' socialist tradition. Titmuss (1971) favoured 'creative' social justice administered by compassionate experts rather than formulaic 'proportional' justice bestowed by rights that are legally prescribed. There have, therefore, been those in both the conservative and the socialist camps who would question the need for social rights that might impair the exercise of benevolent authority in the interests of human welfare.

The history of the capitalist welfare state is in part a story of transition from relief based on charity and discretion to benefits based on legislation and entitlement. Though conservatives resisted the welfare state and Fabian socialists championed it, the common ground they shared was an attachment to the value of discretionary decision-making. The compromise which both were prepared to strike with the liberal ideal of 'rights' can best be understood when it is realised that rights need not extinguish the scope for discretionary decision-making. Dworkin (1977) makes the point that administrative institutions in advanced capitalist societies function in a discretionary 'void', surrounded like the hole in a doughnut by legal rules and principles. Rights created by legislation require the exercise of administrative discretion for the interpretation and application of those rules (Lipsky, 1980/2010). Rights come with strings attached. The creation of rights to welfare extended rather than diminished administrative power and retained a space for populist moral authoritarianism through the refinement of conditionality (Garland, 1981). So it is that the expansion of the discourse of rights into the realm of social policy could be supported or at least tolerated across the board from within the broad swathe of the ideological centre ground.

Perhaps the most potent illustration of the ideological hybridity of capitalist welfare states is the extent to which they all, to a greater or lesser extent, adopt the social insurance principle as a mechanism for funding, regulating and delivering, whether wholly or partly, at least some elements of social provision. It is an internationally supported principle and remains a prominent feature in social policy reforms in several emerging economies and, for example, within the International Labour Organisation's Social Protection Floor initiative (Batchelet, 2011; ILO, 2012). The precedent for this was established not by a liberal administration, but at the end of the nineteenth century in Germany by Bismarck's conservative administration in its successful attempt to outmanoeuvre socialist opposition (Gilbert, 1966). And yet it was a precedent readily adopted by liberal and social democratic administrations across the capitalist world. The point about the social insurance principle is that it appeals both to individualistic and solidaristic ideals. It entails individual contribution and collective risk sharing. It is authoritarian insofar as membership and contributions are compulsory and insurance schemes are rule-bound. But it is also emancipating, since it can create indisputable rights to benefits, pensions or health treatment.

However, social rights, though born of an uneasy consensus, have generated new theoretical and practical concerns about the relationship between state authority and the individual citizen. And insofar as social rights are developing beyond the sphere of established capitalist welfare states, there are concerns as to how far this is feasible or appropriate.

Grand narrative critiques

Challenges to the nature and effects of social rights have come from the radical wings of both the political right and the political left, from the 'grand narratives' (Lyotard, 1984) of both neo-liberalism and neo-Marxism. In each instance, the 'neo' prefix signals a revival or reapplication of an established ideological narrative or critique. Classical liberalism and Marxism provided an analysis and overarching explanation of political economy, contrasting stories about how, in the wake of the Western Enlightenment, the capitalist market economy functioned. The liberal narrative celebrated the achievements of capitalism; the Marxist narrative condemned them. Though each of these classical narratives had things to say about rights, neither provided an account of social rights or the welfare state. Modern thinkers, however, have remedied that (George & Page, 1995).

The neo-liberal challenge

In seeking to recapture and revitalise the classical doctrines of economic liberalism neo-liberals would seek to restrict the rights of citizenship to civil and political rights, and primarily, to the negative liberties by which the free play of market forces may be guaranteed. Though the distributive outcomes of impersonal market forces may be unequal, this is neither intended nor foreseen and cannot therefore be unjust. According to Hayek (1976), the very idea of social justice and of social rights that might compensate for such injustice is no more than a mirage. If the rich and successful have moral obligations, how and to whom these may be discharged is a matter of choice: such obligations are not enforceable and give rise to no implication that those who fail to prosper have rights against those who succeed. Translating wants and needs into rights was once described by Enoch Powell as 'a dangerous modern heresy' (Powell, 1972).

Neo-liberal – or neo-liberal type – arguments are fundamentally sceptical towards the social rights created by capitalist welfare states and espoused within the UDHR. There are two kinds of objection: that welfare rights violate property rights and that social rights do not meet the conditions necessary to qualify as basic human rights. Turning first to Nozick (1974), his argument is based on an interpretation of Kant's 'categorical imperative', namely that respect for other persons depends upon their being regarded as ends in themselves and not as means (see Chapter 5, this volume). This he uses to build a case against any form of social rights requiring redistribution. For Nozick, the inviolability of the individual is synonymous with the inviolability of the property in which their rights are vested. To redistribute any portion of that property to another is to treat that person as a means and not an end. We may not violate persons for the social good because, says Nozick – in words that prefigured British Prime Minister Margaret Thatcher's declaration that 'there is no such thing as society' (*Women's Own* magazine 31 October 1987) – 'there is no *social entity* with a good which undergoes some sacrifice for its own good. There are only individual people with their own individual lives' (1974, p. 32). Individuals may choose to undergo some sacrifice for their own or somebody else's benefit, but they should not be compelled to do so in the name of some other person's 'right'. Such compulsion does not create social rights but rights of the state over the property of its own citizens – rights that violate the principle of respect for persons.

Secondly, there is, for example, Cranston's (1976) denial that social rights can be human rights. From a juristic rather than a political perspective, Cranston, as a legal positivist, draws the distinction we have previously discussed between legal rights (which are 'positively' defined) and human rights (which are 'morally' defined). According to Cranston, human rights have three tests of 'authenticity': practicability, paramount importance and universality (here defined in a strictly legal sense). Civil and political rights by and large meet these criteria insofar as they are relatively easily secured by appropriate legislation, they are fundamentally necessary to the just functioning of capitalist society, and they may be applied to everybody. Social and economic rights, however, are of a different order. The resources required for a social security system, for example, may be beyond the command of governments in the global South; social services and economic security may represent an ideal, but they are not essential; and, he claims, the needs which social rights address are relative, not universal. Therefore,

> the effect of a Universal Declaration which is overloaded with affirmations of so-called human rights which are not human rights at all is to push *all* talk of human rights out of the clear realm of the morally compelling into the twilight world of utopian aspiration.
>
> *(1976, p. 142)*

Onora O'Neill (a distinguished neo-Kantian philosopher who, at one time, chaired the Equality and Human Rights Commission in the United Kingdom) employs a similar logic. Addressing herself to 'The Dark Side of Human Rights' (2005), she observes that while it is clear that the duty to uphold negative rights may be assigned to the state, it isn't in all circumstances clear to whom the duty to uphold positive rights, such as the right to subsistence, can be practically assigned. The former entails claims to the forbearance of identifiable others, while the latter entails claims to performance by agents who cannot be conclusively identified. At this point, neo-liberal libertarian arguments may make common cause with the essentially illiberal and populist rejection of any form of collective altruism such as that espoused, for example, by Ayn Rand and her celebration of 'the virtue of selfishness' (1964). The critique may resonate within both the utilitarian and the survivalist perspectives on social rights.

Objections to these views are rehearsed elsewhere (Plant et al. 1980; Watson, 1980, ch. 4; Pogge, 2007; Ashton, 2011). The two points which need to be drawn out are that what is here broadly characterised as the neo-liberal case against social rights rests: firstly, on an assertion that social rights do not supplement but undermine the liberties necessary to the perpetuation of capitalism; second, on concerns about the costs of achieving social rights and by whom they should be borne. Sen (1999, ch. 4) encompasses the first of these within what he refers to as the 'legitimacy' critique and the second in what he refers to as the 'coherence' critique.

The neo-Marxist challenge

From the opposite end of the ideological spectrum comes a contrasting set of arguments, but arguments that can be just as sceptical about the value of social rights. Firstly, there is a group of academic writers who have sought to interpret Marxist principles in relation to the role which social rights play in regulating labour and sustaining, rather than undermining, capital. Second, there are theorists who have developed the Marxist critique of the form of individual legal rights in order to demonstrate the capacity of social rights for ideological mystification and control. It should be emphasised that what have conventionally been described as neo-Marxist critiques are critiques which draw primarily upon Marx's work on political economy and its essentially economistic elements rather than upon the less-scrutinised philosophical and essentially humanist elements of his writings discussed in Chapter 1 of this volume.

Turning to the first of these approaches, it is necessary to be clear that there are different strands of thought within neo-Marxism. There is an *instrumentalist* strand which adopts the idea that the state under capitalism acts as no more than 'a committee for managing the common affairs of the whole bourgeoisie' (Marx & Engels, 1848, p. 69). There is also a *structuralist* strand which analyses state forms as an expression of the immanent logic of the capitalist system and its class antagonisms. When neo-Marxists came to analyse the twentieth-century welfare state and the significance of the development of social rights, both these strands became, to some extent, intertwined.

The first kind of critique was developed by writers like Saville (1958), O'Connor (1973) and Gough (1979). They began to forge an account of how the welfare state had developed, claiming in essence that it was the product of three interacting influences. The first of these influences was the struggle by the working class for better living conditions. The social policy reforms obtained in this way had the effect of increasing levels of social consumption and general living standards, but they also benefited capital by furnishing an element of 'quantitative regulation' over labour power, partly by reducing the direct costs of labour and partly by having the state look after people whose labour was not required. The second influence was capital's growing need for an efficient environment and a productive workforce. The reforms resulting from this influence amounted to the investment by the state in 'human capital' and the necessary 'modification' of labour power through the provision of health and education services so as to produce better workers. The third influence was a concern for political stability. The policies resulting from this influence involved the discharge of the 'social expenses' necessary for the 'qualitative regulation' of labour power, or, more crudely, for the production of contented workers through the provision of those benefits and services required to secure social order and a degree of ideological control.

The neo-Marxist writer to engage most directly with the idea of social rights was Claus Offe. One of his central arguments was that 'the owner of labour power first becomes a wage labourer as a citizen of a state' (1984, p. 99). Industrial capitalism required more than the passive compulsion of economic forces in order to get people to accept the burdens and risks associated with wage labour and a market economy. To make people actively participate, it was necessary to have systems of political-administrative and normative control. Social policy is 'the state's manner of effecting the lasting transformation of non-wage labourers into wage labourers' (*ibid.*, p. 92). This is the basis upon which Offe challenges Marshall's account of social rights. Social rights were not some optional extra or final refinement to citizenship under capitalism; they are, according to Offe, a necessary part of it. Without such rights, citizens would not 'muster the *cultural motivation* to become wage labourers' (*ibid.*, p. 94). Within Offe's account, social rights were necessary: firstly, as a precondition for the suppression of begging and modes of subsistence which might undermine the wage labour system; secondly, as the medium through which to justify the provision of facilities for improving the quality of labour power (in ways of which individual self-seeking capitalists are incapable); thirdly, as a mechanism by which potentially or conditionally to exempt certain parts of the population from labour force participation (mothers, children, students, disabled people and older people). Social rights are as important as civil rights as a device for articulating labour power with the market.

Turning to the second kind of neo-Marxist critique, this is concerned less with the substance or effects of social rights as with their form. Marx had once argued that law and state apparatuses are no more than 'superstructural' phenomena, supported and indirectly shaped by the economic 'foundations' upon which they are constructed (1859). In *Capital* (1887, 1893, 1894), however, he went further and sought to demonstrate that the form of individual rights within bourgeois liberal ideology is a logically necessary consequence of capitalist production and market exchange. Because under market conditions goods must be exchanged as commodities, the producers and owners of such commodities must recognise in each other the rights of private proprietors and relate to each other on the basis of legal and contractual rules. Under capitalism, it is not only materials, products and services that are traded, but, following the destruction of feudal land tenure, real estate and even human labour are 'freed' to enter the market as commodities. Rights in ownership – of goods, land or labour power – become the universal foundation of human relationships. Unlike Hegel (as observed in Chapter 1 of this volume), Marx dismissed rights in ownership as an illusion, a 'fetishised' form that obscures the fundamentally exploitative substance of the social relations of production under capitalism.

In the course of the twentieth century, these ideas were taken up by other writers, foremost of whom was Pashukanis (1978). Writing in the 1920s, Pashukanis argued that, since it is the exchange of commodities that forms the very basis of social life, even such fundamental legal concepts as equity, restitution and entitlement are all derived from the commodity form. Just as 'value' is a concept that fundamentally defines our understanding of the nature and capacities of commodities, so 'right' is a concept that fundamentally defines our understanding of the nature and capacity of human beings. The individual juridical subject or citizen, as the bearer of rights, is the 'atom' – the simplest irreducible element – of legal and administrative theory. Pashukanis argued that this private form of possessive individual right has been rendered universal by being appropriated into the sphere of public and administrative law. This line of reasoning was developed by later theorists (e.g. Holloway & Picciotto, 1978), who have claimed that the form of the state – and the form of social rights – is 'derived' from capitalism's characteristic commodity form and from the nature of the wage relation as the most exploitative expression of that commodity form. The challenge here is that social rights are not all they seem. To cloak human welfare in an ideological discourse of 'rights' conceals the fundamental nature of relations of power under capitalism. It is nonsense to suggest that civil rights will guarantee that individual employees may bargain on equal terms with corporate employers, and it is nonsense to suggest that social rights will guarantee unemployed people, pensioners or disabled people the power to negotiate their claims with departments or agents of the state. By proselytising the ideal of an abstract universal human individual, human rights discourse continues, it is claimed, to de-politicise the economic processes that give rise to social oppression: such an individual will never 'fully identify the kernel of their being with their particular social situation' (Žižek, 2005, p. 129). Social rights give expression to the ultimate dominance of capital over labour and serve to extend or permeate that dominance beyond the immediate sphere of the wage relation, into the sphere of state-citizen relations, and into everyday life.

Once again, objections to these views are rehearsed elsewhere (e.g. Campbell, 1983; Hall & Held, 1989). There are neo-Marxist or anti-capitalist theorists, such as Lukács (1971), de Sousa Santos (2001), Hardt & Negri (2000) who clearly see an emancipatory role for law – and, by implication, for rights – in a future post-capitalist era (see Fine, 2002). However, in spite of differences between them, the essence of the neo-Marxists' case against social rights is first, that in ameliorating the exploitative impact of capitalism they help ensure its survival; second, that under present circumstances, social rights provide a powerful mechanism for state/ideological control.

A post-grand narrative era?

We have touched in preceding chapters on the crisis that befell the capitalist welfare state towards the end of the twentieth century and the consequences of this for social rights. The era through which we have been living may be described as post-industrial (Bell, 1973), post-modern (Lyotard, 1984) and even post-social (Rose, 1996b). We live, arguably, in a different world than that in which Marshall expounded on social citizenship and the UN first proclaimed its Declaration of Human Rights. However, contrary to the prophecies of some (e.g. Fukuyama, 1992), we have not seen the end of history. The grand narratives have not been superseded. The Marxist narrative appears to be in retreat, and although it is 'increasingly difficult to demarcate the boundaries of what Marxism is and is not' (Fine, 2002, p. 117), its influence is alive in all sorts of current thinking (Callinicos, 2007, ch. 13). The neo-liberal narrative, on the other hand, has been ascendant and enduring (Amin, 1997; Taylor-Gooby, 1994, 2013). Its fundamental premises were reflected towards the end of the twentieth century in the global North, initially through the development of 'new right' approaches and the partial retrenchment of social rights (e.g. Levitas, 1986) and subsequently during the development of 'third way' thinking and the modification of social rights (e.g. Lewis & Surender, 2004). Its impact on the global South has been felt through the pro-market 'Washington consensus' (Williamson, 1990) that informed the development policies of the World Bank and the IMF, policies favouring free market competition and minimal social safety nets. Though it was supposed by some (Stiglitz, 2003) that the implementation of the Millennium Development Goals portended an end to such an approach, some would argue that its influence lives on (Maxwell, 2005; Deacon, 2007; and see Chapter 9, this volume). Neo-liberal orthodoxies, it has been argued, have even survived the crisis of confidence that might have resulted from the global financial crisis that they precipitated in 2007–2010 (Callinicos, 2010; Peck & Tickell, 2012). The implications of this for social rights will be pursued in future chapters. For now, we shall consider other critiques bearing on social rights that have emerged during the transition to the current era.

The transition has fomented alternative insights, theories and critiques. We shall firstly discuss 'emancipatory' critiques associated with new social movements (particularly the feminist, anti-racist and disability awareness movements). Secondly, we shall touch upon some of the 'defensive' critiques emanating from the new political pluralism. The distinction we shall make between emancipatory and defensive approaches owes something to Habermas (1987, p. 393). Finally, we shall touch on theoretical post-structuralist critiques.

Challenges from emancipatory social movements

We refer here to critiques which attempted on behalf of particular constituencies to redeem the universal promises offered by the 'liberal' conception of rights (Hewitt, 1993), which questioned whether social rights did ensure equality and freedom from want for women, for ethnocultural minorities, for disabled people and for other socially or culturally marginalised groups. Reference has already fleetingly been made (see Chapter 3, this volume) to a 'cultural turn' in critical thinking in the global North: a turn towards a politics of identity and recognition; a concern with dimensions of oppression and socially constructed differences other than those associated with socio-economic class.

Foremost, from the 1960s onwards, was the **second-wave feminist movement** (Fraser, 2010, ch. 6). Previous generations of liberal feminists had campaigned against limitations upon women's property rights and voting rights, and more latterly, maternalist feminists began to campaign in favour of rights for citizen-mothers (Lister, 2003). Second-wave feminists, however, began to challenge the underlying form as well as the substance of their 'rights'. As in the sphere of civil and political rights, when it came to social rights, women were 'second class citizens' (Lister, 1990). There remained a liberal feminist strand whose concern was to promote equal opportunities legislation (Williams, 1989, pp. 44–49), but the 1970s witnessed the birth of strands of feminism whose resistance to women's oppression was founded on the critical analysis of patriarchy as a structural characteristic of human society. The central insight of the concept relates to the distinction between the socially constructed public and private spheres (see especially Pascall, 1986, 1997). The public sphere is where civil and political rights reside; it is the domain of the market and the state; it is the site of productive and administrative activity in which, by and large, it was men who colonised the principal roles. The private sphere, in contrast, is not inhabited by rights; it is the domestic domain of hearth, home and family; it is the site for the reproduction of social life, a process in which it was women who were assigned their principal roles. The public/productive sphere is separated from, yet dominates the private/reproductive sphere. Social rights have been important to the articulation between the two. As Pascall puts it, the welfare state was originally forged 'in the void between the factory and the family' (1986, p. 26).

Social rights may have succeeded in redistributing resources from men to women (e.g. Falkingham & Hills, 1995), but women still face a higher risk of poverty than men, both globally (Chant, 2008), and even within capitalist welfare states (Pascall, 2012). Social rights have failed women on two counts: firstly, because they were instrumental in the supervision and enforcement of women's dependency in the private sphere; secondly, because they did not compensate women for their disadvantage in the public sphere. The original architects and subsequent analysts of the capitalist welfare state were inured to the patriarchal norm of the male breadwinner household. They were criticised for failing properly to confront the reality that under capitalism 'men and women are "gendered commodities" with different experiences of the labour market resulting from their different relationship to family life' (Langan & Ostner, 1991, p. 131). As a consequence, many capitalist welfare states incorporated social insurance schemes on the one hand, under which it was predominantly male heads of household who claimed entitlements on behalf of predominantly female dependents, alongside social assistance systems on the other, under which it was predominantly female-headed households – including large numbers of lone parents and single female pensioners – that claimed stigmatised means-tested benefits; the former have been characterised as 'masculine sub-systems', the latter as 'feminine sub-systems' (Fraser, 1989, pp. 111–112). Recent policy reforms across the welfare states of the global North portend a shift away from assumptions based on the male breadwinner household model towards an 'adult worker model' (Lewis, 2000) in which men and women alike are expected to sustain themselves through participation in the labour market. This has resulted in the development of rights to childcare provision and to flexible working arrangements to facilitate work-family reconciliation. In practice, however, such policies may take little account of women's preferences or the opportunities available to them and would seem to be privileging paid employment at the expense of unpaid care (Lewis, 2009). Women's socially constituted roles and identities remain systemically subordinate.

Like the feminist critique, the **anti-racist critique** of social rights claimed that ethnocultural minorities living in capitalist welfare states were 'second class' citizens (see Lister 1990, p. 52). Though there are important exceptions, ethnocultural minorities tend to experience a greater risk of poverty, unemployment, poor health and housing than ethnocultural majorities (for a comprehensive account of evidence from the British case, see Chattoo et al., 2019). This can apply not only to diasporic migrant minorities but also to colonised indigenous minorities (Salomon, 2005; Humpage, 2010). What distinguished the anti-racist critique from liberal democratic concerns about racial discrimination was that it regarded racism not as an illiberal attitude but as an ideology – an ideology that 'racialises' (Fanon, 1967) the relations of power by which social groups and the boundaries between them are defined. Racism first grew out of a mistrust of the 'otherness' of people deemed not to be civilised (Miles, 1989); it is even suggested that the very basis of modern law and rights of citizenship is grounded in a racist mythology

(Fitzpatrick, 1992). Racism, therefore, is more than heterophobia or intolerance, but in the global capitalist context is historically situated in relation to processes of economic exploitation: slavery in the pre-capitalist era and class conflicts set in train as a result of conquests, colonialism, imperialism and global labour migration (Sivanandan, 1990). At the very least, the selective framing of social rights is implicated in the racialisation of the cultural differences through which ethnic identities are defined. Just as the sexual division of labour is rooted historically in the ideological construction of 'the family', so there is a racial division of labour that is rooted historically in the ideological construction of 'the Nation' (Williams, 1989, ch. 4).

The consequences pose peculiar dilemmas for the capitalist welfare state:

- Should migrants enjoy the same social rights as established citizens? There is a tension – the so-called 'liberal paradox' – between individual freedom of movement on the one hand and the principles of national sovereignty on the other. It is claimed that the welfare state 'requires boundaries because it establishes a principle of distributive justice that departs from the distributive principles of the free market' (Hollifeld, 1992). Access to social security benefits, housing and other forms of welfare provision are generally conditional upon citizenship and immigration status, or else social rights can be 'fine-tuned' to include or exclude different social groups (Lockwood, 1996; Morris, 2002). This is an issue to which we shall return.
- Should the members of settled ethnocultural minorities, contrary to liberal-individualist principles, be accorded group rights: for example, rights to the recognition of specific cultural or linguistic requirements? The trend in several capitalist welfare states towards the end of the twentieth century had been towards a variety of 'multiculturalism policies', intended to accommodate ethnocultural diversity rather than attempting to assimilate minorities and violate their right to cultural identity. The implications for social rights and the welfare state are widely debated (Banting & Kymlicka, 2006).

The **disability awareness movement**'s critique of social rights has direct parallels with those of the second-wave feminist and anti-racist movements. Born in the 1970s out of grassroots organisations *of* rather than *for* disabled people in several countries (Barnes & Mercer, 2010; Roulstone & Prideaux, 2012), the movement's primary claim was for self-determination through rights of citizenship (Townsend & Walker, 1981). Disability is something experienced when people are born with a genetic impairment if they suffer illness or injury that limits their functioning, or if they suffer from degenerative conditions as they grow older. The impairments associated with disability may be physical or may entail mental health problems or learning difficulties. While the impairments or functional limitations to which human beings are subject generally relate to biological causes or the effects of physical injury, their impact on people's lives is in large part determined by social context: disability – like gender and ethnicity – is socially constructed. Prior to the development of capitalist welfare states, people adjudged to be physically, mentally or morally 'defective' were often confined in institutions or colonies or otherwise segregated from the 'normal' population. Post-Second World War welfare states developed policies and systems intended to ensure that disabled people should no longer be segregated from non-disabled society, but which succeeded nonetheless in excluding and continuing to 'disable' them. Provision was not necessarily framed as a social right but was shaped by the assumption that people with impairments are not fully competent citizens. The argument championed by the disability awareness movement was that disability should not be addressed as a personal tragedy that has befallen the individual or as an individual medical problem susceptible to medical explanation and management. Rather, it should be understood in terms of the consequences of a hostile social environment that does not, or will not, accommodate the particular needs, or recognise the particular abilities, of people with impairments or functional limitations (Oliver, 1990).

The disability awareness movement has impacted the extension of social rights for disabled people (see Chapters 7 and 8 in this volume), particularly with regard to the right to independent living. Nevertheless, there are enduring issues for the movement insofar as there remains a tension between the goal of enabling people with impairments and functional limitations to live independently and the claim that as vulnerable citizens they also have a right to protective care and support (Shakespeare, 2006).

The emancipatory claims of feminism, anti-racism and the disability awareness movement have contested the basis of social rights. Rather than accommodate their demands to one-size-fits-all universal or general conceptions of rights, emancipatory critics promote the particular needs claims of women, ethnocultural minorities and disabled people, albeit on the basis of universal principles. But should the objective of social rights be to ensure that everybody has effective opportunities and equal life chances regardless of gender, 'race' or disability (an equal opportunities approach) or practically to compensate individuals for the disadvantages that may result from socially constructed differences (a social welfare approach) (see Dean, 2012a)?

The liberal *equal opportunities* approach is concerned with promoting tolerance and fairness. It has been implemented within capitalist welfare states primarily through various forms of anti-discrimination legislation (Bagilhole, 2009). However, equal opportunities approaches are preoccupied with observing formal rights. In so doing, they ascribe fixed, individualised identities on the basis of a person's membership in a particular social group. This may fail to address the fundamental causes of disadvantage and underlying relations of power between dominant and subordinate groups in society. The focus is on discriminatory attitudes and prejudices, not on social structural factors. Anti-discrimination legislation tends to reduce the problem of discrimination to the level of individual instances amenable to individual legal remedies. Second-wave feminists object to the equal opportunities approach when it effectively forces women to compete with men on men's terms. Anti-racists object to the equal opportunities approach if all it does is promote tactical compliance strategies on the part of employers and other bodies, leaving underlying institutional racism untouched. Elements within the disability awareness movement may object to the equal opportunities approach as currently conceived since it does not positively or proactively intervene to ensure that disabled people have autonomy and proper control over their own lives.

The *social welfare* approach is concerned with protecting people and, arguably, promoting solidarity amidst diversity. The danger is that such an approach may perpetuate and consolidate social differences, rather than confront their social implications. This is particularly the case if policy implicitly references differences in relation to some notion of a 'normality' that is, by default, male, white and able-bodied and neglects the extent to which masculinity, majority ethnicity and 'ability' are themselves socially constructed. Compensatory approaches are preoccupied with identifying and meeting substantive human needs but tend in so doing to prescribe the identity of the subject in a top-down fashion. Second-wave feminists may object that rights that support women in their role as mothers and carers or which make it easier for women to combine paid employment and unpaid caring responsibilities may lock women into dependency on men and perpetuate their status as second-class citizens (Lister, 2003). Anti-racists object when rights intended to assist ethnocultural minorities better to celebrate their cultural identities and integrate with the majority communities in which they live in practice trivialise ethnic differences or reify them, thus neglecting the structural root causes of disadvantage (Phillips, 1999, 2007). Activists within the disability awareness movement object that rights to special benefits and services for disabled people, though they alleviate personal suffering, do not necessarily confront the extent to which it is society that is to blame for so many of the disadvantages that disabled people face (Morris, 1991, 2003).

We have focused on three particular social movements that have each sought to re-contextualise social rights in relation to social difference and diversity, but it is important to recognise that similar critiques can be or have been developed by or on behalf of other social groups differentiated by or socially constructed through their sexuality and/or gender identity, their religious beliefs and/or identity and the stage they have reached within their life course (see Box 6.2). The emancipatory demands reflected within all these critiques amount in different ways to a quest for what Ruth Lister (1998) has called 'differentiated universalism' as opposed to the 'false universalism' offered by certain established framings of social rights.

BOX 6.2 SEXUALITY, RELIGION AND THE HUMAN LIFE COURSE

Sexuality and/or gender identity. Feminist critiques have fuelled and informed new debates about the extent to which citizenship rights have been premised not only upon gendered assumptions and supposedly 'traditional' family norms but also on the institutionalisation of heterosexuality (Richardson, 1998; and see Weeks, 1990). Insofar as the rights of gay, lesbian, bi-sexual and trans-gender people are being recognised and defended in some jurisdictions, they are being framed in the context of a heteronormative agenda (Gregory & Matthews, 2022).

Religious beliefs and/or identity. Debates about the rights of ethnocultural minorities may be closely intertwined with issues of religion with regard not only to formal freedoms of belief and expression (Modood, 2013) but also having regard to the effectiveness of social rights for minority religious groups (Torry, 2016). It is also the case that precepts found within all the main world religions have given and may continue – in new or different ways – to give substantive effect to social welfare practices that had preceded the invention of welfare state citizenship (Dean, 2023; Jawad, 2022b; and see Chapter 9, this volume).

Life course stages. The framing of social rights and citizenship status have always been associated with socially constructed assumptions about not only gender and sexualities but also what constitutes a supposedly 'natural' life course, something which in reality is determined not by a person's chronological age but by historically specific social and labour market conventions. Thus, 'youth' is a potentially problematic transitional stage between childhood and adulthood (Coles, 1995), and 'old age' is a stage that begins at a point when a person's labour power may be deemed to have become dispensable (Townsend, 1991).

Challenges from defensive political pluralism

The stirrings of a different kind of movement can also be traced back to the 1960s and 1970s; movements concerned not so much with recognising social differences as with defending humanity against military power (the peace movement), environmental exploitation and degradation (the green movement) and, in particular, excesses of administrative state power. The latter forms of defensive critique have been concerned with the defence of communities, the promotion of civil society organisations and fomenting a different, more inclusive, participative and pluralistic form of politics (Scott, 1990). Social movements – broadly understood – have long had particular pertinence for social rights (Annetts et al., 2009), and, in the context of current struggles for environmental and global social justice, they continue to do so, as we shall see in Chapter 11. It must additionally be borne in mind that movements favouring civil society alternatives to the state can be favoured from across the ideological spectrum, from the neo-liberal right to the social left (Kaldor, 2003; Powell, 2007). However, we are concerned here with a particular radical and nominally non-ideologically aligned shift of thinking that emerged, in part at least, as a backlash against the monolithic capitalist welfare state. The original impetus came from two quarters: the community development movement on the one hand and radical communitarianism on the other, each of which sought to challenge the efficacy of social rights where these have been created through top-down, statist and undemocratic processes.

The 1960s and 1970s witnessed largely unsuccessful attempts to establish poor people's movements, such as the National Welfare Rights Organisation in the United States (Piven & Cloward, 1977) and the Claimants Union movement in Britain (Jordan, 1973), movements that could not achieve formal sustainability in the way that organised labour and the trades unions had succeeded in doing and which demonstrated the limits of informal resistance to the state administration of social rights. Lessons learnt from such experiences informed, on the one hand, techniques of guerrilla-style community organisation (Alinsky, 1969) and, on the other, a variety of professionally organised urban community development and welfare rights projects, which we shall return to discuss in Chapter 10. In the same era, the acceleration of urbanisation in the global South was accompanied by the development of grassroots urban social movements (Castells, 1983) and, for example, an explosion of illegal squatting, a phenomenon to which policymakers were increasingly obliged to accede (Hardoy & Satterthwaite, 1989). Contemporaneously, radical new critiques as to the oppressive or disempowering nature of modern state-organised education and healthcare systems from intellectuals such as Paulo Friere (1972) and Ivan Illich (1971; Illich et al., 1977) began to percolate debate in the global South and the global North alike.

The resulting pluralist critique of the capitalist welfare state achieved a certain level of orthodoxy within parts of the voluntary or non-governmental organisation sector. This was distilled and exemplified in Hadley and Hatch's (1981) attack on the centralised nature of the welfare state and the character this afforded to the administration of social rights. Unitary government, they claimed, is an inheritance that had suited parties of both left and right and was now entrenched by virtue of its own internal momentum. The result was bureaucratic, unaccountable and inefficient. It gave professionals and the officialdom unwarranted power to control the behaviour of clients and service users. The supposedly non-ideological solution was in part a shift to welfare pluralism with a greater role for the voluntary and informal sectors (see discussion in Chapter 2, this volume), but partly also the development of bottom-up 'participatory alternatives' to centralised social services. The nature of such participatory alternatives would have been such as to give clients or service users a more active role in negotiating the nature of the services they received. The performance of such services, it was argued, should be judged with reference to outputs rather than inputs.

This emphasis on results or outcomes, rather than resources or 'rights' represents a theme espoused in common with some radical communitarians, such as Walzer (1983). Walzer has contended that *justice* is more important than 'rights', since distributive justice or equality represents outcomes (which can be assessed) rather than objectives (which cannot). Justice itself, however, 'is a human construction, and it is doubtful whether it can be made in only one way' (*ibid.*, p. 5). Equality, Walzer argues, does not require the elimination of difference, and what justice must entail is egalitarianism 'without the Procrustean bed of the state'. The bed in the Procrustean legend was one to which victims were fitted by being forcibly stretched or butchered, and Walzer's case is that human beings need not be so abused; it is social goods, not citizens, that should be controlled or made to fit. What is required is not universalism but a form of 'complex equality'. This is, incidentally, a rather different sort of communitarianism than that of either traditional conservatives or 'new' communitarians such as Etzioni (1995) or Putnam (1993) and more in tune with elements of the work of Sandel (1982), Taylor (1992), and MacIntyre (2007), who challenge a reductive rights-based understanding of equality.

The common theme of these 'defensive' critiques is a rejection of the generality of the *dirigiste* state and social rights based on prescription. The emphasis on participation, especially political participation, has had particular resonance amongst social movements in the global South in which there has been resistance to ideas premised on the old-style state corporatism of the global North (Foweraker & Landman, 1997) and to social rights as the mere 'politics of demand' (Waterman, 2001).

Post-structuralist critiques

Coinciding with the 'crisis' of the capitalist welfare state, the 'cultural turn' in ideological thinking and the birth of a 'post-modern' era, there have been important developments in social theory and a plethora of new insights into the functioning and limitations of social rights. Foremost among these has been the contribution of post-structuralist thinking. Theorists of post-modernity have called into question whether the Western Enlightenment that gave birth to 'modernity' was ever a dispassionate quest for truth and reason. On the contrary, according to Bauman (1987, p. 80), it was an exercise in two parts:

> First, in extending the powers and ambitions of the state, in transferring to the state the pastoral functions previously exercised by the church, in re-organising the state around the function of planning, designing and managing the reproduction of social order ...... secondly, in the creation of an entirely new and consciously designed mechanism of disciplinary action, aimed at regulating and regularising the socially relevant life of the subjects of the teaching and managing state.

What was obscure under modernity is more transparent within the post-modern world of information technology and new managerialism, in which, for example, scientists are hired 'not to find truth, but to augment powers' (Lyotard, 1984, p. 46). Bauman and Lyotard are echoing here the arguments of Michel Foucault, whose claim had been that modernity was based not on scientific reason and rationality but the 'will to power'; that the legitimacy of modern governance was an effect of power and not truth or justice; and that the reality behind the veil of democratic-welfare-capitalism is that of an inherently 'disciplinary society' (see especially Foucault, 1977).

Foucault's general arguments have also influenced some particular critiques of the disciplinary aspects of social policy (Dean, 1991; Squires, 1990). The basis for such approaches has been a re-examination of the history of the welfare state and of the increasingly sophisticated surveillance and disciplinary processes associated with the administration of social rights. These approaches invoke a relational theory of power, which first holds that the shift from feudalism to capitalism was associated with a shift from coercive to administrative (welfare) state power. Administrative state power has had as much to do with the regulation of human behaviour as the 'dull compulsion' of economic forces. The development of state welfare and social rights has involved new technologies of power and pervasive new disciplinary techniques. The characteristic of these technologies and techniques is that, unlike class power, they bear upon *individual difference*. In place of unbiddable mass movements is the controllable individual subject.

In place of the indiscriminate giving of alms to the anonymous poor, there has been erected the complex panoply of the capitalist welfare state, which scrutinises and documents each individual 'client' or 'case'. In place of careless humanitarianism, there has been inserted meticulous paternalistic control. In place of such practices as the public whipping and branding of vagrants, there have emerged more discreet and gentle forms of coercion based on benefit penalties and disqualifications. In place of an explicit Malthusian desire to punish the poor, there have developed more subtle forms of containment.

In place of crude processes of classification and surveillance associated with the workhouse and the Poor Laws, there have been constructed administrative systems based on legal definitions and regulations to which citizens must submit in order to exercise their 'rights'. In place of the prying concern and moralistic edicts of philanthropists and overseers of the poor has emerged a voluntaristic discourse based on the idea that citizens of the welfare state are juridical subjects with the freedom to exercise their rights and a responsibility to abide by the rules. The history of the welfare state is therefore seen not as a story of progress towards the development of universal social rights but as a story of developing state power and increasingly sophisticated methods of social control. It is additionally argued that, far from dismantling state power, recent policies of welfare retrenchment have often involved subtle refinements to the disciplinary mechanisms which underpin social rights: a new disciplinary logic of 'governmentality' (Foucault, 1991), through which new forms of conditionality and behavioural management may be brought to bear, especially in relation to labour market activation (Henman & Fenger, 2006).

The spectrum of critiques outlined in this chapter reveals, on the one hand, resistances to the development of social rights and, on the other hand, critical analyses of the limitations and contrary consequences of social rights. None, however, expressly consider whether and to what extent social rights have given or can give effective expression to human sociality, a question we shall endeavour to broach in Chapter 11.

PART II
Social Rights in Practice

7

RIGHTS TO HUMAN SERVICES

This book has been addressing social rights and human welfare from a range of different conceptual and theoretical perspectives but will now turn to how social rights work in practice as a means to achieving human welfare. The thread that runs throughout this volume is the concept of sociality as a distinctive characteristic of our species being – a characteristic inextricably implicated in, and which facilitates, human consciousness, creative activity and historical development. Sociality is more than an abstract concept. It refers to an essential component contributing to the sum of human praxis. Where it finds expression through explicit social policy or systemic forms of social provision, it gives birth to what Titmuss (1958) termed 'social services': an expression he applied to the entire spectrum of governmental interventions intended to provide for human needs. However, in the context of a functioning capitalist economy, a distinction may be drawn between, on the one hand, provision intended to provide for human livelihoods by ensuring access to secure incomes that enable people to *purchase* necessary commodities and, on the other, the right to *receive* goods and services that have been to some extent de-commodified or which, having the status of 'merit' goods (Musgrave, 1959), are supplied subject to governmental regulation or oversight. The distinction between these forms of social service can be a fine one since – as will be seen – they may become interconnected, but we shall be discussing the former in the next chapter under the heading 'rights to livelihood' while turning in this chapter to the latter, to which we shall refer generically as 'human services'.

Human services, in this sense, are themselves of various kinds. The provision of healthcare and education might be regarded as 'bedrock' services: these are the services through which our universal life course needs for health

DOI: 10.4324/9781003451518-9

and autonomy (Doyal & Gough, 1991) are met and which provide the foundation of a civilised human existence. Closely connected to health service provision are what may be called 'personal' social services, which are not universally required but reserved for the care and protection of the most vulnerable members of society: specialised social care provision for children, disabled or older people who are at risk or in need of particular forms of support. Finally, the provision of shelter or housing – as seen in Chapter 3 of this volume – was included in the UDHR as part of the right to an adequate standard of living (Article 25 [1]): housing represents a classic merit good in relation to which governments may provide for the planning of the habitable environment and control over the supply of dwellings.

Human services can and have been provided on a *customary* basis as an axiomatic part of everyday life, on a *voluntary* basis by charities or religious institutions and/or on a *contractual* basis by private market-sector organisations. But the giving and receiving of human services are explicitly identified and constituted as social rights at the point when governments intervene not necessarily to provide services directly but to facilitate, oversee or manage such provision. We saw in Chapter 3 that the ICESCR allows for the 'progressive realisation' of social rights, by which it is required that state parties should (see CESCR General Comment 12 and e.g. Shue, 1980):

- firstly, *respect* such rights – for example, by refraining from disrupting or preventing private or non-governmental sector health, educational or social care provision or from forcibly evicting citizens from their homes;
- secondly, *protect* such rights – for example, by regulating private or non-governmental sector health, education, social care or housing provision;
- thirdly, *fulfil* such rights – for example, by subsidising and/or directly providing health, educational, social care or housing provision.

Social rights can be promoted or fulfilled through intervention short of direct public sector provision, in which case, where human services are not free at the point of delivery, contractual arrangements between service providers and service users are entailed. The social rights and the contractual/civil rights agendas interact at the point where policymakers become involved in such arrangements. Where governments are concerned to protect or promote human services, they may be concerned to ensure fair and equal access by providing selective subsidies for those least able to afford the use of services or to ensure equality of opportunity for women and girls and/or for ethnic or religious minorities. Governments may seek to regulate markets in human services or the terms of contractual relationships so as to guard against the consequences of power imbalances between providers and users and the risk that users may be exploited. But, where governments seek to provide directly for human need through public sector institutions, social and civil rights may interact in a quite different way: for example, to safeguard the freedom of the service user lest it be jeopardised through the exercise of over-weaning or paternalistic state power. In the realm of human service provision, social and civil rights cannot easily be disentangled.

We shall, in barest outline, discuss generic issues and principles relating to rights to health, education, social care and housing.

Rights to health

The right to health is one of the two basic needs specified by Doyal and Gough's (1991) theory of human need. Physical and mental health are important for optimal human fulfilment and effective human activity. The preamble to the 1946 Constitution of the World Health Organisation declared that 'the enjoyment of the highest attainable standard of health is one of the fundamental rights of every human being', a principle echoed in the ICESCR (Article 12 [1]), which commits states parties to recognising the right both to physical and mental health. Other than in its constitution, however, the WHO has for the most part avoided the language of rights. Nevertheless, one UN Special Rapporteur on Health has argued that the right to health is to be understood as the right to 'an effective and integrated health system, encompassing both healthcare and the underlying determinants of health' (Hunt, 2006: para. 4). He further stressed that 'an effective health system is a core social institution, no less than a court system or a political system' (para. 20). With this in mind, the principal issues are as follows:

The determinants of health

In the preamble to its Constitution, the WHO defined health as 'a state of complete physical, mental and social well-being and not merely the absence of disease or infirmity'. This sets an ostensibly unattainable standard: nobody can be completely healthy for the whole of their life! The significance of the definition, however, lies in the emphasis on the social context of health, not just the treatment of individual illness (Marks, 2013). Here, the right to health intersects with the right to housing (see below) and to a healthy environment. The ICESCR of 1966 committed states parties to 'the improvement of all aspects of environmental and industrial hygiene' (Article 12 [2]). Two decades later, environmental issues had moved up the global political agenda, and the right to a healthy environment was regarded as a component of a 'third' generation of human rights (Boyle, 2007; and see Chapter 4, this volume). For example, the San Salvador Protocol explicitly declared that 'Everyone shall have the right to live in a healthy environment' (Article 11). It is speculated that Marshall might have added environmental rights as a category of citizenship rights (Newby, 1996; Van Steenbergen, 1994).

But before this, as we have seen, public health had already become a predominant concern informing the development of urban infrastructure in the global North. Indeed, the history of public health technologies –water supply and sanitation – can be traced back further to ancient Egyptian, Greek, Roman and Inca civilisations. And such concerns are now a major preoccupation in many parts of the global South (UNDP, 2022; UN-HABITAT, 2023). Good health is dependent on a variety of preconditions, most immediately, a safe water supply and adequate sanitation. In the current era, it also requires protection against risks from occupational hazards and overcrowded or substandard housing; environmental pollution and degradation, including now pandemics and climate change facilitated or induced by human activities. And beyond the infrastructural and environmental determinants of health, as medical science and knowledge advances, it has become possible, at least partially, to protect human populations from infectious diseases through immunisation programmes, health promotion initiatives and health education (Cahill, 2002; Toebs, 2001; WHO, 2008). Public or environmental health policies may not directly fulfil the right to health, but vitally, they promote it or seek to mitigate factors that threaten human health.

The accessibility of healthcare to all

The ICESCR commits state parties to 'The creation of conditions which would assure to all medical service and medical attention in the event of sickness' (Article 12). As with education, the history of medical practice and the provision of healthcare date from antiquity (Bynum, 2008). In the preindustrial era in the West, it had assumed the form of fee-paying services for those who could afford to pay and informal or charitable provision for those who could not. Industrialisation, however, gave employers a potential interest in healthcare provision (at least for their more highly skilled workers), while the people for whom sickness coincided with destitution placed growing demands on the Poor Laws (Doyal, 1979). What would emerge was a mixture of private and voluntary health insurance arrangements, which in some countries were subsumed into national health insurance schemes; and alongside, a variety of public and municipal healthcare institutions, which in some countries were subsumed into a national health service.

The accessibility of healthcare and the precise content of the right to health are largely dependent on the model of funding that applies within any particular country, of which there are, broadly speaking, three: the private market-based model with a medical assistance safety-net; the social insurance model with state co-ordinated medical provision; and the tax-funded national health service model. (There is a direct conceptual parallel with the distinction between social assistance, social insurance and universal/contingent models of social security provision that we shall discuss in Chapter 8.) In practice, health service provision around the world may comprise elements from more than one model and tends to be in a continual process of flux or reform (Watson, 2013). Inevitably, systems that are more heavily dependent on private provision provide less equal access than national health services that are free to all at the point of use. Nevertheless, even services that are free at the point of use may systemically fail to provide adequately for patients whose health needs are the greatest (Tudor-Hart, 1971; Marmot, 2010). And, where rights of access are conditional on citizenship, the rights of migrants may be denied (Toebs, 2001; Weaite, 2013; and see Chapter 9, this volume).

Rights of patients

An individual person's right to health implies a correlative duty on others. The duties of private healthcare providers will be defined by contracts and service level agreements. The duties of healthcare professionals will be governed by professional doctrines or codes of conduct (of which the most famous is the Hippocratic Oath). The duties of states are defined in human rights instruments and/or are self-imposed through social legislation. For example, the British National Health Service (NHS), founded in 1948, was established on the basis of legislation that placed a clear duty on the Minister of Health to establish a comprehensive health service for the prevention, diagnosis and treatment of illness; a duty modified in 2012 as the government of the day sought to devolve the administration of a largely state-funded, but increasingly fragmentary and marketised, service to local commissioning bodies (Pollock & Price, 2013). Critics contend that this dilutes the right to health, but even prior to this, the courts had ruled that though NHS patients had rights of access to and a choice of providers, they had never had a direct right to NHS resources (Lenaghan, 1997; Weaite, 2013). We shall see below and again in Chapter 10 that disputes over access to expensive medicines and treatments have been a salient issue throughout the world.

But for now, we are concerned with just what a right to health guaranteed by the state can in practice amount to. Returning for illustrative purposes to the British example, the NHS sets out a charter of patients' rights provided in the NHS Constitution for England (see www.gov.uk/government/publications/the-nhs-constitution-for-england#full-publication-update-history). This does not embody an unequivocal right to health, which arguably would be impracticable for any state. It falls short of a right to demand a specific treatment, but one of the important substantive rights afforded in charters of this nature is the patient's right of informed choice and their right to refuse such treatment as is offered. However, in the case of patients with mental health problems, there is legislation in place in many countries to allow treatment, subject to procedural safeguards, to be administered compulsorily (WHO, 2023). The issue of choice, however, is problematic not only for people whose ability to exercise choice may be impaired through mental health problems but for all human beings when they may be suffering from illness because of fundamental disparities of power between patients and healthcare professionals. The fiercest critics of such disparities complain of the risks of iatrogenic medicine; practices that may worsen rather than improve health (e.g. Illich et al., 1977). Critically important to the individual right to health is just who is entrusted with the duty to meet that right and on what terms.

Rationing healthcare

As already indicated, there can seldom in practice be a right of unqualified access to particular drugs or medical treatments. The resources necessary for healthcare are likely to be rationed because, on the one hand, resources may be scarce, while on the other, demand for healthcare can accelerate as a result of population ageing (Grover, 2011) and the multiplication of 'technical needs' generated by scientific discovery and new medical treatments (Forder, 1974). The right to medical intervention may therefore be made conditional, for example, on a prediction of a person's 'quality adjusted life years' (QALYs – a system controversially developed in Oregon, USA) or on generic guidance issued on the basis of an official cost-benefit analysis of different drugs and medical procedures. More generally, there are questions about whether public funds should be allocated to treat potentially avoidable illnesses, such as obesity or diseases attributable to tobacco or excessive alcohol consumption; or to provide fertility treatment, cosmetic surgery or other arguably non-essential procedures that may nevertheless have great significance for those who seek them (Bochel, 2005).

Rights to education

In its broadest sense, education is the process by which human consciousness may be developed. The right to a formal education articulates a number of needs. On the one hand, it gives expression to the basic human need for personal autonomy, though it is necessary here to distinguish between 'thin' and 'thick' understandings of autonomy. Doyal and Gough (1991, p. 67) contend that though 'basic' autonomy of agency may be minimally necessary for human existence, optimal needs satisfaction requires 'critical autonomy' – a level of autonomy that enables a person actively to participate as a fully-fledged social and political actor. On the other hand, a stipulated right to education reflects the need of human society to reproduce itself: to perpetuate skills, knowledge and values. This raises questions as to whether education is more of a social requirement of the individual than a right. With whom should responsibility for that requirement rest? The UDHR requires that

'Education shall be directed to the full development of the human personality and to the strengthening of respect for human rights and fundamental freedoms' (Article 26 [2]). This envisages that the right is concerned in part with the need for autonomy and in part with the need to perpetuate a particular set of values.

Insofar as the right to education is concerned with the human individual's need for autonomy, it has been argued that it is not so much a social right as a foundational right, a precondition for the exercise of civil and political rights (e.g. Nowak, 2001). The capacity to function as a citizen in a democratic-welfare-capitalist society requires a minimum level of literacy and basic knowledge. And to function optimally, it needs a great deal more. A citizen's right to 'decent work' (see Chapter 8, this volume) may very well depend on the education they have received. There is also a sense in which the realisation of cultural rights, which afford a person the right to share in the benefits of scientific and artistic endeavour (see Chapter 3, this volume), are linked with or depend on educational provision. The ICESCR stresses that 'education shall enable all persons to participate effectively in a free society' (Article 13 [1]). It is significant that in 1966 the right to education was incorporated by the Council of Europe, not in the European Social Charter, but in the European Convention of Human Rights, which is primarily concerned with civil and political rights and states that 'No person shall be denied the right to education' (First Protocol, Article 2). This right is cast not as a positive right but in terms of freedom of access to provision that is assumed already to exist; as a declaration of the autonomy that is supposed to define the human subject in the first place: a 'freedom right' (Mehedi, 1999).

Insofar as the right to education is concerned with human society's need to reproduce itself, this will inevitably depend on the form of the society it aims to reproduce. When provision for compulsory elementary schooling was first introduced in England, the declared aim was to underwrite the nation's industrial prosperity and the 'safe working of [its] constitutional system' (Forster, 1870). Education has always had an instrumental function as an investment in what has come to be called 'human capital' (e.g. Giddens, 1998, pp. 47–48) and the means by which children are made ready for the labour market. The development of public educational provision in the global North was regarded as a means to promote national efficiency during the late nineteenth and early twentieth centuries. It was an aim that acquired added momentum following the crisis of the capitalist welfare state in the late twentieth century when there was a renewed utilitarian emphasis on 'vocationalism' (Chitty, 2009). The UDHR, as we have seen, refers to the socially reproductive function of education in rather different terms; it speaks of promoting respect for the noble values expressed in the Declaration itself. There is, inevitably, a fine line to be drawn between promoting respect for particular values and indoctrination. The inter-American 'Protocol of San Salvador' of 1988 (sponsored and adopted primarily by Latin America and not the United States) elaborates on the values which education should promote by including 'respect for ... ideological pluralism', which hints, perhaps, at a challenge to hegemonic liberal-individualist assumptions. However, a very different and morally authoritarian interpretation of the reproductive role of education may be seen in The African Charter on Human and People's Rights, which, in Article 17, having asserted that 'Every individual shall have the right to education', then declares, 'The promotion and protection of morals and traditional values recognized by the community shall be the duty of the State', which hints quite strongly at the possibility that education might serve as a means for behavioural control. The development of state education in the global North – certainly during the early part of the twentieth century – quite explicitly entailed mechanisms for the surveillance of children and the supervision of their physical and moral welfare (Dean, 2000; Donzelot, 1979).

What emerge are four different perspectives on the right to education:

The right to equality of access

Education as a social or 'inter-psychological' process (Vygotsky, 1978) is integral to the human life course, including and especially the processes of informal learning that occur within families during childhood. However, the origins of *formal* education outside the family may be traced to antiquity and the beginnings of human civilisation (Pointer, 1896). Education was implicated in the social divisions and relations of power that were so created, such that formal learning was synonymous with privilege and secular authority, on the one hand, or with religious teaching on the other. Though the Western Enlightenment fomented a spread of learning, education of any substance remained by and large the preserve of the elite. Education for the children of the poor, if it existed, generally amounted to basic instruction provided out of charity or by the Church. This remained the case until it became 'almost a self-evident axiom that the State should require and compel the education, up to a certain standard, of every human being who is born its citizen' (Mill, 1859, p. 175). This realisation, however, did not lead to equality of access.

Expensive private institutions have continued to provide for children of the elite, while the effectiveness of provision in state schools varies in relation, generally, to the socio-economic circumstances of the households from which their students come (Ball, 2008). The current evidence suggests that across OECD countries, the socio-economic background of students and schools continues to have a powerful influence on performance (OECD, 2023). Beyond socio-economic inequalities, there are also issues concerning equality of access for women and girls, for ethnic, religious or linguistic minorities, and for disabled people. Segregated or exclusionary education systems provide conspicuous instances of discrimination and provide an early focus for the criticisms by new social movements (see Chapter 6, this volume). They prompted UNESCO in 1960 to adopt the Convention against Discrimination in Education. Later UN conventions against discrimination (see Table 9.3 in Chapter 9, this volume) were to follow. But inequalities endure. Not only are there still parts of the world where girls are effectively excluded from education (UNESCO, 2013, 2024), but even well-developed education systems may still offer an essentially gendered 'hidden curriculum' (Pascall, 1986/1997: ch. 4). Though systemic racial segregation in schools (for example, in the United States and South Africa) has been ended, effective segregation and educational disadvantage may persist as a result of social exclusionary processes, and the aims and objectives of 'multicultural' education remain controversial (Modood, 2013). Despite demands that children with special educational needs should, so far as possible, be integrated within mainstream educational provision rather than consigned to suboptimal segregated schooling (Warnock, 1978; UNESCO, 1994), progress towards this aim has been uneven. In England, such progress may have been reversed, despite clear evidence of the consequent educational disadvantages for disabled children (Roulstone & Prideaux, 2012, ch. 4; CRAE, 2013: para. 79).

The right to education that is free but compulsory

There is a certain paradox that the right to education is now framed as an enforceable requirement. The moral duty of parents to teach their children or to have them in some manner schooled may once have been policed or supplemented by religious authority, but the encroachment of the state meant that, for it to be compulsory, education had to be free. For households in which subsistence might depend on the labour of children, compulsory schooling imposes a burden to which it is unreasonable or impractical to add by charging school fees. The systematic extension of compulsory education for all children – not only elementary or primary education but in due course secondary education – had already begun in industrialised countries even before the UDHR of 1948 declared that elementary education, at least, should be both free and compulsory (Article 26 [1]). Giving effect to the Declaration, the ICESCR of 1966 (Article 13) clarified that secondary education should also be made 'generally available'; that higher education should be available on the basis of merit or 'capacity'; and that both secondary and higher education should be accessible to all and 'progressively' (i.e. eventually) free.

Internationally, therefore, it is only primary education that is unequivocally a right, though domestic legislation within established welfare states and many emerging economies has extended that right to secondary education, characteristically by imposing an enforceable duty on parents to make arrangements for the education of their children up to a specified age (for overview, see UNESCO, 2011). Arrangements for higher education are highly variable, and in England, for example, free tuition at a higher education level has been withdrawn (Callender, 2010). But, though tuition at primary and (in some countries) secondary levels may be free, education does not necessarily come free of all costs. There are wider issues for all education systems as to whether parents should have to pay for their children to travel to school; for school meals and uniforms; for books, materials and extracurricular activities; or whether there may be undue pressure in some schools upon parents to make 'voluntary' financial contributions; such costs may represent a barrier to educational access (e.g. Smith & Noble, 1995).

The rights of parents

There is some ambiguity as to whom the right to education belongs. In one sense, it is the right of parents to have their children educated. In practice, however, parents' rights are for the most part restricted to 'a prior right to choose the kind of education that shall be given to their children' (UDHR, Article 26 [3]), though the ICESCR makes clear that parents must be at liberty 'to choose for their children schools, other than those established by the public authorities, which conform to such minimum educational standards as may be laid down or approved by the State' (Article 13 [3]). Additionally, both the International Covenant on Civil and Political Rights (Article 18 [4]) and the ICECSR accord parents the right to ensure that the religious and moral education of their children is 'in conformity with their own convictions'. Parental rights of choice may, therefore, enable parents to educate their children independently or privately (subject to regulatory oversight); to send their children to religious schools conforming to minimum educational standards; to choose between single-sex and co-educational schools; to withdraw their children, for example, from any religious or sex education lessons of which they disapprove; and to choose between state schools.

The consequence of this is that it is possible for social segregation or differentiation between schools to occur not by design but through the effects of parental choice and for inequalities between schools to multiply. What is more, parents lacking the resources to pay for private alternatives to state education or the ability to move between neighbourhoods may in practice have limited or no choice as to which school to send their children. Nevertheless, the right of choice between state schools may in some countries be linked to the idea that parents should be encouraged to behave as consumers in a market and that they should have the right to receive published information regarding the performance of the schools between which they must choose. This has been the case, for example, in England, where the introduction of new public management principles was used to drive competition between schools through the production and publication of performance-based league tables, enabling parents to discriminate between schools (Chitty, 2009).

However, though parents may in theory have a right of choice between schools, they generally have no choice but to send their children to school, and they may be liable to prosecution and penalties should they fail to do so and have not made satisfactory alternative arrangements. We shall see (in Chapter 8) that in some parts of the world a right to conditional cash transfers may be provided as an incentive to parents to send their children to school, albeit that this may be withdrawn as a sanction should they fail to comply.

The rights of children

We might suppose that the right to be educated belongs to the child, but we have seen that education up to a certain level is supposedly compulsory and that it is parents, not children, who have the right of choice over the manner of their children's education. As Daniel and Ivatts put it, although education policy is 'in effect ... social policy for children', 'rather than children's needs being placed at the forefront of education policy consideration, a variety of adult concerns and perspectives determine the policy outcomes' (1998, p. 168). Critics of the National Curriculum first introduced to English schools in the 1980s complained that it conformed to a 'factory-farm model of education, in which each child, like a battery hen, is to assimilate as much as possible of the food offered to it' (Kelly, 1994, p. 94). Similar critiques have been advanced in relation to educational systems throughout the world (Friere, 1972). Nevertheless, the UN Convention on the Rights of the Child of 1989 explicitly recognises the right of the child to education (Article 28) and elaborates this broadly in accordance with the principles of the UDHR and ICESCR.

While the notion that children might be regarded as having inalienable rights as autonomous persons is in several respects contentious (for a discussion, see Freeman, 2000) the UNCRC establishes two general principles of particular significance in the context of children's relationships with parents, teachers and educational establishments (not to mention other welfare professionals and institutions): that 'In all actions concerning children, whether undertaken by public or private social welfare institutions ... the best interests of the child shall be a primary consideration' (Article 3); and that a child who is 'capable of forming his or her own views' should be assured 'the right to express those views freely in all matters affecting the child, the views of the child being given due weight in accordance with the age and maturity of the child' (Article 12). In theory, this might give children the right to some say in their education, though in practice the provisions conflict so long as it is adults who are the arbiters of the child's best interests.

Rights to social care

We turn now to social rights that pertain to particularly vulnerable groups in society. Whereas everybody needs the means of subsistence, housing, education and healthcare in the course of their lives, they do not *necessarily* require social intervention to protect them from abuse when they are children, to assist them with physical, mental or intellectual impairments during their life-course, or with frailty during old age. Any of us might very well experience such needs at some stage (especially as we grow older), but they call for forms of care or support that may be specialised and that we might group together using the collective term 'social care'. They are forms of care and support that have been characteristically provided or organised by professional social workers (Glasby, 2022). Insofar as we may speak of rights to social care, such rights were not clearly bestowed either by the legislative frameworks of capitalist welfare states or by the international human rights framework. Though there had been provision for the 'protection' of children, the 'rehabilitation' of disabled persons and the 'welfare' of older people, it is comparatively recently that the specific rights of children, disabled persons and older people have achieved discreet and specific international recognition. And it was only the European Social Charter of 1961 that committed contacting parties 'to promote or provide services which, by using methods of social work, would contribute to the welfare and development of both individuals and groups in the community, and to their adjustment to the social environment' (Article 14 [1]). By and large, therefore, rights to social care had been implicitly inferred from the statutory duties and professional codes of social workers. These are rights that, in a sense, do not fit with the liberal ideal of the autonomous rights-bearing individual because they are rights asserted by or on behalf of persons whose autonomy is or is assumed to be compromised by immaturity, impairment or age and whose claims are rooted in potential or manifest vulnerability. And yet they are social rights precisely because lack of autonomy and vulnerability are in some measure socially constructed. They are artefacts of the ways in which society determines

- the character and effective duration of childhood dependency and when and how responsible adulthood is assumed to begin (Gittens, 1993);
- the social significance and practical implications of physical, mental or intellectual impairment (Oliver, 1990);
- the substantive meaning and lived realities of chronological ageing and the point at which active social engagement is assumed to diminish (Townsend, 1991).

Though they have important issues in common, we shall consider the rights of each vulnerable social group in turn.

Children's rights

We have already touched on the rights of children in relation to education and the significance of the CRC's emphasis on the paramountcy of the best interests of the child (Article 3). It is a principle that sits awkwardly with the idea that children should also be allowed a right to identity (Article 8) and respect for their views (Article 12), but critically, it expresses a right to care and to be cared for. The CRC clarifies the extent to which the social rights proclaimed in the UDHR should apply to children, but it goes further in addressing issues largely glossed over in other major human rights instruments by specifying an explicit duty on the part of state parties to take legislative measures 'to protect the child from all forms of physical or mental violence, injury or abuse, neglect or negligent treatment, maltreatment or exploitation, including sexual abuse, while in the care of parent(s), legal guardian(s) or any other person who has the care of the child' (Article 19 [1]). The significance of this is that it places into a rights-based framework social work practices that had been developing for at least a century. The earliest forms of social work practices in the late nineteenth century in England, for example, had entailed interventions by philanthropic and state bodies who were concerned to rescue the children of the 'perishing classes' while controlling the children of the 'dangerous classes' (Younghusband, 1964). Children and young people at risk were both a worry and a threat – a target not only for care but also discipline. The subsequent development and ethos of professional child protection or 'safeguarding' work have been strongly influenced by contemporary behavioural and social scientific theory and psycho-therapeutic methods (Halmos, 1973; Howe, 2009). But its practical functions are the support and supervision of families in which children are in need or at risk and of children engaged in dangerous or illegal activities; and the provision of alternative care for children deprived of, or who have been removed from, their families.

Children's rights to social care arise when their families may be judged to be dysfunctional. In recent years, the scope of this right has been extended to embrace a particular concern with early childhood care and education programmes, which are believed to enhance children's cognitive development, improve their subsequent educational attainment, economic productivity and prospects for social mobility (Allen, 2011; UNESCO, 2007). This raises complex issues. In much of the global North, there has been pressure to extend early years' childcare so as to facilitate greater labour force participation by mothers, but there remains some controversy regarding the boundary between care and education and just how to define the best interests of the child (Moss, 2005). Also implicit in the linking of early childhood care and education with the aim of enhancing social mobility is a suggestion that it is parental neglect or incompetence rather than the material disadvantage experienced by poorer families that accounts for enduring social inequalities: the best interests of children might better be served through rights to higher living standards (Morabito et al., 2013). Social care, in its literal sense, must be understood in its broadest context.

Disabled persons' rights

Every human being is subject to some degree of vulnerability during childhood, but any human being may also experience vulnerability – sometimes from childhood, sometimes later in life – as a result of a disability associated with a physical or mental impairment or dysfunction. We have already discussed disability and its meaning in Chapter 6, in the context of the critiques of social rights emanating from the disability awareness movement. Disability may be evaluated and understood not as a direct effect of biological impairment or dysfunction but of society's response: as a consequence of the substance, character and adequacy of social care. For so long as disability is regarded as a medical problem, disabled people may be accorded rights:

- to social security – though subject (as we shall see in Chapter 8, this volume) to whether they might be adjudged capable of paid employment;
- to housing – though this may depend on the extent of structural adaptations and personal supervision this might entail;
- to education – though subject, as we have seen, to how their 'special needs' might be accommodated;
- and to healthcare – though this is likely to focus on measures to rehabilitate or 'normalise' the patient (Wolfensberger, 1972).

The UN's adoption in 2006 of the Convention on the Rights of Persons with Disabilities is comparatively recent. It addressed itself to the extent to which the impairments experienced by disabled people 'in interaction with various barriers may hinder their full and effective participation in society on an equal basis with others' (Article 1).

This emphasis accommodates the 'social model' of disability, but the emphasis throughout the document is very much on individual autonomy and choice, independent living and the principle that disabled people should, so far as possible, enjoy equal access to the built environment, the labour market, and to commercial and public services. This rather elides the right to respectful care and a reasonable quality of life for those disabled people with limited agency and extensive needs (Shakespeare, 2006). Article 19 of the Convention expressly endorses the existing drive towards social inclusion and care in the community: the right to 'have access to a range of in-home, residential and other community support services, including personal assistance necessary to support living and inclusion in the community, and to prevent isolation or segregation from the community'. Social workers and other care workers engage increasingly in the organisation and/or delivery of residential or domiciliary care for disabled people within or as near as possible to the community. But critics have long questioned whether care *in* the community can be the same as care *by* the community (Bornat et al., 1993). It is difficult to legislate for 'community' or social care in this last sense. Legislation in Britain, for example, has for some years entitled disabled people (including children with special educational needs) to an assessment and statement of their needs, albeit that the resulting statement does not statutorily oblige social care, health or educational agencies to provide for the needs identified (Balloch & Hill, 2007). The problem, in part, is that social care in its widest sense necessitates a holistic understanding of needs. If public resources are scarce and responsibility is fragmented between separate often relatively specialised agencies, planning and co-ordination are difficult.

Older people's rights

Human beings generally expect or at least hope to grow old. The process has implications for their autonomy and for their health. As with childhood and disability, the experience is shaped by social context, specifically, by customs and expectations relating to 'retirement', to which Townsend once referred as a 'kind of mass redundancy' (1991, p. 6), and with regard to housing and living arrangements. Rising living standards and medical advances mean it is possible for people not only to live longer but also to remain healthy and to live independently for longer than ever before, albeit the extent to which this occurs is highly unequal around the world (WHO, 2008). It remains the case that the need for care arising from disabling degenerative disorders is likely to be at its greatest during the final years of life. Relative frailty during old age entails needs for care and support that may be broadly similar to those of younger disabled people that we have discussed above, and in general, the needs of these two groups ought not to be considered entirely separately. There are, however, particular largely untreatable degenerative illnesses associated (especially but not exclusively) with ageing, such as dementia, in which institutionally drawn boundaries between what constitutes medical healthcare and what constitutes social care become problematic (Gauthier et al., 2021).

The UN has not adopted a Convention on the rights of older people, but as part of an International Plan of Action on Ageing, it did adopt certain 'Principles for Older Persons'. These might be inferred as a statement of rights, and they include a specific set of 'principles' under the heading of 'Care' (see Box 7.1). While acknowledging that family and community care may accord with a society's cultural values, pronouncements as to the freedoms, autonomy and respect that should be accorded to older people set

BOX 7.1 THE RIGHTS OF OLDER PERSONS TO CARE

According to the United Nations Principles for Older Persons, adopted by the General Assembly on 16 December 1991, older persons should:

- benefit from family and community care and protection in accordance with each society's system of cultural values;
- have access to health care to help them maintain or regain the optimum level of physical, mental and emotional well-being and to prevent or delay the onset of illness;
- have access to social and legal services to enhance their autonomy, protection and care;
- be able to utilise appropriate levels of institutional care, providing protection, rehabilitation and social and mental stimulation in a humane and secure environment.
- be able to enjoy human rights and fundamental freedoms when residing in any shelter, care or treatment facility, including full respect for their dignity, beliefs, needs and privacy and for the right to make decisions about their care and the quality of their lives.

certain standards of care, and there is a clear reference to 'appropriate levels' of institutional care. The ability of families in advanced or post-industrial societies to provide sustained and intensive care for frail elderly relatives is much diminished as a result of demographic, economic and cultural factors, and some countries have sought to establish social insurance arrangements to assist with the costs of long-term social care for older people (Peng, 2002; Barr, 2010). More broadly, however, it is particularly in the sphere of social care for frail older people that the right to care as a social good (Daly, 2002) and the distribution and management of that good become contentious. In what circumstances can social care be care that is – as of right – supervised, assisted or even provided by the state?

Rights to shelter

Like nourishment and raiment, shelter is one of the most elemental of human needs. As with food and clothing, 'housing' is a need that will be met in different ways depending on climatic and cultural conditions. Before human beings ever built 'houses', they will have established customs or rights as to how spaces and structures for human habitation should be allocated. The idea of what constitutes a 'home' and a 'household' is entirely socially constructed, but so too is the concept of property. We saw in Chapter 2 how the invention of property and the commodity form shaped modern understandings of rights. The commodification of land has been fundamental to framing the right to housing. But like labour, land cannot be an ordinary commodity. Land, whether initially occupied by settlement or conquest or arbitrarily bestowed as the gift of a ruler or despot, is not only an essential livelihood resource but also, potentially, a source of power and profit. To establish land as private property required a doctrine not of tenure but title: inalienable and exclusive ownership, with protection against expropriation, the foundations for which were laid in the Fifth Amendment to the US Constitution of 1791 and the French Declaration of the Rights of Man of 1789, the substance of which would be encapsulated in 1948 in the UDHR, which provides for the permissive right to own property and not to be arbitrarily deprived thereof (Article 17) (and see Jacobs, 2013). This does not confer a right to housing, but it does furnish the terms on which people may or may not establish the tenure of their homes: as owners, as lessees or tenants, as licensees, or as bare occupants or trespassers. The rights that flow from this – where they exist – are civil, not social rights.

At the same time as land – and thereby the housing on which it stands – was turned into a commodity, so the way in which human beings house themselves began to change. Industrialisation depended on the mobility of labour, and this was facilitated as freedom of movement was afforded to agricultural workers who had in previous eras been tied to the land. In 1800, barely 2 per cent of the world's population lived in cities. By 2000, three quarters of the 'developed' world's population and nearly half of all humanity were urban dwellers (UN-HABITAT, 2003). The rapid urbanisation associated with economic development necessitates local governmental intervention to secure the supply of housing and urban infrastructure and to prevent or control the emergence of the 'slums', 'shanty towns' or *favelas* in which the poorest urban inhabitants are likely to find housing. This is the context in which rights to or in relation to housing, as substantive social rights, have emerged. Broadly speaking, such rights fall into four categories:

Consumption subsidies

As will be seen in Chapter 8, of this volume, social security or income maintenance provision can be extended explicitly to enable citizens to pay for housing. This may take a variety of forms: as supplements to means-tested social assistance or as separate social assistance-based housing benefit schemes. Such provision, axiomatically, is specifically targeted to low-income households: to provide public-sector tenants with rent rebates; to support private or voluntary-sector tenants with the payment of rent; to assist homeowners with mortgage interest payments. Such assistance is likely to be conditional not only on a test of means (with all the implications discussed in Chapter 8) but on a variety of other factors. Assistance may be withheld or reduced depending on the age and status of applicants; whether there are members of applicants' households (such as adult sons and daughters) who can be called upon to contribute to housing costs; whether applicants' housing costs are deemed to be excessive, or their accommodation is deemed to be larger than they require. In Britain, attempts to limit the eligibility of low-income households for assistance in high housing cost areas and of public sector housing tenants with 'spare bedrooms' resulted in the displacement of tenants and a condemnatory report by the UN's Special Rapporteur on Housing (Rolnik, 2013). Alternatively, fiscal benefits may be made available to homeowners in the form of tax relief, though this is likely indiscriminately to benefit higher income groups; a practice that in Britain, for example, was discontinued in 2000.

Controls over landlords

The history of measures against forcible eviction can in England be traced back to the fourteenth century, when the concern was to prevent summary dispossession. In more recent times, landlord and tenant law has developed – both through common law and statute – to maintain principles that protect legitimate tenants and homeowners from eviction without due process, though protection for illegal occupants or 'squatters' may be limited. There is insufficient space in this chapter to address the Byzantine complexities of landlord and tenant law in jurisdictions around the world, but it is possible for governments by way of legislation:

- to impose certain minimum obligations upon landlords as implied covenants – for quiet enjoyment and the conduct of repairs – in any or every tenancy agreement;
- to define categories of residential tenancy with specific terms as to security of tenure;
- to supplement remedies available in civil law by the creation of criminal sanctions for illegal eviction or harassment;
- to regulate the rents that landlords may charge (e.g. McQueen, 2022).

By and large, however, such legislation does not create social rights, so much as support or supplement them through modifications to civil rights.

Environmental protection

The process of urbanisation has provoked governmental concerns with a wide range of spatial governance activities (UN-HABITAT, 2003), including public health controls on the one hand and strategic and regulatory planning on the other. Public health intervention evolved in industrialised countries when, in the nineteenth century, overcrowded and insanitary conditions in growing metropolises and conurbations threatened the health of rich and poor alike. Formal processes of urban planning emerged when the unsustainable consequences of unregulated development and land use became self-evident. The resulting interventions, including slum clearance schemes past and present, may indeed promote social rights by raising general living standards, but they do not directly bestow social rights. And, for example, where slum clearances lead to enforced evictions, they may even violate rights (as in the celebrated case of Irene Grootboom before the Constitutional Court of South Africa in the 1990s) (see Liebenberg, 2008; and Chapter 8, this volume). However, public or environmental health legislation may directly benefit people living in sub-standard conditions when it includes, for example, the imposition of fitness for habitation and overcrowding standards on landlords, especially when rights of the complaint are extended to tenants, or provision for home improvement grants for homeowners on low incomes (e.g. Stewart & Lynch, 2018).

Social or public sector housing

Governments can fulfil the right to housing through direct provision. Practices among established welfare states over time have varied enormously. There are some fundamental issues: whether social housing is to be provided to meet general needs or whether it is a form of residual and potentially stigmatised housing tenure reserved for poor and vulnerable people; whether rents chargeable for social housing should be market rents or whether they should be subsidised; whether and how access to social housing should be rationed; whether people should 'qualify' for social housing on the basis of the length of time they have been waiting to be housed, or the nature and strength of their connections to the locality in which they are seeking to be housed, or simply the urgency of their need? Some welfare states have legislated for the right of homeless persons to be housed (Fitzpatrick & Stephens, 2007), though definitions of 'homelessness' differ and there are no instances in which citizens enjoy an unconditional right to housing. In the British case, for example, the right has long been restricted to households with children or who are vulnerable and who can establish that their homelessness is genuine and unintentional (e.g. Burrows et al., 1997). A country's decision or self-imposed duty to provide housing may be met by funding voluntary housing bodies to provide suitable accommodation, but it is to be expected that social sector housing – whether provided by a public or a voluntary sector body – will be let subject to a tenancy that affords similar rights and protections to those afforded to private sector tenants.

8

RIGHTS TO LIVELIHOOD

If one considers the fundamental human needs that may be translated into rights, one might start from the idea of a right not merely to life but to livelihood and to the *means* of achieving human personhood. Human beings interact symbiotically with Nature in order to satisfy their needs. The basis of humanity's 'species-being' has been conceptualised as a process of social-ecological metabolism – a consciously organised 'exchange of matter between Man and Nature' [*stoffvechsel*] (Marx, 1887). Human beings lay claim to natural resources in order to survive and flourish. It has already been argued in this book that in the earliest forms of human society, what we now identify as social rights would, in effect, have been constituted through the customary expectations and practices by which human beings self-consciously engaged with Nature and, in the process, with one another. The 'work' human beings do and their essential sociality are all of a piece, though the relationship between these facets of our humanity and the ways in which it is understood has become more complex.

In a bid to theorise the causes of famine, Sen (1981, p. 2) has suggested that there are four categories of 'entitlement' to food (and here he is talking not about rights but effective command over resources): production-based entitlement, own-labour entitlement, transfer entitlement or trade-based entitlement. In other words, we can *work* in order to feed ourselves from Nature by growing food or earning it in kind, and/or we can *subsist* by receiving gifts of food in kind (from family, community, charity or the state) or by buying food (if we have the means, which may be obtained through paid labour or through transfers). Development theorists have since introduced the concept of 'sustainable livelihoods' to define the processes by which people mobilise resources – natural, human, financial, physical and social – in order

DOI: 10.4324/9781003451518-10

to sustain themselves from generation to generation (Chambers & Conway, 1992). There has been a proliferation of alternative approaches to analysing 'livelihood frameworks', encompassing the diverse ways in which such frameworks may be culturally as well as materially constituted (see Gough et al., 2004). But for the purposes of reflecting on *rights* to livelihood, we shall for the moment focus on those rights that are premised on needs-based claims in relation to work on the one hand and subsistence on the other. Human personhood is achieved through a person's practical doings and material well-being; a person's '*work*' (broadly understood in the terms outlined in Chapter 1 of this volume) and their level of *subsistence*, accepting that the latter may directly or indirectly depend on the former. But both may be considered in the context of human sociality and the part played by social rights as collectively mediated (and partial) guarantees in relation to work and/or subsistence.

The right to work

If we are to regard work as purposeful and constructive human activity – as socially engaged metabolism with Nature – it amounts to more than just paid labour. It includes unpaid care work, domestic labour and voluntary work; community, political and religious activism; studying; and all kinds of artistic and creative pursuits. Even recreational activities or 'amateur' pursuits, necessary to human well-being, may entail effort, training and the application of skill. Work is what people *do*, and, insofar as we *need* to work in order to be fully human, we may argue for a right to work. In practice, however, the rights we shall now discuss relate narrowly to rights to, or in, paid labour. We shall first discuss such rights as are defined under the human rights framework before turning to the ways in which rights relating to work tend to be constituted within nation-states when defined as rights of citizenship.

International labour rights

As will be seen in Chapter 9 of this volume, the International Labour Organisation (ILO), which sets international labour standards through Conventions and Recommendations, was originally founded after the end of the First World War as an agency of the League of Nations. Its constitution (1919: Preface) did not speak of rights but of the extent to which world peace could be imperilled by social injustice and, specifically, by unjust conditions of labour. Towards the end of the Second World War, the ILO's Declaration of Philadelphia (1944) explicitly situated the aims of the organisation within a human rights context while also declaring controversially that 'labour is not a commodity' (Article I [a]).

The context for the post-Second World War human rights agenda had been set not so much with the aim of de-commodifying labour as by principles fostered in the course of the preceding century by the international campaign for the abolition of slavery and the prohibition of *forced* labour (Drescher, 2009), a campaign that had culminated in the League of Nations' Slavery Convention of 1926. The primary emphasis within much of the subsequent international human rights agenda has been on the principle that 'work' should be freely chosen and justly remunerated.

- The UDHR declares that 'Everyone has the right to work, to free choice of employment, to just and favourable conditions of work and to protection against unemployment' (Article 23[1]).
- The ICESCR 'acknowledges' the right of everyone to the opportunity to gain their living by work, which they freely choose or accept (Article 6) but also (under Article 7) to 'fair wages' (including equal pay for equal work as between men and women) and a 'decent living', safe working conditions, equal opportunities for promotion at work and (reiterating UDHR Article 24) reasonable working hours and paid holidays.
- The Council of Europe's Social Charter of 1961 (revised 1996) provides for a person's right to earn their living in an occupation freely entered upon, but more generally to the benefits of economic and social policies designed, inter alia, to ensure full employment (but also, for example, vocational training and free employment services). Additionally, in the European context, the European Union's Charter of Fundamental Rights of 2007 provides more cautiously for 'the right to engage in work and to pursue a freely chosen or accepted occupation' and 'the freedom to seek employment [and] to work'.
- The American Convention on Human Rights of 1969 (to which most Latin American nations are a party but which the United States never fully ratified) includes provision for freedom from slavery (Article 6) and a provision (Article 26) for the progressive development of economic, social, educational and cultural standards set out in the Charter of the Organization of American States of 1948 (as amended in 1967), which refers in general terms to 'Fair wages, employment opportunities and acceptable working conditions for all' (Article 34 [g]). The Additional Protocol of San Salvador to the American Convention (not signed by the US) includes ambitious and detailed provisions (under Article 7) for 'Just, Equitable and Satisfactory Conditions of Work', including the abolition of night work and the right of every worker to follow their vocation.
- The African Charter on Human and People's Rights of 1981 states simply that 'Every individual shall have the right to work under equitable and satisfactory conditions and shall receive equal pay for equal work' (Article 15).

Of course, the implementation of human rights may not be fully realised at the domestic level. But in any event, it appears there is no unequivocal obligation on state parties under any of the above instruments actually to provide a citizen with a job. While the right to work is established as a human right, its availability as a right of citizenship may not necessarily or unequivocally be guaranteed. And even in developed welfare states, some have been more willing than others to protect citizens by mitigating the potentially or inherently exploitative character of wage labour through, for example, intervention to regulate wages and the terms and conditions of employment.

National labour rights

Mention was made in Chapter 6 (this volume) of Claus Offe's argument that in industrial capitalist societies, people became wage labourers as citizens of a state. The terms on which they sell their labour power and the conditions under which they are supposedly free to do so can be shaped in part by social legislation. But ultimately, they will be governed by market forces. Though citizens are supposedly free to sell their labour, Polanyi (1944, p. 6) has suggested that because labour cannot be separated from the person who labours, labour should be regarded as a 'fictitious' commodity. By the same token, we might regard the right to labour (as opposed to a right to work in its broader sense) as a fictitious right. We shall see in Chapter 9 that jobs were, after a fashion, guaranteed under Soviet communism, but the availability of employment in the context of a capitalist market economy is subject ultimately to market forces.

Macroeconomic and local development policies may aim to create jobs, but employment for all cannot necessarily be guaranteed unless governments themselves are prepared to act as employers of last resort (Sawyer, 2003). Relatively high levels of public sector employment have in the past assisted Social Democratic welfare states to maintain near full employment, but insofar as such states had also relied on the fiscal, active labour market and wage policy to maintain full employment, this would have been an incidental effect (Kananen, 2014). Counter-recessionary public works programmes, such as those in the US following the global financial crisis of 2008–2011 under the so-called Obama Jobs Act and following the COVID crisis of 2020–2023, Biden's Inflation Reduction Act, have never guaranteed jobs for all. There has been an attempt in India to introduce a National Rural Employment Guarantee Scheme: a programme that offers up to 100 days of unskilled manual labour per year on public works projects for any rural household member who wants such work at a stipulated minimum wage rate. Initial implementation of the scheme was partial and selective, and there remains considerable unmet employment demand in all parts of the country (Dutta et al., 2012).

If work equates with paid employment, a right to work under capitalism will remain elusive. Welfare states provide rights to social security protection for workers, and these we shall consider in the next section of this chapter. However, welfare states have developed a significant array of rights *at* work for citizens who are in employment. It is to these that we shall now briefly turn. Though it may be difficult or impossible to ensure a right to work, it is arguably reasonable to demand a right to 'decent' work, which was the aim of the campaign mounted by the ILO (1999).

The first thing to be said about the rights of citizens who are in employment is that their employment is governed in law by a contract with their employers, whether that be written or implied. The employees' rights are primarily civil rights, not social rights. Workers have the freedom and a right – in theory – to negotiate the terms of their contracts of employment, though the disparity of power between workers and employers may make this practically impossible. Through social legislation, however, policymakers can impose certain terms and conditions on such contractual arrangements. And in a democracy, workers can – in theory, once again – exercise their political rights in an attempt to influence policymakers, though bringing influence to bear on the policy-making process can be difficult.

There is a variety of possible employment protection or social regulation measures, some of which are expressly required of those states parties that have ratified human rights treaties or the Conventions of the ILO, though some of these measures evolved over time in advance, or independently, of international human rights frameworks. These are some of the more important forms of regulatory intervention that give rise to rights at work:

- *Minimum wage* regulation may be applied on a nationwide basis or selectively in different regions and/or in different employment sectors within a country. Over 190 countries worldwide claim to fix minimum wages (ILO, 2022). The rates set and methods of enforcement are highly variable. In some countries, such as Brazil, the level of the national minimum wage is used as a benchmark for fixing a range of other social entitlements. Countries that don't have minimum wages, including the Nordic countries, consider that to do so would undermine the principle of free wage bargaining. Britain abandoned a fragmentary system of wage regulation in the 1980s, only to re-instate a modest national minimum wage in 1999. Neo-liberal opponents of minimum wages assert that they increase unemployment, a claim that was shown to be largely unproven (Coates, 2007).
- The regulation of *working hours* became a concern of policymakers in the first industrialised countries during the first half of the nineteenth century, as factory-based production systems began to develop (e.g. Fraser, 2017), culminating in Britain in 1844 with a restriction in the working hours of

women and children to 10 hours a day. The very first ILO Convention in 1919 established the principle of 8 hours a day and 48 hours a week, and the UDHR in 1948 specifically demanded the 'reasonable limitation of working hours' (Article 24). Working hours legislation has been identified in over 100 countries worldwide, with a trend towards a dominant, but by no means universal, standard of 40 hours per week (Lee et al., 2007), albeit that actual working hours vary considerably. The European Union Working Time Directive provides for a maximum 48-hour week, from which certain professions may be excluded and individual employees may opt out, though France, for example, has legislated for a 35-hour week. Working hours regulations may include provisions for rest periods, holiday entitlements and night work restrictions.

- Occupational *health and safety* standards similarly developed because of concerns about the hazards associated with industrial production methods, which resulted, for example, during the second half of the nineteenth century in Britain in a series of Factories Acts and legislation relating to safety measures and compensation for workplace injury. The right to safe and healthy working conditions was included in the ICESCR (Article 7 [b]), and, as with the regulation of working hours, ILO Conventions and EU Directives have evolved. Legislation and systems of enforcement have been instituted in more than 120 countries worldwide (ILO, 2009). Such systems generally provide for inspection regimes with penalties against employers for non-compliance, rather than specifically defined rights for workers, other than regulated rights to civil compensation after the event for industrial injuries or diseases.
- Protection against arbitrary or *unfair dismissal* is something that developed more recently. The relevant legislation was first introduced in Britain in 1971, and the ILO later agreed to a Convention in 1982 (developed from a prior recommendation in 1974). Some forms of regulation relating to the termination of employment were subsequently identified in more than 100 countries (ILO, 1995). The right not to be unfairly or unjustifiably dismissed is to be distinguished from the civil right not to be wrongfully dismissed insofar as it is a right established by legislation which specifies the grounds on which a dismissal can be fair or justifiable. These characteristically include grounds associated with the worker's capability or conduct or because of redundancy (where the worker's job has ceased to exist), in which case there is a provision in some countries for statutory redundancy compensation.
- Rights to equal opportunity or *non-discrimination* have their origins in the UDHR, which declared that everyone has the right 'without any discrimination, to equal pay for equal work' (Article 23 [2]), explicitly interpreted in the ICESCR as discrimination on the grounds of sex, albeit that the right was extended by the International Convention on the Elimination of

All Forms of Racial Discrimination of 1965 and subsequently, the Convention on the Rights of Persons with Disabilities of 2006 (Article 27). The ILO's Discrimination (Employment and Occupation) Convention of 1958 had defined discrimination as including 'any distinction, exclusion or preference made on the basis of race, colour, sex, religion, political opinion, national extraction or social origin, which has the effect of nullifying or impairing equality of opportunity or treatment' (Article 1 [a]). The convention has been ratified by an unusually high proportion of ILO member states (169 out of 183), and there is evidence that legislative and institutional initiatives continued to develop worldwide (ILO, 2011).

- Initiatives to promote *work-life balance* or work-family reconciliation are ostensibly of more recent provenance. Capitalist welfare states had been initially constructed with the male breadwinner model in mind (see Chapter 5, this volume), but since the 1990s, policymakers in the global North have been driven to facilitate the mutual accommodation of labour markets and household living and earning strategies by introducing extended parental leave schemes, the enhancement of childcare and the promotion of 'family friendly' employment practices (Lewis, 2006). However, the foundations for some such initiatives had in part been laid in the form of maternity leave provision (introduced in several countries in the mid-twentieth century and specifically required by Article 10 of the ICESCR); and, for example, the extension of non-discrimination principles in the European Social Charter (Article 27) and the ILO Convention 156 to Workers with Family Responsibilities.

Of critical relevance to the right to work is the role of trade unions. The right to form and join a trade union stems from the right to freedom of association and might therefore be considered to be as much a political right as a social right. Nevertheless, it is explicitly present both in the UDHR (Article 23 [4]) and the ICESCR (Article 8 [1]), which includes the right to strike, as a component of the right to work. Trade unions have been and are important for their role in negotiating the framing of workers' substantive rights, whether formally (as in corporatist and social democratic welfare regimes) or through lobbying and campaigning activity (as in liberal regimes), and in defending their members' rights, whether collectively or through support provided to individual workers. However, though trade unions remain resilient in some countries, the effects of neoliberal economic globalisation were reflected in a decline in union power and recruitment (Visser, 2006). What is more, despite their importance, trade unions have been subject to criticism for their 'labourist' approach (e.g. Standing, 2009): their adherence to an institutional model of industrial capitalism, favouring protection for labour market insiders, often at the expense of marginalised, precariously employed and informal sector workers. What were once called 'atypical' workers – part-time, temporary, casual or agency workers – who in many instances tended to be legally excluded from the protections outlined above have seldom been represented by trade unions. However, the polarisation and flexibilisation of labour markets around the world (Doogan, 2009) have meant that what was once 'atypical' has become the norm for large numbers of workers, even within the formal economy. Increasingly, those workers with limited skills and qualifications are consigned to low-paid, insecure work with little or no prospect of advancement. As mentioned in Chapter 3, Guy Standing has referred to this emerging class of workers as the 'Precariat'. Though legislators in established welfare states have sought to extend protection to 'atypical' workers, employers have found new devices – zero-hours contracts, bogus self-employment arrangements, etc. – to circumvent protection. And as we shall see in Chapter 9, in many parts of the world, much if not most work is not formalised and enjoys no protection.

The right to subsistence

In discussing rights to livelihood, it is difficult to disentangle work and subsistence. A subsistence farmer may achieve subsistence through their own work but cannot satisfactorily do so in the absence of transactions with other human beings; they are likely to barter or sell some part of their own produce or labour in order to obtain food stuffs, tools or materials they cannot themselves produce. As suggested above, in the absence of any formal legal framework, this might require the implicit development and exercise of what would amount to customary rights. But when it comes to formal rights in the context of a market economy, the relationship between work and subsistence becomes more problematic. If a right to work for wages cannot be guaranteed, to what extent can a right to subsistence be ensured? Once again, we shall first discuss such rights as are defined under the human rights framework before turning to the ways in which rights relating to subsistence tend to be constituted within nation-states when defined as rights of citizenship.

Human rights framework

A general right to subsistence or to an adequate standard of living was established in the following terms by the UDHR:

> Everyone has the right to a standard of living adequate for the health and well-being of himself and of his family, including food, clothing, housing and medical care and necessary social services, and the right to security in the event of unemployment, sickness, disability, widowhood, old age or other lack of livelihood in circumstances beyond his control.
>
> *(Article 25 [1])*

This wide-reaching statement begs a variety of questions, of which the most obvious is whether the right is to be established through the provision of goods in kind or cash. In the case of the right to food, is this a right to a food parcel or to a cash transfer? Insofar as the world faces enduring challenges from hunger and malnutrition, the UN's World Food Programme, established in 1961, has continuing responsibility for international food aid in order to protect livelihoods in emergencies (World Food Programme, 2022). At the national level, there are past examples of a right to food being provided through food stamps in the US (a scheme dating from the 1930s – see Elsinger, 1998; Sen, 1981) or through various experiments with food parcels or food tickets under Brazil's Zero Hunger Programme during the 1990s (da Silva et al., 2005). Supporters of a right to food in kind would argue that it is more redistributive than cash transfers; it can be used to support local agricultural production and to promote adequate nutrition. Opponents complain that it is paternalistic and potentially stigmatising: people should be allowed to choose what they eat, and by and large – with the exception of emergency provision – a right to food for citizens without the means of subsistence is usually met by way of cash transfers.

A right to food may be underwritten by state parties not directly through provision to individual citizens but more generally. The San Salvador Protocol to the American Convention on Human Rights of 1988 sets a high standard for the right to adequate nutrition, insisting it should guarantee 'the possibility of enjoying the highest level of physical, emotional and intellectual development' (Article 12 [1]). But the protocol also suggests that state parties must 'undertake to improve methods of production, supply and distribution of food, and to this end, agree to promote greater international cooperation in support of the relevant national policies' (Article 12 [2]). We see here an example of rhetoric that links social rights to a wider international social development agenda (cf. Chapter 9, this volume).

Article 25 [1] of the UDHR also provides for rights to clothing, housing, medical care and necessary social services. The right to clothing appears to be largely a 'forgotten right' (James, 2008), except in so far as it is indirectly provided for through cash transfers. Housing, medical care and social services have been discussed in Chapter 7, since these may be considered human services as opposed to subsistence goods. These too may be provided in kind – through public sector provision – or their cost to the individual may be met through cash transfer schemes specifically intended to cover rents, fees and charges.

Social security systems

We move therefore to consider the complex realm of cash transfers, or, the term we shall now be using, social security. The term social security is mired in a certain amount of misunderstanding since it can refer to different things in different parts of the world. However, by social security, we are alluding to the UDHR's reference in Article 25 to 'security in the event of unemployment, sickness, disability, widowhood, old age or other lack of livelihood'. Curiously, the provision relating to social security in the ICESCR is startlingly brief. It says only that the state parties 'recognise the rights of everyone to social security, including social insurance' (Article [9]) – a clumsy compromise reflecting unresolved disagreement as to the meaning of social security (Davy, 2013).

Michael Hill (2006, p. 67) has provided what is perhaps the simplest definition of social security: 'collective action to protect individuals against income deficiencies'. Collective action may take a variety of forms: social assistance funded through general taxation; social insurance funded through specific contributions; universal social allowance schemes; tax allowances; or the public regulation of private provision. We shall be considering each in turn. The complexity of social security and the different mechanisms or systems it can entail stem partly from the different contingencies or circumstances in which a right to social security might arise, but partly also from the proviso that the right does not arise other than in circumstances where individuals' lack of livelihood is 'beyond their control'. Rights to social security are, to a greater or lesser extent, conditional.

- Social assistance is the term applied to forms of relief that are conditional on proof of need, usually a test of means. 'Traditional' forms of social assistance have their roots directly in the Poor Laws: forms of poor relief characteristically to be found in Western countries prior to the development of welfare state regimes. The receipt of relief under such schemes had been based not on rights but upon the exercise of administrative discretion. The Poor Laws superseded charitable forms of relief with organised relief, funded from local rates or taxes. Relief was at best judgemental, being reserved only for those deemed to be sufficiently deserving; and at worst punitive, requiring supplicants to submit to incarceration in workhouses, where they were subject to conditions that were deliberately contrived to be worse than those endured by even the poorest independent labourer (e.g. Fraser, 2017). Social assistance schemes under capitalist welfare regimes can vary in terms of the degree of discretion vested in those who administer them, but they are usually framed as a right for the poorest in society and as a social safety net. Subject to conditions, social assistance may be dispensed for the maintenance of persons and the households of such persons where the household has no or insufficient income from any other source. It is a characteristic feature of 'liberal' welfare regimes (to be discussed in Chapter 9), though usually not as the only form of social security provision (the exceptions here being Australia and New Zealand).

The advantage of social assistance is that it can target assistance where it appears to be most needed. Its disadvantages are that it can stigmatise those who receive it (because they are identified by their poverty); it is inevitably complex to administer (because the household circumstances of every recipient must be assessed); and because it can create perverse incentives (since relief is withdrawn should recipients receive other income from earnings or savings). In the US, social assistance is not thought of as a form of social security but as 'welfare' – a term that has acquired distinctly pejorative associations, wholly distinct from social insurance. But in Australia and New Zealand, where means-tested benefits are the mainstay of social security, they attract less stigma.

Social assistance programmes have emerged in the global South: the *dibao* system in China (Yan, 2014); and the Child Support Grant in South Africa (Lund, 2008). But the most prominent have been 'new' forms of social assistance, known as conditional cash transfers (CCTs) (Bastagli, 2009). These were first developed in Latin America – e.g. *Opportunidades* in Mexico and *Bolsa Familia* in Brazil – but schemes have proliferated elsewhere. Characterised as a form of 'social citizenship for the global poor' (Leisering & Barrientos, 2013), these locally based schemes provide cash incomes to poorer households on condition that mothers report with their younger children to health clinics while older children attend school. The explicit aim was not merely to relieve current poverty but to underwrite investment in human capital so as to ensure higher levels of productivity among future generations. The schemes have generally been popular with recipients, though there have been practical issues relating in some instances to the inaccessibility of health clinics and the poor quality of education available in schools. There is also, potentially, a matter of principle at stake because of the way such schemes make the household's right to subsistence interdependent with their children's rights to healthcare and education. Whereas 'traditional' social assistance, with its roots in the Poor Laws, reflects elements of the survivalist perspective on social rights (see Figure 5.1 in Chapter 5, this volume), the 'new' form of social assistance, which is strongly supported by the World Bank, reflects elements of the utilitarian perspective.

- Social insurance may be remembered as one of the big ideas of the twentieth century. The point made in Chapter 6 of this volume is that social insurance entails a principle that can be embraced from either an individualistic or a solidaristic perspective: the term may encompass a fully funded scheme where individual entitlements are strictly dependent on individual contributions, and which is 'social' only in the sense that it is state administered (or administered as a provident fund on behalf of the government as it was, for example, in Hong Kong); or a scheme where the state itself maintains a fund on behalf of workers from which benefits and pensions are paid, and which is insurance-based only in the sense that everyone has 'assured' protection (though it was only under Soviet communism that any such scheme existed). In practice, contemporary social insurance schemes can represent compromises that sit somewhere between these extremes: they are 'pay-as-you-go' (PAYG) schemes into which workers and employers pay contributions, while the state underwrites the ability of the scheme to meet current liabilities for benefits and pensions. But globally, some have feared that the social insurance principle may be marginalised in favour of social assistance safety nets on the one hand and regulated private insurance schemes on the other hand (e.g. Rys, 2010).

Nevertheless, social insurance against life's risks – including and especially the risks of unemployment; sickness, injury or disability; and old age – continues as a substantial and resilient component of most established social security systems and has been incrementally adopted by some newer ones, including China (Chan et al., 2008). The essence of social insurance is that membership and therefore contributions are compulsory, but that risks are shared. Statutory social insurance arrangements sometimes subsumed voluntary schemes, begun by civil society organisations in the nineteenth century. However, the ranges of risks or contingencies and the populations or employment sectors covered by such insurance vary from country to country. Contributions and benefit rates also vary, and the redistributive effects of such schemes will depend on just how such rates are set. The advantage of social insurance schemes is that they provide benefit recipients with a clear sense of entitlement, and they are usually, therefore, popular. Their disadvantage is that they may tend primarily to benefit only certain workers: labour market 'outsiders', especially women, can be excluded. Social insurance schemes characteristically reflect elements of the communitarian perspective on social rights (see Figure 5.1 in Chapter 5, this volume). However, fully funded forms of social insurance reflect elements of the utilitarian perspective, while generous and universally inclusive forms reflect elements of the universalist perspective.

- Universal social security schemes, sometimes called 'social allowances', are universal in the sense that they are non-means-tested and non-contributory. In practice, schemes are not so much universal as 'categorical': they are benefits payable in some welfare states to or for particular demographic groups or categories, including:

    ◊ Children or families with children. The right to social security for children (specifically re-stated in the UN's Convention on the Rights of the Child) can be realised through social assistance provision to the low-income households in which children reside or through child additions to social insurance benefits payable to parents. Alternatively or additionally, however, provision can be made through universal family allowances or child benefits payable to all households with children.

- ◊ Disabled people and carers. People who become disabled in the course of their working lives may have previously 'earned' an entitlement to benefits under social insurance schemes, and those who have been disabled from birth or since childhood may be entitled to relief under social assistance schemes. Additionally, however, social security provision may be made by way of universal benefits, intended to compensate not for lack of earnings but for the additional living costs experienced by a disabled person. Entitlement, however, will be subject to medical assessment criteria. Universal social security may also be instituted for people who provide full-time unpaid care for a disabled relative.
- ◊ Older people. For people above a specified retirement age, social assistance schemes may provide a safety net or else social insurance schemes may pay retirement pensions. However, it is also possible for governments to provide a universal state-funded retirement pension to all older citizens.

There has been long-standing debate around the idea of a fully universal Basic Income, Social Dividend or Citizen's Income (Fitzpatrick, 1999; Torry, 2018), and limited experiments with such ideas have been attempted in Namibia (Haarmann et al., 2009) and India (Standing, 2013). The advantages of universal benefits schemes are that they are simple to administer (since they involve no means-testing or contributions) and they are symbolically highly solidaristic. The perceived disadvantages are that unless benefits are set at a low level, the levels of progressive taxation required to pay them would be high and that people with high incomes would pay high taxes while receiving a benefit they do not need. Depending on *exactly* how they are designed and implemented, universal benefits schemes can appeal either to a universalist or a utilitarian perspective on social rights (see Figure 5.1 in Chapter 5, this volume): in theory, at least, they can help to underpin either a substantively or a formally egalitarian society.

Richard Titmuss (1958) coined the terms 'fiscal welfare' and 'occupational welfare' to refer to systems that run in parallel with the kind of social security systems outlined above. By fiscal welfare, he was referring to systems of tax allowances or tax credits that can be of benefit to people who already have taxable incomes. And by occupational welfare, he was referring to the panoply of perks and benefits that can be made available by employers to their employees. Titmuss' particular concern was that such systems were more likely to be of benefit to individuals and households with higher incomes and better opportunities, and it was important that state administered social security should not be reserved primarily for the poorest or least advantaged in society. Nevertheless, fiscal and occupational welfare have played a part in providing social security. Of particular importance in many countries has been the development not only of occupational pension schemes operated by employers but also the range of private savings schemes and financial products that governments can both actively promote and regulate with a view to ensuring optimal security for older citizens. The World Bank (1994; and see Holzmann & Hinz, 2005) recommended that all countries should establish pension systems based on three 'pillars':

- first pillar: a guaranteed, publicly funded minimum safety net; whether means-tested, flat-rate social insurance-based or universal. (Possibly, an earnings-related social insurance scheme might provide for an intermediate 'pillar' above the first pillar and the next one.)
- second pillar: a mandatory savings scheme, either an occupational or a personal pension plan, subject to government regulation.
- third pillar: voluntary additional private insurance or savings. (Arguably, informal intra-family or inter-generational transfers represent a final 'pillar'.)

The right to social security may be interpreted as a right to secure subsistence across the life course, but its most problematic aspect relates to its intersection with the right to work.

The subsistence rights of workers

We have seen that the UDHR provides a right to social security for individuals and their families in the event of unemployment. It additionally provides that 'Everyone who works has the right to just and favourable remuneration ensuring for himself and his family an existence worthy of human dignity, and supplemented, if necessary, by other means of social protection' (Article 23 [3]). The prevailing assumption is that human beings will normally sustain themselves within families and through paid employment, but if they cannot, they should have a claim upon the state for protection. It is not said, but perhaps implied, that it is a person's reciprocal responsibility to sustain themselves in such a manner. The bearer of rights is primarily constituted as a potential wage labourer who, during their adulthood, should work to sustain themselves, their children and, as needed, their spouse or adult partner. In the two preceding sentences, I have deliberately used the plural/gender-neutral possessive pronoun, though the instruments by which rights are declared or instituted have classically been framed using the male possessive pronoun; in the minds of those who framed such instruments, the bearer of rights would have been envisaged primarily as male (e.g. Lister, 2003). The foundational assumptions upon which such rights had been framed have long since been challenged by such trends as the increase in women's labour market participation and, in the global North, the changing dynamics of family life. These trends have cast new light on how the rights of men and women, as workers and carers, breadwinners and homemakers, may be interpreted.

The normative ambiguity of the social rights agenda was exposed in other ways by the critical backlash that began in the 1970s (see Chapter 6, this volume): in particular, a hardening neo-liberal consensus among the capitalist welfare states of the global North that the responsibilities of citizens-as-workers should be more explicit. The mantra that achieved a virtual consensus by the turn of the Millennium was that there should be 'no rights without responsibilities' (Giddens, 1998, p. 65). In the global South, meanwhile, the fragmentary nature of formal labour markets and state administration meant that the nexus of rights and responsibilities within families and in relation to work were differently understood (Gough & McGregor, 2007; and see Chapter 9, later in this volume). Nevertheless, welfare programmes developing in some emerging economies – for example, South Korea's Self Sufficiency Programme (Jo & Walker, 2014; Kim, 2011) – demonstrate clear similarities with trends in the global North.

This section of the chapter will focus on transitions that have occurred in the welfare states of the global North: transitions variously described in terms of a transition from passive to 'active' welfare states (Esping-Andersen, 2002), from welfare states to 'workfare' states (Jessop, 2002), from protective to 'enabling' state models (Gilbert, 2004). It is important, however, to note firstly that such transitions often entailed changes of emphasis rather than substance; secondly, that some of the principles informing such transitions can already be seen to be informing developments in emerging economies. The fundamental issues for welfare states, whether established or incipient, are: how to make workers work; how to make work pay; and how to make workers' families self-sustaining.

Labour market activation

There has undoubtedly been an increase in the degree of conditionality attaching to the receipt of benefits or cash transfers for welfare state citizens of working age (Dwyer, 2004). Conditionality, however, is nothing new. Since unemployment benefits were first introduced in industrialised countries around or even before the early part of the twentieth century, the right to benefit was invariably conditional. In the British case, benefit could be withheld if the claimant had become unemployed voluntarily or through misconduct, and entitlement was in any event conditional on the claimant's continued availability for work (Gilbert, 1966). The subsequent evolution of social security for unemployed people – or 'job-seekers' as they came to be known in the 1990s – entailed a relentless tightening of rules, procedures and sanctions intended to encourage, assist or compel people to engage or re-engage with the labour market (Lødemel & Trickey, 2000). The trend was consistent with a shift from Keynesian macro-economic orthodoxies to supply-side economic measures, whereby governments sought to attract private investment by maximising labour market participation and 'driving up' the skills and motivation of their domestic labour force.

The initial impetus towards 'welfare-to-work' schemes has been associated with developments in the US (Mead, 1997), but such provisions rapidly spread to Britain and other welfare states (Peck, 2001). However, there were significant variations in the approach taken (see Dean, 2007 and Box 8.1).

BOX 8.1 VARIETIES OF WORKFARE[a]

Work-first. Policies that seek to move unemployed people rapidly into available employment, however low-paid or insecure, on the premise that any job is better than no job and may provide a stepping stone to a better job. Characteristically, claimants will have benefits immediately withdrawn if they refuse a job offer. The approach is consistent with a survivalist perspective on social rights (see Figure 5.1).

Human capital. Policies focused directly on the labour market supply side that emphasise the need for skills training and making people job-ready. Characteristically, claimants will be allowed time to engage with the labour market, though claimants may have benefits withdrawn if they refuse appropriate training or work experience or if they fail to co-operate with employment services staff. The approach is consistent with a utilitarian perspective on social rights.

Insertion. Policies that seek to 'insert' marginalised or hard-to-place workers into the labour market, often in temporary jobs, with minimum coercion on the one hand and taking care not to disrupt existing labour relations on the other. The approach is consistent with a communitarian perspective on social rights.

Flexicurity. Policies that seek to adapt social security provision to a flexible labour market by coupling relatively generous short-term social protection measures for unemployed people with supportive labour market activation measures on the one hand and policies to promote life-long learning and work-family reconciliation measures on the other. The approach is consistent with a universalist perspective on social rights.

[a] **NOTE:** This is a heuristic taxonomy. Models can overlap, and actual workfare regimes generally combine elements of more than one model. For these reasons, the terms used above may be used in slightly different ways in different contexts.

Part and parcel with labour market activation measures have been policies to 'make work pay'. Such measures are not wholly new. In England, towards the end of the eighteenth century, at a time when the Poor Laws were less draconian than they would later become, a system of relief known as the Speenhamland system (after the name of the parish in which it was first instituted), was introduced in parts of the country where agricultural wages had fallen beneath subsistence level. Under the Speenhamland system, local Justices supplemented workers' wages from the Poor Rates (de Schweinitz, 1961). The system was later abolished, but since the 1970s, a number of countries have introduced a variety of means-tested wage top-up or tax credit schemes in order to sustain the functioning of low-wage economies (Dean, 2012b), sometimes as an alternative, but often in addition, to minimum wage regulation. Though framed as a right of low-paid workers, such schemes function in effect as an indirect subsidy to their employers. The rationale, however, is that supplementing low wages in this way provides an incentive for citizens to engage with the labour market while enabling employers to employ them on wages beneath subsistence level.

Labour market activation has not only been intensifying but also extending to new groups of citizens, including lone parents and disabled people. Each group in its own way has been problematic for the capitalist welfare state. Lone-parent households, which tend to be female-headed, are hardly a new phenomenon: in any era and community in which average male life expectancy is relatively low, the numbers of widowed mothers are likely to be relatively high. Such circumstances applied prior to and during the early part of the Industrial Revolution (and still apply in some parts of the world today). But despite increased longevity associated with rising living standards, greater diversity and fluidity in patterns of family formation were associated in the last part of the twentieth century with an unexpected growth in the incidence of different kinds of lone parenthood throughout the global North (Lewis, 2001). As divorced, separated and never-partnered lone parents with the care of dependent children became a major component of social assistance caseloads, attempts were made to encourage, assist or coerce them into the labour market by incorporating them into the various kinds of the scheme outlined in Box 8.1 while simultaneously seeking ways to provide or to subsidise childcare provision to enable them to do so (Knijn et al., 2007). Practice between countries varies as to how soon after the birth of their youngest child a lone parent (or, for that matter, any non-working parent in a household supported by social assistance) should be expected or required to substitute the unpaid work of full-time parental childcare for paid employment.

Disabled people, similarly, would once have been a more or less accepted part of any human community, though in the early part of the modern industrial era there had been a trend towards the development of institutional care for disabled people, on the premise that they were a burden if not a threat to the productivity of the labour force (Slorach, 2016). But following the formation of modern capitalist welfare states, there had been a new trend – driven in part by the disability awareness movement (see Chapter 6, this volume) – towards greater integration of disabled people in society. However, growing concern in recent decades about the numbers of long-term sick and disabled people in receipt of social security benefits has driven some capitalist welfare states to tighten eligibility tests for such benefits and/or to evaluate disabled people's capacity for work with a view to incorporating them into the kinds of scheme outlined in Box 8.1 (e.g. Roulstone & Barnes, 2005).

Enforcing family responsibilities

The other prevailing assumption implied in the way that rights to social security are framed is that workers are responsible for maintaining their families. In most jurisdictions there is legal liability established by statute whereby parents may be held *financially* responsible for dependent children, spouses are held responsible for each other, and, in some instances, adult children may be held responsible for their aged parents. Whether statutorily defined intrafamilial liabilities give rise to intrafamilial rights is a moot point. The evidence suggests that attempts by legislators to interfere with the complex ways in which responsibilities within families are negotiated can be ineffectual at best and counterproductive at worst (Finch, 1989). The moral rationality of, for example, those parents who see virtue in caring for their children rather than working for wages is at odds with the utilitarian logic of the prevailing policy environment. Welfare state societies have been experiencing changes in cultural expectations with regard to what people seek in familial and intimate relationships (Beck & Beck-Gernsheim, 1995). Nevertheless, there are certain instances in which it is through conditions imposed on a working-age citizen's right to social assistance that the state may seek to impose its interpretation of where material responsibilities lie.

The first of these arises in the administration of household means tests conducted for the purposes of assessing social assistance entitlement. These characteristically assume that all members of a cohabiting household unit will maintain one another. In calculating a household's entitlement, the account is taken of every household member's resources (including savings and income from part-time employment, child maintenance, pensions and other social security benefits). The assumption applies not only to adults' responsibilities to child dependents within a household but to mutual responsibility between adults, whether they are married, in a civil partnership or cohabiting *as if* they were in such a relationship. The implication, when this arises, is that adults in a conjugal relationship are required to be financially interdependent, whether or not they are so in reality, or would choose to be

(McLaughlin, 1999; Tranter et al., 2008). The consequence of this constraint on citizens' rights to social assistance is that they might lose their right to benefit upon entering a cohabiting relationship. In Britain, when concern about the rising numbers of lone parents in receipt of social assistance began to surface in the 1960s and 1970s considerable administrative effort was invested into the intrusive investigation of lone parent claimants suspected of cohabiting relationships (Fairbairns, 1985; Dean, 1991).

The second instance relates to the provision by absent parents for the financial support of their children. In Britain this was a matter of perennial concern to parish authorities during the Poor Law era but in more recent times such matters had been regarded as private matters and had been left by and large to the civil courts to administer (Wikeley, 2006). However, where a lone parent with care of a child is in receipt of social assistance, the state has a direct interest in the enforcement of such liabilities so as to limit claims upon the state. Arrangements vary between countries, but in recent decades there have been attempts in several Anglophone countries (including Britain, the US and Australia) to introduce specialised child support schemes specifically intended to enforce the liabilities of what in the US were called 'deadbeat dads': feckless fathers who had walked out on their children (Garfinkel et al., 1998). Though a parent with the care of children could file for support from an absent biological parent, the state itself could also institute action directly against such a parent to recover child support. In Britain at one stage, lone parents in receipt of social assistance could be penalised with a reduction in benefit if they failed to co-operate with the authorities in tracking down an absent parent (Garnham & Knights, 1994). The British scheme has since been modified, but fundamental issues remain with all such schemes: should parents with care (predominantly women) be *forced* to depend on absent parents (predominantly men) for the means to sustain the children, or should they and their children have a right to subsistence regardless of such relationships as they may have had in the past?

A related question has arisen in relation to whether a lone parent's right to assistance – or indeed, that of any household – should be conditional on their not having any more children. The US applies 'family cap' policies, which restrict a lone parent's social assistance entitlement so as to exclude additional help in relation to children conceived while they remain in receipt of state assistance (Walker, 2005). And more recently, the United Kingdom introduced a 'two child limit' which denies means-tested benefit increases to families having a third or subsequent child while in receipt of benefits – a policy described by one commentator as 'the worst social security policy ever' (Bradshaw, 2017).

9

SOCIAL RIGHTS IN GLOBAL CONTEXT

We have seen that social rights were initially framed as rights of citizenship through substantive social legislation by capitalist welfare states of the global North but also formulated as general principles within the Universal Declaration of Human Rights. This chapter will consider to what extent social rights as expressions of essential human sociality have developed globally, to which they have not necessarily been 'spreading' from North to South but have in any event emerged throughout the world. We shall start by building on the discussion begun in Chapter 4 of this volume regarding the contested role of social rights in human development before providing a brief overview of the uneven ways and varying extents to which social rights have in practice been developing in different parts of the world. We shall then turn to consider whether it is appropriate to introduce social rights as they have been framed in the global North into all societies and cultures and whether it is possible to protect and promote human wellbeing without recourse to concepts and discourses of rights.

Finally, we shall discuss globalisation: the ways in which social rights are being promoted on the global stage and the implications of global trends affecting social rights, including trends in migration. Chapter 1 of this volume cited Charles Darwin's observation that human beings' 'social instincts and sympathies' towards members of their species who are not personally known to them might eventually transcend 'artificial barriers' of race and nation. This implied, perhaps, the prospect of global social rights and human welfare provision that reaches beyond national boundaries – a potential 'scaling up' of our human sociality, albeit one constrained by barriers posed by dehumanising ideological schisms and geo-political forces.

DOI: 10.4324/9781003451518-11

Social rights and human development

It was shown in Chapter 3 of this volume that social policy-making and rights declarations have not succeeded in ensuring that all human needs are met; manifestations of social inequality and poverty remain evident globally and even within established welfare states. The UNDP's Human Development Index attempts to measure human progress around the world by means of a composite index, the Human Development Index, which combines within single-integer measures of standard of living (Gross National Income per capita), health (life expectancy) and education (mean and expected years of schooling). Countries can then be ranked in terms of their 'performance'. The results imply a correlation between national wealth and development, but a more complex picture emerges when account is taken of the extent of inequality, poverty and, for example, public social expenditure within each country (see Table 9.1). We have already, in Chapter 4 of this volume, discussed important debates about the meaning of 'development' and in particular the relative importance of, and interaction between, economic and social development as components of social development. In this chapter, we shall consider how the contested relationship between economic and social development plays out in practice.

When development was held to be synonymous with industrialisation and explanations of relative wealth and poverty at the international level were framed in terms of development and underdevelopment (George, 1988), the world was divided into the Western 'First World' of industrialised capitalist nations, an Eastern 'Second World' of partly industrialised communist nations, and the 'Third World' of supposedly underdeveloped nations. Such terminology has been rendered obsolete by a variety of global factors: the acceleration of economic globalisation and the international mobility of capital; the eclipse of industrial manufacturing; the rise of the service sector (so-called 'tertiarisation'); and the proliferation of new information-based technologies; the collapse of Eastern bloc communism and rapid economic growth across much of East Asia and Latin America.

However, we have yet to develop entirely satisfactory terminological alternatives. In this book, we have on occasion adopted the shorthand convention of referring to the world of capitalist welfare states as the global North (whether or not they are situated in the northern hemisphere) and the rest of the world as the global South. This is far from satisfactory, not least, because there appears to be little agreement or consistency about the criteria by which countries are deemed to achieve global North status. The club of capitalist nation states has been joined, on the one hand, by post-communist countries in which social rights had developed quite differently than in Western welfare states; and, on the other, by countries which – though they have moderately or even *very* high HDI rankings (e.g. South Korea) and have attained

TABLE 9.1 Human Development data: Selected countries[1]

	HDI ranking (out of 191 Countries) 2021[2]	*GNI per capita ($US at PPP) 2021*[2]	*Inequality adjusted HDI ranking 2021*[2]	*Gini co-efficient measure of income inequality 2010–2021*[2]	*% pop^n^. 'in poverty' (by differing criteria)*	*Social protection expenditure as % of GDP*[5]	*Government health expenditure as % GDP*[5]
Germany	9	54534	8	31.7	10.1[3]	19.4	4.9
UK	18	45225	17	35.1	11.1[3]	15.1	7.9
USA	21	64765	26	41.5	17.8[3]	18.4	8.5
Russia	52	27166	51	36.0	14.6[3]	13.4	3.2
China	79	17504	82	38.2	28.8[3]	7.2	3.0
Brazil	89	14370	109	48.9	20.9[3]	15.7	4.0
South Africa	109	12948	131	63.0	27.0[3]	5.5	4.5
India	132	6590	130	35.7	21.9[4]	1.4	1.0
Kenya	152	4474	149	40.8	36.1[4]	1.0	2.2
Nigeria	163	4790	170	35.1	40.1[4]	0.7	0.6
DRo Congo	179	1076	172	42.1	63.9[4]	1.8	0.8

Notes

1 All having populations in excess of 50 million. NOTE: the highest and lowest HDI ranking countries were Switzerland (population 9 million) and South Sudan (population 11 million) respectively.

2 Source: UNDP, 2022

3 % below 50% median equivalised disposable income (2016 or nearest year) – source: OECD, 2019

4 % below national poverty line (2009–2019) – source: UNDP, 2022. (NOTE: this does not necessarily provide a meaningful comparison with the data for the countries listed above and UNDP statistics based on a Multidimensional Poverty Index which takes into account factors other than income provides a far more nuanced account of poverty in 'developing' countries.)

5 Latest available years – source: ILO, 2022

membership of the Organisation of Economic Co-operation and Development (OECD) and the G20 group of nations, have welfare states that are recently instituted and as yet comparatively immature. The anomalies are legion, but the difficulties entailed in defining and measuring 'development' speak to a deeper problem.

The data assembled for early versions of the UNDP's annual Human Development Reports demonstrated that there is no automatic link between economic growth and social development (UNDP, 1993). Later, it was observed that the association between income and non-income dimensions of human development was weakening over time (UNDP, 2010); in other words, rising per-capita income does not necessarily translate into better social outcomes.

Even in the European context, the evidence can be interpreted as suggesting that measures to enhance 'social quality' through social rights may assist rather than impair economic competitiveness (Gough, 1997). But regardless of whether social rights help or hinder economic development, opponents of Wilensky's (1975) once-celebrated contention – that social rights are a spin-off from economic prosperity – have long argued that it takes insufficient account of the part that political processes play in determining the level of spending on things like social security provision (Castles, 1982). Social rights clearly can arise as political achievements and not as an incidental outcome of the capitalist development process. The historical and political context matters.

Regimes and regions

In Chapter 2, we considered Esping-Andersen's influential taxonomy of capitalist welfare state regimes, which had been based, in part, on an empirical evaluation of the extent to which different welfare states had sought to moderate or regulate the commodification of labour under capitalism. That taxonomy has been critiqued, elaborated and reapplied in myriad ways, generating a body of theory relating to the formation of welfare state regimes. However, the primary purpose of this chapter is to consider the evolution of social rights and the wide variety of potential paths to social development to be found *beyond* the predominantly Western capitalist welfare states, where this body of regime theory may or may not have any relevance (Midgley, 2013).

Alternative legacies

To that end, let us go back to the negotiations that took place between the state parties represented on the Commission on Human Rights during the drafting of the UNDHR in the 1940s (see Chapter 3, this volume). The dominant, essentially liberal, conception of social rights proposed by the United States and broadly supported by European representatives was confronted by two alternatives: the developmental view expressed by Latin American countries and the statist view from the Soviet Eastern bloc.

What is here described as the developmental view stemmed from a belief in development as a process that was both economic and social and which represented an explicit policy goal – a goal already expressed in the national constitutions of several Latin American countries. Development and social rights were regarded as all of a piece. At that time, the region sought to transcend the corporatist-conservative traditions of its colonial past and was infused by a heady if conflictual blend of both liberal and socialist influences. The Latin Americans pushed for the specification of collectively guaranteed individual social rights in greater detail than the US and Western European nations wished to countenance.

In the event, Latin American ambitions were thwarted, not so much with regard to the drafting of the UDHR's final text – on which they had some influence – as with regard to the substantive development of social rights within their own region. Latin American economies were destined to grow spectacularly, if erratically, on the back of unregulated inward investment, but the extension of social rights provision lagged behind. Characteristically, Latin American countries already had partially developed welfare states, dating from earlier in the twentieth century, based on highly stratified and fragmented social insurance arrangements, quite extensive employment protection measures, and reasonably well-developed public health and education provisions. Provision, however, was largely restricted to the formalised employment sector and urban areas, whereas substantial swathes of Latin America remained, and still are, economically informal and rural. Uneven economic growth was accompanied by substantial increases in poverty and inequality. In the 1980s, the region was gripped by an economic recession and was dependent for recovery on assistance from international financial institutions, conditional on neo-liberal 'structural adjustment' policies. These led to extensive privatisation of social insurance arrangements, the de-regulation of labour markets and the decentralisation of health and education provision. The end result, according to Barrientos (2001, 2004), was a transition from what had once been a conservative-informal welfare regime to a kind of liberal-informal welfare regime. From the 1990s onwards, the attitudes of international financial institutions began to change, favouring support for social safety-nets based on conditional cash transfers (see Chapter 8, this volume). At the same time, several Latin American countries elected left-leaning political leaders committed to poverty reduction within the constraints to which the region remained subject. And often policy steered by left-leaning leaders could be negated when they were succeeded by right-leaning leaders. Poverty has been somewhat reduced, but social inequality remains stubbornly high. Nevertheless, Latin American countries may be defined as welfare state regimes, in which social rights are recognised, albeit that they are incompletely or unevenly implemented.

The statist view, expressed by the Eastern European countries (led by the USSR), stressed a different interpretation of social rights. Initially, they had abstained from participation in debates about social rights and did not join the discussions until the third session of the Commission. For them, the issue was not that of achieving a balance between state powers and individual freedoms but of ensuring state guarantees of work and social security. They sought to strengthen the obligations of other state parties to prevent unemployment and to fund social insurance, not through individual contributions by workers but directly. Their influence on the final text of the UDHR, and later in the framing of the International Covenant on Economic, Social and Cultural Rights turned out to be negligible (Davy, 2013).

Prior to 1989, Soviet-style communism in Central and Eastern Europe represented a distinctive welfare regime that provided extensive social rights through guaranteed employment, subsidised prices and extensive state-enterprise-based social benefits. The demands that led to the eventual fall of that system were for the political and civil rights that such a regime had withheld. For their part, the architects of such regimes had believed they were forging a new form of civilisation, premised on transformative social rights and services by which, according to the slogan of the Moscow Sports Clubs, they were 'mending the human race on scientific principles' (cited in Webb & Webb, 1935, p. 805).

Towards the end of the Soviet era, however, state-guaranteed jobs were often highly unproductive, and the guaranteed minimum wage had fallen below the poverty line: workers joked, 'they pretend to pay us, we pretend to work' (cited in Standing, 2009, p. 43). The real value of insurance benefits and pensions had dwindled and the quality of health services and state housing had declined, with access to the best provision reserved for party *apparatchiks* (George, 1993). After 1989, the countries of Central and Eastern Europe, under the guidance of Western 'shock therapists', withdrew price subsidies and exposed state enterprises to market competition, but without first ensuring that alternative forms of social protection were in place (Standing, 1996). The immediate result was staggering increases in poverty and social inequality and a decline in health and life expectancy. The process of recovery entailed a contest between economic liberalism and the legacy of state paternalism (Deacon, 1993; Deacon et al., 1997), in the context of fragmentary social provision by burgeoning numbers of NGOs (Stephenson, 2000). As in Latin America, living standards for many were sustained only through a resilient and extensive informal economy (Jordan, 1998, p. 165). What has since emerged within the Soviet bloc is a variety of post-communist welfare states with different kinds of social rights, with a divide between the more Easterly states, most notably Russia, and the Central European and Baltic states. The former had tended towards post-communist corporatism (albeit Russia's recent oligarch-led economic recovery has been accompanied by selective marketisation of social provision) (Davidova & Manning, 2009). The latter are now mostly members of the EU, albeit that these have tended to varying degrees towards liberal welfare regime characteristics (Fenger, 2007; Cerami & Vanhuysse, 2009).

Outwith the rights agenda?

Asian and Arab states, though they contributed, did not exercise a concerted influence during the original deliberations over social rights by the Commission on Human Rights (Davy, 2013). They remained by and large marginal to the central debate. The explanation for this might in part be cultural, and this we shall consider in a moment. But there are other explanations.

The fundamental conditions for the development of social rights in the Marshallian mould were, on the one hand, a formalised economy and labour market and, on the other, an effective and legitimate state apparatus. Where these conditions do not apply, conventional welfare regime theory loses relevance (Gough et al., 2004), and the conventional concept of social rights has little foundation. Even in the case of Latin America and Eastern Europe, we have seen that the existence of a substantial informal sector could displace or inhibit social rights development. In the Latin American context especially, the term 'social exclusion' has been applied to refer not as in Western societies to the marginalisation of aberrant minorities but to the wholesale exclusion of entire populations in rural areas or 'slum' settlements from social rights of development and the 'social project' (Rodgers et al., 1995; Munck, 2005). However, for regions of the world that had little semblance of a formal economy or a modern state apparatus, the social rights debate was a secondary or remote concern of limited or no immediate relevance. Within some regions, this still applies (see Kennet & Retief, 2022).

The South Asian subcontinent consists largely of countries defined by Gough et al. (2004) as 'informal security regimes', denoting that practical provision for human need stems not so much from state-administered rights as from family, kinship and community. India, the largest country in the region, had had a pervasive but often dysfunctional state bureaucracy, bequeathed from its British colonial past (Townsend, 1993, ch. 8); and the country has more recently incorporated 'directive' social rights principles into its written constitution (Muralidhar, 2008). Despite this, in the 10 most populous cities of India, one in four children have been found to have stunted growth and development due to chronic nutrition deprivation (Naandi Foundation, 2018). Across the South Asian region as a whole, social protection programmes, education and healthcare provision are at best uneven or fragmentary, and, in rural areas, they may be non-existent. There have been initiatives, such as locally co-ordinated food for work schemes, national work guarantee schemes and micro-credit schemes, which, even with NGO involvement, have sometimes been subverted by patronage and clientalism at the community level (Davis, 2004).

As a region, Sub-Saharan Africa is the poorest in the world. It may be noted that all three of the lower HDI ranking countries included in Table 9.1 are in sub-Saharan Africa. The region consists largely of countries that have been defined by Gough et al. (2004; and see Bevan, 2004) as 'insecurity regimes', denoting that practical provision for human needs depends not necessarily on state-administered social rights but in many instances on local leaders, warlords, mafia bosses, corrupt officials or benign aid workers. In much of the region, colonial domination was succeeded not so much by Western-inspired models of governance as by a form of modernity without development, in which, outside urban areas, the populations are not so much citizens as subjects (Mamdani, 1996). Despite some progress in relation, for example, to education and healthcare, there has been a tendency for temporary measures to become institutionalised, creating what Cerami (2013) characterised as 'permanent emergency welfare regimes'. In recent years, substantial strategic economic investment across Africa by both Russia and China may to some degree have facilitated social development, but without addressing geopolitical fragilities across the region (Ramani, 2021).

In contrast, the Arab countries of the Middle East/North Africa include several spectacularly rich oil producers, as well as some poorer nations. In generalised terms, its welfare regimes may be described as 'corporatist/residual' (Jawad, 2022a). Though based in lands hailed as ancient cradles of civilisation, these countries are all as nation-states relatively modern creations. They have tended until lately to encompass relations of power that remain in some respects pre-modern, if not semi-feudal. Destremau (2000) had characterised some such countries as 'rentier states': lacking productive economies, they are heavily dependent on external revenues from oil exports, financial revenues and tourism. The wealth so created has enabled their rulers to develop public services, including healthcare and educational provision, but shares in the nation's 'rent' may be unevenly distributed and are not rights-based. The characteristically patrimonial form of capitalism to be observed across the region has tended towards a kind of welfare regime that has been 'neither democratic nor socially inclusive and [whose] developmental role has been limited' (Karshenas & Moghadam, 2006). In recent times, parts of the region – which is more complex and diverse than can be conveyed in any thumbnail sketch – have been variously subjected to external military intervention, internal civil strife and inter-factional tensions based on sect, religion and ethnicity. The so-called 'Arab Spring' of 2011 witnessed insurgent demands for democracy, but this has been followed by counter-revolution, chronic instability and, in some instances, violent extremism. It is difficult to predict whether and in what form social rights may now develop.

Emerging economies

Finally, in this section, there are places around the world where economic development has more recently been especially evident and where the conditions for the evolution of Marshallian-type social rights might have been anticipated.

Foremost, have been countries in East Asia. It should, of course, be noted that Japan, as an established industrialised power, had already developed a welfare state, albeit one difficult to categorise using Esping-Andersen's typology. In the 1960s, a group of smaller East Asian countries (South Korea, Hong Kong, Taiwan and Singapore), the so-called 'Tiger Economies', began to take off. Their approach to social provision and social rights was pragmatic, involving selective copying of policies from Japan or other industrialised countries, but with comparatively low levels of social spending and with particular emphasis on human capital development (i.e. education and healthcare). More recently, the rapid growth of the original East Asian Tigers, where economic growth slowed in the 1990s, has been replicated by so-called 'Tiger Cubs', like the Philippines and Indonesia, with a similarly modest approach to the extension of social rights (e.g. Comola & de Mello, 2010). Goodman and Peng (1996) once argued that the emerging model should be characterised as 'Japanese style welfare-systems', but other commentators have preferred to define these new capitalist nations as 'productivist' regimes (Holliday, 2000; Gough et al., 2004), reflecting the extent to which they prioritise economic production over social rights.

Also, within East Asia is what is now the world's second most populous country, China, a country which, in many ways, defies categorisation. China is the last major communist nation, albeit that, following market liberalisation, it is best regarded as 'state capitalist' (*The Economist*, 2012). The People's Republic of China in the 1950s had nationalised most land and industry, giving it over to collectives and co-operatives, creating an 'iron rice bowl' by which to ensure life-long employment and 'five guarantees': enough food, clothes and fuel, education for children and an honourable funeral. Market liberalisation began in 1978, leading according to some critics to a dismantling of the iron rice bowl (Leung, 1994). A revised constitution in 1982 identified certain social rights: to work, education, rest, retirement and 'material assistance' in the event of illness and disability. As economic growth accelerated, new forms of state social provision have been introduced, often based on Western-style state welfare models but on a limited scale (Chan et al., 2008) and with extensive variations around the country (Shi, 2012), including disparities between affluent urban coastal regions and largely impoverished rural Western China.

It should always be borne in mind that there can be significant diversity and differences between countries within the same region, and the above account is crude. If indeed it is economic growth that drives social rights development, we should perhaps review the prospects of the largest and most rapidly developing economies. At the turn of the twenty-first century, the economist Jim O'Neill (2001) first coined the acronym BRIC for a group of leading emerging economies and G20 members: Brazil, Russia, India and China. The countries thereafter formally established themselves as a co-operative grouping and were joined in 2010 by South Africa. More recently, the acronym MINT (Fraser, 2011) was coined for a further group of nations with large populations and rapid economic development: Mexico, Indonesia, Nigeria and Turkey. Economic performance of the BRICS and MINT countries, though fluctuating, appeared generally to be outstripping that in North American and Western European, and the diversity of their trajectories challenges orthodox analyses of how social rights development might occur.

Russia is an oligarchic capitalist/post-communist welfare regime. Brazil and Mexico are Latin American liberal-informal welfare regimes (Mexico is an OECD member). China and Indonesia are radically contrasting East Asian countries: the former being set potentially to become the mightiest economy in the world; the latter being one of the vibrant young capitalist Tiger Cubs; but each has uneven social rights provisions. South Africa and Nigeria are radically contrasting African countries: the former is an exceptional case in the African context, which, despite its legacy of Western-style industrial development during its apartheid era, suffers entrenched poverty and inequality; the latter with very high levels of poverty and simmering social divisions, despite its expanding, largely oil-based, economy. Turkey might until recently have been characterised as a Middle Eastern regime, subject to authoritarian paternalist rule, but with an incipient welfare state it had been moving towards democratic-welfare-capitalism (and an EU 'partner' but not a full member), albeit subject lately to strong neo-liberal policy tendencies (Boratav & Özuğurlu, 2006; Manning, 2007). These clearly are rapidly changing countries, but there is no discernible pattern as to the prospects or the most likely manner in which social rights will develop.

The cultural critique

The third of three broad critiques of the human rights agenda identified by Sen was the *cultural* critique (the other two being the *legitimacy* and the *coherence* critiques – see Chapter 4, this volume), the essence of which is that concepts of 'rights' forged during the Western Enlightenment and developed within democratic-capitalist-welfare states are inimical, for example, to Asian cultures. Attempts to impose them in the name of development amount to ethnocentrism (e.g. Polis & Schwab, 1979), if not cultural imperialism. There are two questions we might ask: is this true and just why does it matter?

Cultural values and practices

We have explored how the ethical foundations of rights discourse lie in Western philosophy and value systems, but there are Eastern philosophies and value systems – Confucian, Hindu, Buddhist, Muslim – through which other cultures and traditions have been shaped and which may, for example, prize loyalty, self-reliance and obedience above individual rights. Early attempts to characterise welfare state regimes emerging in East Asia sought to characterise them as Confucian welfare regimes constructed on principles of hierarchical community building and in the manner of a traditional extended Confucian family (Jones, 1993). This characterisation has since been questioned, not only because it oversimplifies complex influences but also because it can be 'a convenient excuse, with a persuasive historical and cultural camouflage, to filter responses to social welfare needs' (Walker & Wong, 2005). It is a characterisation that also sidesteps the fact that even China has written certain social rights into its Constitution, as do, for example, a number of Islamic states (Jung et al., 2013). The Organisation of the Islamic Conference in 1990 adopted the Cairo Declaration on Human Rights in Islam. The Declaration insists that the roots of such rights lie in Sharia, not Western law, but it includes, for example, the statement that 'The State shall ensure the right of the individual to a decent living which will enable him to meet all his requirements and those of his dependents, including food, clothing, housing, education, medical care and all other basic needs' (Article 17[c]). And though the Association of Southeast Asian Nations' (ASEAN) Declaration of Human Rights, which was adopted in 2012, has been held by Amnesty International, Human Rights Watch and the UN High Commissioner for Human Rights on several grounds to be flawed, it does contain an explicit array of social rights.

Sen (1999, pp. 231–238) suggests that allusions to non-Western values may not be used to explain or justify authoritarian policies or systemic inequalities. He claims that values associated with tolerance and equality have deep-rooted counterparts within several Asian philosophies, pointing by way of example to parallels between the ancient teachings of Kautilya, the Indian philosopher and royal adviser, and Aristotle, with whom Kautilya would have been a chronological contemporary. Kautilya was a strong advocate of personal liberty for the privileged elite in Indian caste society, as was Aristotle for the Athenian city elite, but like Aristotle, he advocated no such thing for slaves or the members of lower castes, for whom nevertheless he advocated paternalistic governmental assistance to relieve their misery. Historical trajectories vary, but cultural constructions may at times concur.

A case can be made for the existence within a variety of non-Western philosophies of ethical or moral principles that, it may be argued, are implicitly or even explicitly consistent with the idea of shared responsibility for meeting individual needs and therefore with some sort of basis for social rights as articulations of shared human needs (though not necessarily framed in the language of rights):

- The Confucian idea of *Rén* (or *Jen*), which translates as human-ness and is the ultimate state to which all should aspire through the observance of such values as filial piety and loyalty (Chan, 1999). There is, perhaps, a tenuous resonance between *Rén* and the Aristotelian notion of *eudaimonia*, as a state of fulfilment as a *social* being, concerned not with personal pains and pleasures but with one's harmony of existence with other beings.
- The ancient pan-African belief system, *Ubuntu*, whose essence is captured in the aphorism, 'a person is only a person through other persons'. It implies an inherently solidaristic, albeit potentially conservative philosophy, that

can nonetheless inform caring and sharing practices between and within human generations (Ramose, 2003; Whitworth & Wilkinson, 2013).

- The Islamic principle of *Zakat*: one of the pillars of the Muslim faith based on a religious obligation to share a portion of one's individual wealth with needy members of the *Ummah* (the worldwide community of the faithful). At the heart of Islam lies a quite particular conception of social justice (Dean & Khan, 1997).

It is not suggested that we should romanticise the manner in which these ideas have over the centuries been interpreted and reinterpreted. The point is that 'non-Western' value systems are by no means incommensurate with social rights. They entail implicit theories of personhood and alternative expressions of human sociality that have implications for the way in which human needs are to be understood and provided for, whether or not the framing of needs-based claims involves an explicit discourse of rights. However, elusively, the examples given potentially resonate with elements of the communitarian and/or even the universalist perspectives outlined in Figure 5.1 in Chapter 5 of this volume.

The cultural critique, however, has relevance not only for the real or imagined tensions between Western and Eastern philosophical traditions but also for the very practical tension between the social standards that are promoted in the global North and the social customs that apply in the global South. A well-intentioned attempt in 2000 to establish a set of 'Global Social Policy Principles' distilled from the raft of relevant UN conventions and declarations (see Ferguson, 1999) foundered at the UN's 'Copenhagen plus 5' Social Summit, amidst charges of hypocrisy against its proponents by representatives from the global South (Deacon, 2007, pp. 139–40). The proposals were resented as an unacceptable interference with the sovereignty of nations in the global South, and, without a transfer of resources from North to South, they would amount to an unachievable imposition. The imposition of ILO labour standards has long been a thorny issue for many countries (Ferguson, 1999). It has been claimed that the protection of highly exploited women workers and the abolition of child labour in certain parts of the world cannot necessarily be achieved without endangering the limited sources of income available to women (Kabeer, 2004) and without imposing Western cultural conceptions of childhood and of children's legitimate role in social and economic life (Edmonds & Pavcnik, 2005).

Conflicting epistemologies

There is a problem with transposing notions of rights constructed largely within the capitalist North to other parts of the world, but is this a cultural problem or an epistemological issue? Culture, undeniably, is dynamic, syncretic and evolving (Phillips, 2007). In a riposte to the cultural critique, Donnelly hones in on precisely this argument, asserting that 'Culture is not destiny' (2013: 88). At the same time, however, he also dismisses the possibility that there can be, or ever were, non-Western conceptions of human rights. He suggests that just as cardinal principles of mathematics have universal validity even though they were invented in the Arabic world, so the principles of Human Rights have universal validity even though their origins are 'Western'. His argument is redolent of Meyer's 'World Society' idea: the idea that systems of management and governance around the world conform to increasingly similar assumptions (Meyer, 2007; Meyer et al., 1997). When conceptions of individual rights are alien to culturally established welfare traditions, states may pragmatically adopt the world cultural language of rights, albeit that there may be a 'decoupling' between talk and action (Meyer, 2009, p. 182): their relevance in relation to practical policy implementation may be superficial (Leisering, 2022) and conceal nuanced differences of perspective.

For Donnelly, however, human rights are a modern epistemological triumph, and just because older philosophies defined that which was 'right', it did not mean that they satisfactorily conceptualised the 'rights' that inhere to the individual human being. Though certain margins of appreciation may apply when it comes to differing interpretations of human rights, cultural relativism, according to Donnelly, should be confined within proper limits. Donnelly is right about culture, but mistaken, it may be argued, about the epistemological status of human rights.

So far as social rights are concerned, these may have been incorporated into the UDHR and subsequent international covenants, but we have already seen: firstly, that social rights in the Marshallian sense had already been substantively formulated as legislative entitlements within various types of welfare states; secondly, that the terms on which they were incorporated as human rights were not discovered or deduced but *negotiated* by representatives from many nations. They are not eternal verities. They might yet be re-negotiated. So far as human rights more generally are concerned, the issue is not a conflict of cultures so much as an epistemological or ideological conflict between what was referred to in Chapter 3 in this volume as a hegemonic liberal-individualist conception on the one hand and the critical minority conception on the other: the former is premised on what Arendt described as the 'arrogant myth' (1951, p. 439) of inborn individual dignity; the latter on an understanding of the shared vulnerability that is the human condition (e.g. Turner, 2006). In an increasingly multi-polar world' (Held, 2010, p. 2), it isn't so much that Western and Eastern assumptions and beliefs converge or that the global South must adapt its understanding of rights to that of the global North; but that East and West, South and North can and will, it is to be hoped, mutually negotiate and together evolve broader understandings as human sociality historically unfolds.

Reflecting on the significance of the global justice movement in general and the deliberations of the World Social Forum in particular, Boaventura de Sousa Santos has suggested that their potential role is to supersede the hegemonic mono-cultural and technocratic epistemology of the global North with an insurgent epistemology of the South. The former entails an axiology of progress through capitalist development; the latter, an 'axiology of care' (2006, p. 31). In the process of framing future alternatives for the articulation of human needs and claims, such an axiology (or theory of value) might draw on insights or precepts from the past and present. We shall return to these issues in Chapter 11.

Globalisation

The emergence of what was originally described as an *anti*-globalisation movement was testimony to the extent to which globalisation, like development, is a contested concept (Held & McGrew, 2007). The processes that both concepts purport to define are interconnected. Supporters of globalisation regard the process as coterminous with that of human development. Some opponents fear that the hegemonic neo-liberal form of the globalisation process promotes a socially and environmentally damaging form of economic development at the expense of effective and inclusive social development, contending that the age of neo-liberal globalisation 'has now superseded the age of development' (Sachs, 2010: vii). The direction and pace of global change and human development are affected by global events: acts of terrorism, military interventions, financial crises, pandemics and a human-induced climate emergency. But the extent of the interdependence and interconnectedness of countries, regions and transnational corporations is ever more intense as they interact within a social space that is increasingly de-territorialised: 'globalization is synonymous with a process of time-space compression - literally a shrinking world - in which the sources of even very local developments, from unemployment to ethnic conflict, may be traced to distant conditions or action' (Held & McGrew, 2007, p. 3). It must also be acknowledged that there is a converse form of anti-globalisation movement represented by populist authoritarians, who, with their supporters, would resist globalisation, deny climate change and value national and territorial supremacy above global collaboration. The paradox, perhaps, is that populist authoritarian resistance to globalisation seeks to damage the global institutions that might ameliorate the adverse consequences of economic globalisation and climate change, and it is to those institutions that we now turn.

Global institutional framework

The consequences of globalisation have provided the context in which social rights have been changing. Bob Deacon once argued that we have been witnessing 'the globalisation of social policy and the socialisation of global politics' (2007, p. 3). The spirit of optimism that followed the end of the Cold War led some commentators to envision a global community and a form of global citizenship based on shared objectives of peace, social justice and ecological sustainability (Falk, 1994). The reality has been less harmonious, not least because of a drive towards the 'securitisation' of citizenship and concerns with risk containment rather than socially inclusive development processes (Nyers, 2009). Nevertheless, there is an increased awareness that social policy in one country or region cannot be made without reference to the global context and that global poverty and social inequalities have potential implications for every country and region. Neo-liberal globalisation (as a process entailed by the ascendancy and contradictions of the Washington consensus) obliged its supporters and opponents alike to think systematically about what Deacon calls the three 'Rs': global redistribution, global regulation and global social rights (2007, p. 1).

The Byzantine panoply of UN agencies and organisations includes several of direct relevance to social rights. Figure 9.1 identifies the key agencies, though there are many others. Under the overarching authority of ECOSOC, these agencies between them are responsible for providing or overseeing financial aid to countries in need of assistance; for developing regulatory frameworks or codes of conduct in relation to social protection and international trade for state parties and, for example, multinational corporations; and for promoting and monitoring the observance of social rights. Within the UN Secretariat, there is a department dedicated to social rights matters (the UNDESA), and the promotion of human rights in general is overseen by a High Commissioner through her/his office (the OHCHR). A group of

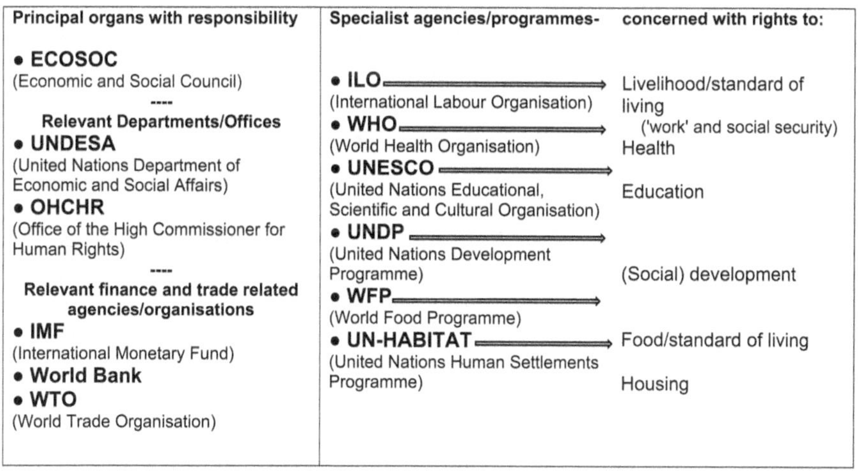

FIGURE 9.1 Social Rights at the United Nations

agencies, originally proposed in 1944 by the Bretton Woods Monetary and Financial Conference, provide a contextual framework by attempting to ensure global monetary stability (the IMF), finance social and economic development projects (The World Bank) and regulate world trading systems (the WTO), which prior to 1995 had been known as the General Agreement on Tariffs and Trade. Three specialist agencies that had existed in some form since 1919 under the auspices of the erstwhile League of Nations have responsibility for labour standards and social security (the ILO), for public health and healthcare standards (the WHO) and for educational, scientific and cultural development (UNESCO, previously the International Committee for Intellectual Co-operation). Finally, there are several more recently created specialist agencies, including, as already mentioned, the UNDP (founded in 1966), the WFP (founded in 1961 and responsible for food security) and UN-HABITAT (founded in 1996 and the only UN agency with a brief explicitly focused on housing standards).

The world over which the UN system presides is very different from that for which it was created in the aftermath of the second of the world wars to have occurred in the twentieth century. However, the relevance of a supranational perspective on the promotion and implementation of social rights is, arguably, greater now than ever before.

Global consumers and regulatory standards

Nicola Yeates (2001) has suggested that a distinction may be drawn between a 'strong' and a 'weak' globalisation thesis. Clearly, there is a spectrum of interpretations as to whether globalisation is an inevitable process and as to what its implications are for the future of social rights. At the 'strongest' end of the spectrum of beliefs, it is supposed that globalisation has ushered in a wholly new era (Fukuyama, 1992), in which markets will rule supreme and in which our rights to income security and pensions, to health and social care, education and housing will all be met on the basis of our rights as consumers of financial products and human services offered competitively by private and/or transnational providers in a global market place. Insofar as there may be supposedly aberrant minorities or communities who cannot access such provisions, there should be publicly provided safety-nets, but these should be selective, conditional and temporary. Though this is something of a caricature of the neo-liberal perspective, it is arguably consistent with the free-trade agenda of the WTO, which has developed mechanisms by which to open the provision of public social services to competition, a process which could unfold globally if established welfare states start to relinquish overall public control over key services (Holden, 2022). At the 'weaker' end of the spectrum, it has been contended that the significance of globalisation can be overstated (Hirst & Thompson, 1996). The process of internationalisation in trade, technology and ideas is a long-term secular trend, and welfare state development is pretty much an irreversible phenomenon: mature welfare states are durable and can survive even in the context of a more pluralistic welfare mix (Mishra, 1990; Rieger & Leibfried, 2003). Such a perspective is broadly consistent with, for example, the ILO's promotion of an international social protection floor (see Chapter 8, this volume) and commitment to social insurance-based rights and corporatist principles of social partnership.

If indeed these were the models imposed by globalisation on existing and emerging welfare states alike, the trend to a neo-liberal US-style solution would entail a 'race to the bottom' as existing welfare states compete to establish the lowest levels of publicly funded social protection. The trend to EU-style social protection, on the other hand, would entail a hard climb to the top for countries with limited or incipient welfare states – a fear, as we have seen, often voiced by such countries. Globalisation does not necessarily entail a straightforward transfer of social policies and the rights they supposedly impart from the global North to the global South (Hulme & Hulme, 2008). Social policies are not necessarily popularly equated with rights. And the framing of social rights as concessions to an international human rights agenda can have the effect, especially for vulnerable and marginalised people, of making rights seem abstract and distant from immediate needs and concerns (e.g. Soysal, 1994). We have seen in Chapter 4 of this volume that international regulation of social development is inclined to establish, not rights but social standards.

Measures taken by the UN to promote social development have fallen short of direct regulation but have included, significantly, the introduction in 2000 of the Millennium Development Goals (the MDGs) (UN, 2000), a range of important, if relatively modest, targets set for achievement by 2015 and against which some progress had been made (McArthur & Rasmussen, 2017). The MDGs resonated distantly with earlier social development approaches premised on the Basic Needs Approach, while influenced by the capabilities-oriented human development approach (see Chapter 4, this volume), yet bearing the stamp of a neo-liberally inspired form of managerialism. By setting measurable performance targets, the MDGs reflected the application of an essentially managerialist technique and exhibited elements of New Public Management thinking scaled up to the global level (see Chapter 2, this volume) and incorporated as a component of a World Society conception (see Meyer et al. 1997 and discussion above). While the language of rights retained some rhetorical purchase, the social development agenda was in practice premised upon a marginalisation of social rights (e.g. Porter & Craig, 2004).

The MDGs were succeeded in 2015 by a set of 'Sustainable Development Goals' (SDGs) (UN, 2015) to be achieved by 2030 – see Box 9.1.

BOX 9.1 THE UNITED NATIONS' SUSTAINABLE DEVELOPMENT GOALS

Declared in 2015, each goal has a detailed range of specific targets, many specifically set for achievement by 2030. The goals are interconnected, but for the purposes of this book, they may be regarded as falling within the following four groups:

1 Goals of direct relevance to the spectrum of social rights to human services and livelihood, discussed in Chapters 7 and 8 of this volume.

Goal 1. End poverty in all its forms everywhere (includes targets for the implementation of nationally appropriate social protection systems and measures for all)
Goal 3. Ensure healthy lives and promote well-being for all at all ages (includes target for the achievement of universal health coverage)
Goal 4. Ensure inclusive and equitable quality education and promote lifelong learning opportunities for all
Goal 8. Promote sustained, inclusive and sustainable economic growth, full and productive employment and decent work for all
Goal 11. Make cities and human settlements inclusive, safe, resilient and sustainable (includes targets for access for all to adequate, safe and affordable housing)

2 *Goals associated with the water-energy-food nexus* (see Schmidt & Matthews, 2018), *contextually essential to the right to an adequate standard of living* (see Article 25, UDHR 1948)

Goal 2. End hunger, achieve food security and improved nutrition and promote sustainable agriculture
Goal 6. Ensure availability and sustainable management of water and sanitation for all
Goal 7. Ensure access to affordable, reliable, sustainable and modern energy for all

3 *Goals relevant to the implementation and enforcement of social rights (see Chapter 10 of this volume)*

Goal 5. Achieve gender equality and empower all women and girls (includes targets for recognition and valuing of unpaid care and domestic work through the provision of public services, infrastructure and social protection policies)
Goal 10. Reduce inequality within and among countries (includes targets for promotion of social and economic inclusion of all, for equality of opportunity and the reduction of inequalities of outcome)

Goal 16. Promote peaceful and inclusive societies for sustainable development, provide access to justice for all and build effective, accountable and inclusive institutions at all levels

Goal 17. Strengthen the means of implementation and revitalize the Global Partnership for Sustainable Development (includes targets for mobilisation of additional financial resources for developing countries)

4 *Goals relating to the economic and environmental context in which social rights may effectively apply*

Goal 9. Build resilient infrastructure, promote inclusive and sustainable industrialization and foster innovation

Goal 12. Ensure sustainable consumption and production patterns (includes targets for achievement of efficient use of natural resources, reduction of food waste, the management of chemicals and all waste materials)

Goal 13. Take urgent action to combat climate change and its impacts (includes targets for strengthening resilience and adaptive capacity to climate-related hazards)

Goal 14. Conserve and sustainably use the oceans, seas and marine resources for sustainable development (includes targets for action on marine pollution and fish stock management)

Goal 15. Protect, restore and promote sustainable use of terrestrial ecosystems; sustainably manage forests; combat desertification; and halt and reverse land degradation and halt biodiversity loss

By and large, the SDGs represented a continuation of technocratic colonisation or de-politicisation of the social development agenda. Nevertheless, the SDGs were in some respects more broadly framed and sought to promote more extensive collaborative activity in support of the goals at the international level and for a Global Peoples' Assembly for civil society representatives to evaluate progress in 2023 at the midpoint of the 15-year programme (see www.peoplesassembly.global/en/). However, many of the targets set were less well defined and/or less measurable (Vandermoortele, 2015). Like the MDGs, while incidentally acknowledging the relevance of the human rights agenda in their preambles, the SDGs are nowhere substantively framed in terms of rights (see Köhler & Pogge, 2014).

As suggested in Box 9.1, the goals may, for our purposes, be grouped under four broad headings, having regard to their relevance for social rights. Several goals are directly relevant to the right to social security, healthcare, education, work and housing and right-based approaches can have a role in meeting such goals. Other important goals relate to rights that may be subsumed within the overarching social right to an adequate standard of living, including the rights to food and water/sanitation (effectively acknowledged as social rights by ECOSOC in 1999 and 2002 under Comments 15 and 17, respectively) and the right to energy, widely demanded by NGOs (Walker, 2015). There are further goals that are indirectly relevant to social rights since they relate, on the one hand, to the redress of inequalities in which social rights can potentially play a role and, on the other, to institutional arrangements relevant to the extension, implementation and enforcement of social rights. Finally, there are goals which are contextually relevant to the space in which social rights and human welfare may be allowed to develop by explicitly addressing the issues of economic and environmental 'sustainability'.

There remains, however, a fundamental tension between the goals of economic and environmental sustainability. We observed in Chapter 1 of this volume how Marx encapsulated the interaction between humanity and Nature as a form of social-ecological metabolism and had suggested there was a risk under capitalism of a 'metabolic rift' should the side-effects of intensive agriculture and industry damage, degrade or disrupt the natural environment at humanity's own expense. In the late twentieth century, that risk was eventually recognised as an existential threat, most notably by the World Commission on Environment and Development (Brundtland, 1987), which concluded that 'Development cannot subsist upon a deteriorating environmental resource base; the environment cannot be protected when growth leaves out of account the costs of environmental destruction' (para. 40). The targets currently set by the SDGs remain aspirational and are far from practically enforceable; they are premised on the assumption that development requires continued economic growth while the environmental changes of the Anthropocene era are to be accommodated through moderation, adaptation and resilience. It has been expressly acknowledged that progress towards achieving SDG targets has been significantly undermined by 'The COVID-19 pandemic, rising conflicts and a global cost-of-living crisis, compounded by the already relentless and inequitable effects of climate change' (Guterres, 2023, p. xiii).

Rights of migrants

Migration has been integral to the history of humanity, but it has acquired particular significance for social rights and human welfare in the context of current often intersecting trends, including globalisation, persistent geopolitical instabilities and violence and, increasingly, climate change. International migration affects a range of countries and regions, and there is considerable diversity and complexity to migration flows as people move around a rapidly changing and sometimes volatile world in pursuit of employment opportunities or better living standards, or as they flee from hunger, poverty, danger or persecution (de Haas et al., 2019).

The UNDHR provides that everyone has the right to leave any country and the right in other countries to seek asylum from persecution (Articles 13 and 14), while the 1951 Geneva Convention Relating to the Status of Refugees accords persons granted refugee status certain rights to work, housing, healthcare, basic education and public relief/social security, and it requires states parties as far as possible to 'facilitate the assimilation and naturalization' of refugees. Other than for asylum seekers, however, there is no prescribed right for a person to enter a country other than their own (save that citizens of the EU enjoy a degree of freedom of movement between countries within the EU).

It was observed in Chapter 6 of this volume that one of the dilemmas facing capitalist welfare states is whether and in what circumstances economic migrants, once admitted to a country, should enjoy the same rights as settled citizens to state welfare provision. The issue has particular pertinence when it comes to rights that require access to limited jobs and scarce public resources and/or when there is populist xenophobic or racist hostility towards migrants (Craig, 2008). Lockwood (1996) identifies the way in which social rights can be 'fine-tuned' to exclude or include different social groups, a process leading to 'civic stratification': stratification based not on class, but civic status constituted through differential entitlement to public goods. Lydia Morris extends this analysis to consider how the granting and withholding of social rights become 'a valuable tool in the management of population and society' (2006, p. 54). This is something that may apply especially in the case of the social rights that individual nation-states may selectively accord to economic migrants as opposed to refugees, whose social rights are, in principle, internationally assured and overseen by the UN High Commissioner for Refugees. Also, the UN Children's Fund has specialised oversight in relation to the rights of migrant children.

The categorical distinction to be drawn between economic migrants and refugees can in practice be tenuous. Globe-trotting entrepreneurs and skilled professionals for their part may settle in foreign countries without any immediate call upon social welfare provision, but lower and unskilled migrants seeking an escape from destitution rather than persecution have welfare needs much in common with refugees. The UN's International Organisation for Migration has no specific remit in relation to social rights provision, although the ILO is concerned with labour standards and social protection coverage for migrant workers where the migrant workforce is highly represented (Yeates & Piper, 2022, p. 190). The SDGs do pay some attention to migration issues insofar as they aim to 'Take immediate and effective measures to eradicate human trafficking' (Target 8.7), which addresses in principle issues facing the most vulnerable 'economic' migrants whose persecution may have crossed national boundaries and to reduce the transaction costs of migrant remittances (Target 10c), which acknowledges that many economic migrants play a vital role in providing for the needs of transnational families and of the important part played by informal social welfare provision within diasporic communities that straddle national boundaries.

We have been using the term social rights to encompass what is referred to in the UDHR as economic, social and *cultural* rights, yet we have not so far discussed cultural rights. Cultural identity and expression might be thought of as being a 'private' rather than a public or civic issue. As individual human rights, they appear to have been included, according to Eide (2001, p. 289), 'almost as a remnant category'. Specifically, the ICESCR (Article 15) provides for the right to take part in cultural life and the right to enjoy the benefits of scientific progress and its applications. The intention is ambiguous. Insofar as we are concerned with social rights as articulations of human needs, the socio-cultural component of social rights is concerned with participation, identity and knowledge. Migrants may be inferred to have a right to participate in the life of the society to which they have migrated; to have access to educational opportunities; to take part in creative and leisure activities; and to share equally in the benefits of technological progress enjoyed by that society, whether this relates, for example, to having access to the latest advances in medical treatment or more generally to prevailing living and housing standards. Migrants might also claim the right to preserve their own language, religion and customs, and it is on this basis that cultural rights may be regarded as an element of collective or group rights to self-determination (e.g. Kymlicka, 1995). But that is conceptually distinct from the contention that a migrant has a right to cultural inclusion in the life of a 'host' society and, by implication, to be protected from discriminatory treatment.

A full discussion of immigration policies and debates surrounding multiculturalism lies beyond the scope of this book, but it behoves us nevertheless to consider how the different perspectives on social rights, human needs and responsibilities – as outlined in Figure 5.1 in Chapter 5; this volume – play out in terms of competing approaches to migrants (this analysis is developed from Dean, 2011):

- The utilitarian perspective will be accepting of the right of free movement by migrants, who can expect to experience some degree of civic inclusion and cultural tolerance. Their social rights may well be conditional in nature. But the migrant is socially constructed as a potential settler.

- The survivalist perspective is likely to be actively hostile to the admission of migrants, who can expect to experience civic exclusion and cultural rejection. Their social rights are likely to be minimal in nature. The migrant is socially constructed as an unwelcome alien.
- The communitarian perspective will be accommodating to migrants, who can, however, expect to experience restricted civic status and cultural isolation. Their social rights are likely to be sufficient, but not necessarily equivalent to those of a citizen. The migrant is socially constructed as a transient guest.
- The universalist perspective will ostensibly be openly welcoming of migrants, who can expect to experience the benefits of full civic status and cultural inclusion. Their social rights are likely to be universalistic in character. The migrant is socially constructed as a new citizen.

This model, once again, is no more than a heuristic device with some value for the interpretation of approaches to the social rights of migrants, particularly those moving from the global South to the global North, though most international migration in fact occurs between countries in the global South (e.g. Shutes, 2016). Liberal welfare regimes such as the UK and the US have in the past actively encouraged inward migration at times when cheap labour was required, but, in the case of the UK, this was restricted to migration from former colonies and since the 1960s has been closely regulated. Practices in social conservative regimes have varied: Germany, for example, once restricted citizenship to the indigenous ethnic group, and migrant labour was admitted as 'guest workers' (with separately defined rights), though reforms to immigration and citizenship laws have now changed this. Social democratic Nordic countries, which had long been welcoming towards migrants, have lately come under pressure to restrict the social rights of migrants. Populist moral authoritarian tendencies can come into play within any substantive welfare regime.

Humanity is more interconnected than in Darwin's day, and yet the 'artificial barriers' posed by national boundaries can still impose constraints on human sociality and the development of social rights.

10

RIGHTS OF REDRESS

Rights that remain unfulfilled or that are dishonoured do not necessarily cease to *be*. But to exist in any meaningful sense, rights must be effective. They cannot be effective unless they are recognised and observed. To survive once established, rights-based claims must continue to be systematically sustained. It must be possible for people who have been denied rights to seek some form of reparation. This applies as much to social rights as any other kind. If we are to understand social rights as articulations of need and as expressions of human sociality, they are constituted through an ongoing interactive process of bottom-up claims-making and top-down prescription – a social process of challenge and concession. We have seen that social rights are not the same as legal or civil rights, yet when constituted as citizenship rights, they depend for their formal definition on national law-making processes, and in many instances, they necessarily intersect with civil law. The legal and administrative machinery of a welfare state will generally provide the individual with at least some means of redress if they cannot obtain or enforce those rights. But the notion of 'enforcement' may be problematic when it comes to the functioning of social rights. When internationally constituted as human rights, the enforceability of social rights is altogether less certain, though the international legal framework provides the context in which the interpretation and development of social rights can and does occur. Legal frameworks are premised on concepts of legal redress rather than social reparation. This entails, as we shall see, an unresolved tension, if not a fundamental contradiction.

The chapter will first critically consider the relationship between social rights and the law. It will discuss the process by which social policy provision has been 'juridified'; the issue of access to legal expertise and the role of

DOI: 10.4324/9781003451518-12

lawyers; and the enduring debate as to whether social rights can or should be justiciable. We shall then turn to examine the different levels at which redress in relation to social rights may be obtained, focusing on international monitoring arrangements, the role of the courts at the national level and the significance of administrative mechanisms of redress. It is a chapter of interest both to legal scholars and to community activists.

Social rights and the law

Albeit in different ways, the founding 'fathers' of the sociological tradition – Durkheim, Weber and Marx – had regarded the evolution of modern law and the administrative state in the post-Enlightenment period as integral to the emergence of capitalist societies (Hunt, 1978). But they had not foreseen the emergence of the welfare state and the manner in which social rights of citizenship might be framed. We have seen in Chapter 6 how contemporary theorists have adapted the Marxist critique of rights to an analysis of social rights, but other thinkers have also considered the relevance of law and jurisprudence to social rights in capitalist welfare states. The discretionary relief once administered under the Poor Laws assumed a new form, a legalised form, whereby official decisions were subjected 'to the governance of predetermined rules' (Jowell, 1975, p. 2). This legalisation and the consequent juridification of social administration presented what Teubner (1987) describes as a 'regulatory trilemma'. As a systems theorist, Teubner regards the law and social administration as separate 'autopoietic systems', each with its own integrity and distinctive self-regulatory knowledge. The framing of social rights as rights of welfare state citizenship brought these two systems into collision with one another, and in the process, three things could happen.

Firstly, the systems might prove *incongruous*. In Britain, for example, even before the consolidation of the post-second world war welfare state, policymakers had deliberately and systematically attempted to frame social policy provision in ways that insulated it from judicial scrutiny (Cranston, 1985, pp. 287–288). Secondly, the process might lead to the *over-socialisation* of law. This was the outcome feared by lawyers adhering to the classical legal theory, famously exemplified by Dicey's (1885) insistence on judicial purity – the principle that the law must be kept above politics and policymaking. The supposition was that the judiciary, far from being a constitutional check upon the legislature and the executive, might be reduced to an overstrained political instrument (Harden & Lewis, 1986). Third, the process might alternatively lead to the *over-legalisation* of social administration. This is the outcome identified by Habermas, who contends that juridification is part of the process by which technical welfare systems can colonise the life world of the individual subject (1987; and see Tweedie & Hunt, 1994).

These three possible outcomes can be presented as a hypothetical trilemma or simply as three ways of problematising the relationship between social rights and law.

A related sociological interpretation is that the relationship between the state and the individual becomes 'fundamentally depoliticised - referenced in terms of welfare instead of power' (Garland, 1981, p. 43): social rights, in other words, become an expression of inviolable legal principles, not negotiable social policies adapting to real lives. Processes of legal enforcement entail intervention by an external judicial or quasi-judicial authority; the invocation of a power that is alien to people's lives and popular demands (Foucault, 1980, ch. 1). Certainly, it may be argued that legally framed modes of redress are potentially alien to the workings of human sociality. Alternatively, presenting the argument in the terms introduced in Chapter 1 of this volume, human sociality can be obscured by legal fetishism.

We shall consider the development of legal remedies in the second part of this chapter, but for now, we shall discuss, on the one hand, how it is that lawyers have been drawn into the realm of social rights and, on the other, whether or not that is a realm that can appropriately be subject to judicial oversight.

Access to justice

When Marshall delivered the lectures on which the ground-breaking paper setting out his concept of social rights was based, he used the occasion to mark the publication of the Legal Aid and Advice Bill by which the British government was to extend the provision of state-funded legal aid, subject to a means-test, to civil legal matters (1950, pp. 29–31). This he plainly regarded as an extension of social rights. Legal aid might alternatively be regarded as a civil right since it guarantees effective access to the courts; as a foundational right that is 'conservative of all other rights' (e.g. Durbach, 2008, p. 59); or even as a 'fourth right of citizenship' (NCC, 1977). In practice, as we shall see, legal aid is not necessarily available directly to support litigation in relation to disputes concerning *social* rights, but it is worth a moment to discuss the provenance and development of legal aid. As with other social services, the origins of legal aid are to be found in philanthropic provision and, for example, the English 'dock brief' system by which litigants and defendants coming before the court without means might have counsel assigned from any willing to take on their cases 'pro bono', or free of charge (Zander, 1978, ch. 1). Public funding for the defence of criminal prosecutions in which the liberty of the subject was at stake has become a human rights obligation (Article 14 of the ICCPR), though it is a right extended in several jurisdictions to assistance in civil cases involving, for example, risks of domestic violence or homelessness (Durbach, 2008).

The definition of legal aid adopted by a UN global report – generated in the context of the Sustainable Development Goals and which calls for 'access to justice for all' (see Goal 16, see Box 9.1, this volume):

> encompasses services provided by lawyers and paralegals in criminal as well as in civil and administrative matters to individuals who are poor, marginalized, or otherwise in need of special legal protection, to enable them to exercise their rights. This includes the provision of legal advice, representation in courts or proceedings under other State tribunals, assistance in drafting of documents and pleadings, mediation, assistance in navigating the rules and procedures of State administrative agencies, along with a range of other services.
>
> *(UNDOC/UNDP, 2016, pp. 8–9)*

The findings of the report show that legal aid provision around the world has been expanding, and around two-thirds of the 106 countries studied had established some level of provision, albeit focused for the greater part on criminal justice matters rather than civil and administrative law, especially in 'less developed' countries. Where civil legal aid is available, it is concentrated primarily around family, property and labour disputes; for example, claims relating to state services or disputes with state agencies feature less prominently. Legal aid systems generally direct state funds to underwrite the costs of lawyers in private practice, to whom the poorest and least advantaged in society are unlikely to turn (e.g. Mameli, 1997); alternatively, the provision of specialist legal and paralegal assistance – with or without state aid – remains in substantial part the provenance of the voluntary/civil society sector. The global report shows that across the world, the foremost challenges identified by country experts arise because 'lawyers are paid very little for legal aid work' and 'people are not aware that legal aid services are available', closely followed by concerns that 'people lack confidence in the quality of legal aid services' or that 'people may not understand how legal aid services can help them' (UNDOC/UNDP, 2016, p. 63). Certainly, demand for civil legal aid outstrips availability in lower income countries, while in high-income countries, official estimates as to the extent to which civil legal aid is in theory available are, by and large, belied by low levels of actual take-up (*ibid.* p. 123), suggesting that practical constraints on access, together with misunderstanding and mistrust, may inhibit demand. Austerity measures in established welfare states have been associated with increasingly severe constraints on legal aid spending and the reach of legal aid provision (especially, for example, in England – see Law Society, 2023; ALA, 2014; WBG, 2023).

Nevertheless, a UN Task Force on Justice continues to declare that 'Without increased justice the world will not be able to end poverty [or] reduce inequality'. Justice, in this context, appears as a synonym for law, but without ever expressly alluding to social rights, the Task Force asserts that justice systems should work 'in collaboration with other sectors' such as health, education, housing and employment (Task Force on Justice, 2019, p. 17). Legal aid aimed at vulnerable social groups appears as part of a wider drive to promote people's consciousness of their legal rights and their engagement with legal institutions. However, the use of the law for the advancement of social rights had its beginnings in a welfare rights movement that may arguably be traced back to the 1960s and such developments as the pioneering approach adopted by neighbourhood law firms in the United States, staffed by radical young lawyers. This was in part, a self-funded activity fuelled by the civil rights movement but also sponsored for a while under the Economic Opportunity Act of 1964 as part of President Johnson's 'War on Poverty'. The first director of the Office of Economic Opportunity had described these legal services as the 'heavy artillery' in the war on poverty (Carlin et al., 1967). Britain, in the 1970s, witnessed the emergence of its own Law Centre movement, based on the US example (Stephens, 1982); a variety of community-based projects undertaking welfare rights casework, often grant aided by local government; and campaigning charitable bodies, such as the Child Poverty Action Group, committed to 'test case strategies', whereby they would take social rights cases for rulings before the higher courts (Prosser, 1983).

It was an era in which the legal profession and an emerging breed of paralegal welfare rights experts went out into the world as 'secular missionaries ... to do important ethical work' (Gearty, 2011, p. 34); to bring new 'counter-hegemonic strategies' to bear in support of the welfare rights movement (Hunt, 1990); to empower the powerless. The secular missionaries were not without their critics. Neo-Marxist and 'critical' legal theorists agonised that, far from being counter-hegemonic, such strategies channelled or co-opted working class resistance into bureaucratic and legal modes of participation. The welfare rights movement, while seeking to undermine the abstract 'high bourgeois image' of the law, succeeded in bringing it closer to people (Bankowski & Mungham, 1976). In so doing, lawyers and welfare rights workers, far from empowering their clients, were dehumanising them by negating people's own understanding and experience of how problems might be solved. Contemporary sceptics continue to express concern lest social rights activists carry with them a partiality for the law that eclipses the necessarily open-textured nature of social rights and the 'necessity of politics' (Gearty, 2011, p. 52). The risk was fully realised by at least one such secular missionary (this author) when he wrote:

> The illusion created by a society whose complex laws and bureaucratic procedures isolate and oppress the individual is that people's problems appear to be 'personal' and that the only possible solutions to those problems appear to be those that are that professionally administered.
>
> *(Brixton Advice Centre, 1976, pp. 13–14)*

TABLE 10.1 The pros and cons of legal strategies in the field of social rights activism

Pros	*Cons*
• Empowers individuals and groups	• Can individuate and disempower
• Harnesses and extends social rights	• Cannot secure substantive resources
• Raises awareness and informs debate	• May unintentionally create inequality
• Delivers evidence of policy failure	• Victory can be negated by legislation

There are undeniably pros and cons to legalistic strategies in the field of social rights activism (see Table 10.1). They can succeed in securing social security benefits for people who are entitled to them, in curbing bad employment practices and in improving local housing conditions. They can raise awareness of social injustice and/or demonstrate to policymakers where policy is failing. However, the improvements they can bring to the living conditions of poor people are likely to be marginal. This is firstly because individual casework cannot improve the levels at which social security benefits are set, and they cannot create new jobs or homes. Secondly, when the resources required to fulfil social rights are scarce and must be rationed, those who exercise their rights successfully may do so at the expense of others. Third, the gains made as a result of ground-breaking test cases may be short-lived if the legislature has the power to change the law and effectively nullify the victory.

The justiciability debate

This leads us to what has been called the 'justiciability' debate (Hunt, 1996; Langford, 2008; Gearty & Mantouvalou, 2011). Is it possible – is it right – that social rights should be subject to judicial scrutiny? We might argue that social rights, though equal in standing to civil and political rights are, different in character. It is not simply that they are self-executing or ill-suited to processes of judicial scrutiny, but that as articulations of human need, the transactions they entail are not legal but fundamentally social. They are expressions of sociality – of the mutual recognition of claims made both by and upon other human beings. For the most part, however, the basis for such claims has generally been framed and negotiated remotely – both temporally and spatially – by political representatives or beneficent experts, and their administration and legal adjudication will be undertaken by relatively powerful and socially distant personnel. There are issues here to which we must return in Chapter 11, but in the meantime, let us consider the established contours of the debate.

The first problem is that the judicial process is primarily framed as the resolution of contests between disputing parties. The roots of this problem may be traced back to the ancient practice of trial by combat. This is, perhaps, less manifest in legal systems based on the Roman legal tradition (premised on inquisitorial procedures and legal codification) than in those now based on the English tradition (premised on adversarial procedures and common law principles) (e.g. Watson, 1990). In the contemporary world there is considerable overlap between systems, and the concept of the *inter partes* trial has universal symbolic significance. Though the judicial duel could assume a variety of forms, its most pertinent manifestation entailed a petition to the King by nobles requiring a resolution to some dispute between them. Resolution was achieved through armed combat, presided over by the King, between the appointed champions of the contesting parties. The King would specify the rules of combat and determine which of the champions had won. The dispute was thereby settled without regard to substantive considerations of truth or justice in favour of the party whose champion was declared the victor. Combat now takes place by way of formal argument between appointed advocates on behalf of the disputing parties, and the role of the judge is not to intervene in the contest but – like a sovereign of old – to ensure the rules of combat are observed and (except in jury trials) determine who has won. Even with the safeguards that can be provided by, according to the judge, a more active inquisitorial role in the proceedings, any dispute resolution procedure is likely to disadvantage weaker parties at the expense of the powerful. Parties without access to expert advice and assistance are likely to suffer some element of disadvantage relative to those with the resources to hire the best. We shall see in the second part of this chapter that legal justice and social justice are not just inevitably incommensurable, but there is also a fundamental issue about framing the pursuit of justice as the resolution of a dispute. Social rights disputes, by their nature, are likely to pitch vulnerable citizens against powerful governmental agencies, and the strategic role of the welfare lawyer or social rights advocate becomes that of 'party upgrading' (Galanter, 1976); of compensating for the inherent inequality of the contest.

The second problem lies with, on the one hand, the expertise of the judiciary and its attitudes on the other. The charge made against the judiciary has been that it is ill-equipped to consider matters of social policy (Harden & Lewis, 1986) and that its members are likely to be drawn from a privileged stratum of society with little understanding of, or sympathy for, the problems of the most needy in society (Griffiths, 1997). These tendencies are clearly more evident and more entrenched in some countries than in others, but in principle, both problems are remediable. Judges' principal expertise, axiomatically, is in matters of law. Nevertheless, procedural rules could be adapted better to harness that expertise (Lewis & Birkinshaw, 1993). And there is no reason why judges should not be advised as occasion demands by social policy experts or why they should not receive specialist training as they might in relation to any specialist area of jurisdiction (e.g. Alston, 1990). Certainly, there is evidence, for example, of extreme conservatism and inconsistency on the part of the British judiciary in the era when social rights cases were first brought before them (Griffiths, 1997), but there is more recent evidence from around the world where judges have displayed considerable understanding and sympathy for the plight of people in need (Mantouvalou, 2011, pp. 118–121; and see Sachs, 2009). What is more, steps can be taken to ensure that judges are not necessarily drawn only from the upper echelons of society (see, for example, Neuberger, 2010).

The next problem has to do with the legitimacy and the potentially undemocratic nature of judicial intervention. Checks and balances on the exercise of power within a liberal democracy are supposedly provided by the division of powers between the legislature, the executive and the judiciary. We have already seen that judicial purists were afraid that allowing the judiciary to adjudicate on social rights risked drawing them into tasks more properly fulfilled by the executive, particularly with regard to the allocation of public resources. The concern arises because social rights, unlike civil rights, are costly, and it is not for the judiciary to impose costs on the government. However, as Plant (1992) among others have argued, the costs of social security, healthcare and education systems are no less legitimate than other forms of public spending, including the costs of the judiciary themselves, the administration of the courts, and the civil and criminal justice systems as a whole. But related to this is the extent to which an unelected and unaccountable judiciary ought not to be allowed to tread on the toes of the democratically elected legislature. This is especially the case in jurisdictions using the English common law system, where principles of interpretation established by higher courts set precedents for lower courts to follow and can so 'make' law independently of the legislature, for example by reinterpreting its meaning and effect. In some jurisdictions, such as the US, the courts have the power to strike down legislation as unconstitutional. Constitutionality and democracy can be uneasy companions. The judiciary is accountable for overseeing the conduct of the executive and the legislature, and if within a majoritarian electoral democracy, it should act to protect the social rights of powerless or unpopular minorities, it can fulfil a significant democratic function (e.g. Mantouvalou, 2011, p. 125).

Finally, we have already alluded to the possibility that social rights activism can have unintended effects and may even fuel inequalities. This is a criticism that can be aimed at such judicial decision-making as results from such activism, though it is as much a criticism of unequal access to the courts, which can result in sharp-elbowed middle classes using the courts to secure access to public goods and services unavailable to their poorer compatriots: an issue of recent concern, for example, in countries such as Brazil and Columbia (Piovesan, 2008; Landau & Dixon, 2019). The extension of the provision for collective complaints and class actions has a part to play in this respect (see below). Nevertheless, whatever the limitations of the remedies available through judicial scrutiny, litigation can be a means of providing a voice to the voiceless. Though Schiengold (1974/2004) had once dismissed as a 'myth' the very idea that social rights can be defined or realised through the pursuit of legal enforcement, he nevertheless conceded that recourse to litigation and individual rights can be a *tactic* within a broader mobilisation for change. It continues to be argued that in the field of social rights:

> Litigation is a political act and can have multiple consequences for policy, politics and perceptions. As far as possible, it is important that advocates are oriented to maximising broader impacts as much as compliance in individual cases.
>
> *(Langford et al., 2017, p. 35)*

The juridification debate has generated a great deal of heat, but its importance lies in the light it casts on those mechanisms of redress that are available in relation to social rights matters.

Levels of 'redress'

We therefore turn to relevant rights of redress. Rights of redress in themselves have a long history, and to tell a chronological story of their relationship with social rights, we would need to revert to the beginnings of the capitalist welfare state. In this instance, however, it is more sensible to consider social rights in a global context and to consider the different levels at which redress may be sought. The human rights framework has provided supranational monitoring mechanisms; nation-states have provided a variety of mechanisms for judicial supervision through the courts; and finally, given the peculiar nature of social rights, there is also, apart from the courts, a myriad of specialised, quasi- or non-judicial administrative mechanisms of redress.

International mechanisms

The effective cornerstone of social rights within the international human rights framework is the ICESCR of 1966 (Craven, 1995; Hunt, 1996; Ikawan, 2020). Chapter 4 in this volume draws attention to two fundamental differences between the ICESCR and its sister document, the ICCPR. Firstly, the latter required state parties immediately to take steps to ensure that their constitutional and legislative arrangements complied with the covenant; the former required that countries take steps within their available resources progressively to realise compliance with the covenant; we are therefore forever waiting for the realisation of social rights (Young, 2019). Secondly, whereas the ICCPR established the Human Rights Committee, an independent body of experts, to oversee the implementation of the covenant and receive complaints about violations, the ICESCR entrusted oversight to the standing

UN body, the Economic and Social Council (ECOSOC), composed of government representatives, a responsibility that ECOSOC initially delegated to a Sessional Working Group. It was not until 1985 that ECOSOC appointed a specialist committee of independent experts (prominent lawyers and human rights specialists), the Committee on Economic, Social and Cultural Rights (CESCR), to function in parallel with the Human Rights Committee.

The CESCR receives quinquennial reports from state parties as to their progress in realising social rights. The reports are subject to pre-sessional scrutiny, followed by plenary discussion with state representatives. The Committee is empowered to undertake missions to visit countries in the event that it should wish further to investigate particular concerns, as occurred twice in the 1990s in the case of alleged housing rights violations in Panama and the Dominican Republic. The Committee seeks to characterise its engagement with state parties as a 'constructive dialogue' (Hunt, 1996, p. 20). Since 1992, the Committee has invited submissions from NGOs in order that they might contribute to its deliberations, but the response from NGOs has been described as 'disappointing' (Hunt, 1996, p. 234). Nevertheless, in 2008, following a process of consultation and debate that had gone on for 18 years, an Optional Protocol to the ICESCR was adopted to allow the Committee to consider individual complaints or communications by or on behalf of persons aggrieved by violations of social rights. The Protocol finally came into force in 2013 (Langford et al., 2016). It has an advisory jurisdiction, with the power to express views and make recommendations but not to make directly enforceable orders against state parties. It is able to issue General Comments as to the interpretation of state parties' obligations under the ICESCR, and though these represent a form of jurisprudence, they do not have the status of case law.

The 'linchpin' (Craven, 1995, p. 107) of the ICESCR and, arguably, its critical weakness, is the progressive realisation principle contained in Article 2 and already alluded to above. The International Commission of Jurists has twice convened groups of experts to consider the meaning and scope of Article 2, giving rise to the promulgation in 1986, of the Limburg Principles and in 1996 the Maastricht Guidelines (both are reproduced as appendices in Eide et al., 2001). The Limberg Principles are broadly reflected in the CESCR's General Comment No. 3 of 1991, which sought to define the core obligations of state parties to ensure minimal essential levels of social provision, the widest possible enjoyment of such provision as can be achieved and that particular attention be paid to the needs of vulnerable members of society. The subsequent Maastricht Guidelines included a call for lawyers, judges and the legal community generally to 'pay far greater attention' to violations of social rights (paragraph 28). The principle that social rights are to be progressively realised signals that social rights may not in practice be inviolable; it is a principle born of political pragmatism, not legal exactitude.

And yet the legal community has laboured valiantly to provide a coherent understanding of the principle (Alston & Quinn, 1987; Langford & King, 2008). But, harking back to the justiciability debate, one can see that critics might object that in the process, the lawyers have rather taken ownership of the principle and its interpretation (Gearty, 2011).

This is the context in which three regional supranational systems of adjudication in relation to social rights have also developed, each instituted under the terms of one of the three regional charters identified in Chapter 3 of this volume. The Council of Europe, under the Social Charter of 1961, created the European Committee of Social Rights with parallel functions to the UN's CESCR (Conant, 2010; Chenwi, 2020). The Charter was revised in 1996 to include provision for collective complaints from trade unions and NGOs regarding alleged social rights violations. The complaints procedure eventually came into force in 2007, and the Committee has, for example, considered complaints on behalf of Roma minorities and disability groups (Harris, 2009), but, like the CESCR, it lacks the power to make binding judgements. Nevertheless, the Social Charter's sister document, the European Convention on Human Rights of 1950, had constituted the European Court of Human Rights (ECHR). The ECHR ostensibly has jurisdiction only in civil and political rights matters but has on occasions ruled in matters where social rights could be 'read across' from civil rights: the so-called 'integrated approach' explained in Table 10.2 (Palmer, 2007; Mantouvalou, 2011). Additionally,

TABLE 10.2 Illustrations of the 'integrated approach': reading across from civil rights to social rights

The civil right:	*Potential relevance to social rights:*
• to life itself	• where – in extreme circumstances – a person is systematically denied any means of livelihood
• of equality between men and women	• where men and women may be treated differently with regard to social benefits (for example, carers' allowances or pensions)
• to protection against inhumane or degrading treatment	• where, for example, asylum seekers or prisoners are denied the means of basic subsistence or necessary healthcare
• to private and family life	• where a person is denied the means to maintain themself independently of others and/or the opportunity to share an adequate home with members of their family

Note

These are loosely based on specific legal cases cited in jurisprudential literature referenced throughout this chapter, but it is important to stress that they are drawn from diverse civil rights jurisdictions – both national and supranational – and are based on unique and often complex individual circumstances, which cannot here be fully explained. These should therefore be regarded as illustrative instances, not as statements of universal principle.

elements of the European Social Charter have been incorporated into the European Union's Charter of Fundamental Rights of 1989 and 2000 (later incorporated in a protocol to the Lisbon Treaty of 2009), in relation to which the European Court of Justice has jurisdiction.

The other two regional supranational systems are those relating to the American Convention on Human Rights of 1969 (and its Additional Protocol of San Salvador) and the African Charter of Human and People's Rights of 1981. The former is overseen by the Organisation of American States' Inter-American Commission on Human Rights and the Inter-American Court on Human Rights, and the latter by the Organisation of African States' African Commission on Human Rights and the African Court on Human Rights (Chenwi, 2020). In each instance, the Commission was entrusted, broadly speaking, with an advisory jurisdiction and the Court with an adjudicative role. In the African context, this is further complicated by the intersecting jurisdiction of the African Union's Court of Justice (now set to be superseded by the African Court of Justice and Human Rights). It has been suggested that 'the needs of the peoples of Africa seem to have been rather lost in the designing of successive frameworks of ever grander human rights architecture' (Gearty, 2011, p. 45).

Some of the supranational bodies identified above have made important contributions to the interpretation and development of social rights. They are, however, remote from the everyday workings of rights workers and the everyday experiences of the world's most vulnerable people. Additionally, treaty-related complaints procedures can only be implemented against countries that are full parties to the relevant treaty and such protocols as may apply. There is insufficient scope in this book to detail the many instances of countries which have not signed or ratified social rights treaties, or the related protocols relating to complaints procedures, or which have done so subject to reservations. Significantly, some established welfare states are not full parties to all such treaties and protocols. For example, neither the UK nor the US have signed the Optional Protocol to the ICESCR; the UK had, in any event, opted out of the social rights Protocol to the EU. The Lisbon Treaty has since left the EU and has not signed up to the complaint procedure under the Council of Europe's revised Social Charter; the US never fully ratified the American Convention on Human Rights and is not a party to the social rights provisions of the San Salvador Protocol. Though it was, paradoxically, a US President and his widow (Franklyn and Eleanor Roosevelt) who were so vitally instrumental in ensuring the incorporation of social rights into the international human rights framework, the US has consistently resisted attempts to make such rights binding (Sunstein, 2005).

The Human Rights Commission, whose oversight extended to all the rights proclaimed in the UDHR, had operated a confidential complaints procedure until it was superseded by the Human Rights Council (HRC) in 2006.

BOX 10.1 UN SPECIAL RAPPORTEURS WITH SOCIAL RIGHTS-RELATED RESPONSIBILITIES

- Special Rapporteur on adequate housing as a component of the right to an adequate standard of living
- Special Rapporteur on the right to education
- Special Rapporteur on extreme poverty and human rights
- Special Rapporteur on the right to food
- Special Rapporteur on the right of everyone to the enjoyment of the highest attainable standard of physical and mental health
- Special Rapporteur on the human right to safe drinking water and sanitation

The Council operates an open complaints and representations procedure, which may encompass complaints that cannot otherwise be addressed to a treaty body or similar regional complaints procedure in the field of human rights. However, the Council is concerned to investigate only such cases as appear to reveal a consistent pattern of gross and reliably attested violations of human rights. The Council also has the power to appoint and receive reports from Special Rapporteurs (OHCHR, 2013), Independent Experts and Working Groups who may report to the HRC. This provides a non-judicial mechanism for promoting social rights, and there are currently several Special Rapporteurs with investigative responsibilities in specific social rights-related fields (see Box 10.1). In 2006, the HRC introduced a process of Universal Periodic Review (see www.ohchr.org/en/hrbodies/upr/pages/BasicFacts/aspx) under which, at four-yearly intervals, UN member states are required to submit for critical examination national reports relating to their compliance with human rights obligations. Human rights bodies and NGOs have the opportunity to submit independent reports as a part of the Periodic Review process, providing yet another avenue by which failures to respect, protect or fulfil social rights may be highlighted.

National courts

It will be clear from our discussion of the justiciability debate that the role of the courts in relation to social rights has been controversial, and, unsurprisingly, there is considerable variation between countries as to the extent to which courts can or do in practice engage with social rights matters. The basis of a court's jurisdiction may depend on whether social rights arise from a national constitution or from specific social legislation. And, in either case, the role of the courts in interpreting social rights may vary depending on legal traditions (e.g. whether a country operates with a predominantly common-law or a civil/codified law system). The account that follows is general and much simplified: it will mention the role of constitutional courts on the one hand and ordinary courts on the other and will offer a brief discussion of judicial discretion.

Most countries have a written constitution, though a few (including the United Kingdom) do not. Most national constitutions incorporate at least some social rights, such as the right to education, but the inclusion of a comprehensive range of social rights is rare (Jung et al., 2013). Of those constitutions that include social rights, there is a distinction to be drawn between, on the one hand, those that regard them as aspirational or express them to be 'directive principles' (e.g. India and Ireland) and, on the other, those that explicitly provide for the justiciability of social rights (e.g. South Africa and Finland). Broadly speaking, post-communist and Latin American countries are rather more likely than Western European and North American countries to make social rights justiciable, though there appears to be little by way of regional norms in other parts of the world. Several developing countries have established separate constitutional courts to adjudicate on alleged constitutional violations (Gargarella et al., 2006; Gauri & Brinks, 2008), but in other jurisdictions, it may fall to a supreme court to oversee the interpretation and observance of the constitution. And in Germany, for example, there is a specialist Federal Social Court to oversee the provision for social rights specifically provided under the national constitution.

Social rights, however, are the rights of everyday life, and it is in the ordinary courts that they are likely most frequently to surface. Long before the concept of social rights was established, courts of law exercised a role in relation to dealings between employers and employees, or landlords and tenants, that had a bearing on what we might now identify as the social rights of the employees or tenants. In capitalist welfare states, this has continued, albeit subject to social legislation that may have developed, modified or circumscribed the workings of the law or conferred particular responsibilities on the courts. In some instances, as we shall see, specialist areas of jurisdiction have been removed or withheld from the courts and conferred on quasi-judicial or administrative bodies or tribunals. Nevertheless, the decisions of these bodies and tribunals will usually remain subject to appeal or review by the courts. And in liberal democratic societies, decisions by administrative and executive bodies ought in any event to be susceptible to judicial review, whether governed by prerogative or constitutional convention.

From a positivist perspective, the fundamental significance of rights is that they are ostensibly determinate. The significance of social rights as conceptualised by Marshall was that they constituted the transition from the Poor Law to the modern welfare state, from capricious charity to guaranteed support, from discretionary poor relief to defined rights. In practice, however, social rights are seldom rigidly defined. Specified as human rights, they are loosely defined, as we have seen. Specified as rights of citizenship, they may appear to be precisely defined, but however exactly framed a statute or regulation they might seem to be, they will always (as discussed in Chapter 6 of this volume) leave some space for discretion as to its implementation or interpretation. This is the space within which administrative and judicial decision-makers alike may exercise their power. In the judicial context, they may have room to decide whether or not to intervene in response to a complaint or else to decide just how a specified right is to be interpreted.

We have already seen how in Britain in the 1960s and '70s social rights activists first began to take test-cases before the ordinary courts. The outcomes revealed trends in just how the judiciary exercised its discretionary power. In social security cases, when asked to review the decisions of administrative tribunals, they would decline to intervene in cases of claimants whom they appeared to regard as undeserving, while sympathetically invoking principles of administrative justice in support of claimants whom they appeared to regard as deserving. In housing cases, they used their power to protect property owners against the claims of tenants on the one hand and the interventions of public authorities on the other, while sympathetically defending public authorities against the claims of those whom they appeared to regard as the undeserving homeless (Griffiths, 1997). Nevertheless, there are many examples from around the world where judicial innovation has played an important role in advancing social rights. The 'integrated approach' (see above), whereby judges, when constrained to adjudicate solely on the basis of civil and political rights charters but confronted by social injustice, have read across from those charters in support of social rights (see Table 10.1 above). Such a practice has been important even in the British context, where the Human Rights Act of 1998 'domesticated' the civil and political rights provisions of the European Convention on Human Rights on terms that allowed British courts to comment on whether British laws were compliant (King, 1999; Mantouvalou, 2011, p. 142).

It has been suggested that in the past two decades, social rights jurisprudence has been 'emerging from the shadows' (Langford, 2008, p. 1) and most certainly there is a considerable volume of reported cases from around the world (Langford, et al., 2019). This book is not a legal text, however, and will refrain from citing an array of illustrative cases. But we should mention what has become one of the most celebrated cases, not least because it arose in an era of promise in post-apartheid South Africa. It is known as the Grootboom case, the story of which is told in Box 10.2. The story speaks to a number of issues concerning the role that courts can play, most particularly regarding the limitations imposed by the progressive realisation principle, not just in housing cases but in relation to all social rights.

BOX 10.2 THE GROOTBOOM CASE

[Official Report reference: *Government of the Republic of South Africa and Others v Grootboom and Others* [2000] ZACC 19, 2001 (1) SA 46 (CC), 2000 (11) BCLR 1169 (CC)]

The background

Irene Grootboom lived in Wallacedene, an informal squatter settlement in the eastern suburbs of Cape Town in South Africa. The settlement had been established during the 1980s after a relaxation of the apartheid pass laws made it easier for rural populations to migrate to urban areas. The residents of Wallacedene lived in severe poverty and without basic services. Many Wallacedene residents had their names on a waiting list for low-cost housing. Eventually, a group of about 900 people, including Irene Grootboom, began to move from Wallacedene onto adjacent, vacant, privately-owned land that had been earmarked for low-cost housing. The landowner obtained an eviction order, and the sheriff was ordered to dismantle and remove any of the makeshift structures remaining on the land. The magistrate granting the order said the community and the municipality should negotiate in order to identify alternative land for the community to occupy on a temporary or permanent basis. In 1999, having nowhere to go, the community moved onto the Wallacedene sports field and began to erect temporary structures.

In the high court

With legal assistance, the community demanded that the municipality provide temporary accommodation. In the absence of a satisfactory response, the community – in the name of 'Irene Grootboom and 900 others' – applied to the Cape High Court, arguing firstly that on the basis of the South African Constitution of 1996, everyone had a right of access to adequate housing and the state had a duty to take reasonable measures, within its available resources, to make sure that right was progressively realised; secondly, that under the Constitution their children had an absolute right to shelter. The High Court rejected the first argument, asserting that the government's housing programme was reasonable and fulfilled the requirements of the Constitution. It was conceded, however, that there was an obligation on the state to provide shelter for the children, and it was in the best interests of children that they should not be separated from their families.

In the constitutional court

Unhappy with this decision, the government appealed against it before South Africa's Constitutional Court. Hearing the case afresh in 2000, the Court concluded, unlike the Cape High Court, that, in fact, the government's housing programme had fallen short of the state's obligation to provide relief to people in need and that an insufficient proportion of the national housing budget had been devoted to that purpose. The court's judgement set out the state's obligations to devise and implement a comprehensive and coordinated short-, medium- and long-term programme for the provision of adequate housing, ensuring along the way that this would not exclude any significant segment of society. An order was made in terms then agreed between the parties, by which the national and provincial governments were to provide for the needs of Irene Grootboom and the 390 adults and 510 children in the informal settlement.

The aftermath

It should be noted, however, that the Constitutional Court also ruled that Irene Grootboom had no right to demand immediate housing and, notwithstanding their intolerable living conditions, that the Wallacedene squatters had no right to resort to land invasion, a form of self-help the Court found to be unacceptable. In the event, Irene Grootboom was never rehoused and later left Wallacedene. Eight years later, in 2008, at the age of just 39, she died penniless and living in a shack. It has become an iconic case. Its significance is that it was the first clear ruling by a national constitutional court in support of a claim based on social rights. However, the case also illustrates the limitations of social rights premised on the progressive realisation principle. Irene Grootboom, despite the fame the case brought her as a housing rights activist, never benefited from the court's ruling.

Administrative mechanisms

More important still than the courts, perhaps, in terms of their day-to-day impact on people's lives are the various administrative and quasi-judicial mechanisms and procedures by which social rights are, or might be, safeguarded or promoted. Inevitably, there is enormous variation between countries as to the nature and extent of the mechanisms that may be deployed. It is also quite difficult to summarise the different types of redress that may be available. There is a spectrum, ranging from specialised tribunals chaired by lawyers, which are courts in all but name, to processes by which disputed decisions are merely double-checked by administrative officials. However, it is not simply a question of the degree to which a mechanism is legal or administrative in character. It is a question of just how social rights are conceived and where the focus of the procedure lies. A tentative taxonomy of the different forms and mechanisms of redress is presented in Table 10.3. It may be seen

TABLE 10.3 Forms of administrative redress

Conception of rights	*Focus of redress*	*Form of redress*	*Implied status of the individual*	*Typical mechanism of redress*
Doctrinal	Obligations of the state	Appeal	Juridical subject	Tribunal (quasi-judicial forum)
	Demands of the individual	Personal complaint	Heroic consumer	Complaints procedure (managerial process)
Claims-based	Obligations of the state	Petitionary complaint	Aggrieved citizen	Ombudsperson (*or* public forum)
	Demands of the individual	Review	Passive client	Case committee/Panel (*or* supervisory check)

that this draws on the distinction initially explained in Chapter 2 between doctrinal and claims-based conceptions of rights and, on the other hand, a distinction between procedures which are focused on the obligations of the state as opposed to those focused on the demands of the individual. The resulting model draws out the different ways in which the form of redress and the status of the individual may be constituted. The specific mechanisms or fora for redress may be variously described, using terms such as 'tribunal', 'ombudsperson', 'complaints procedure' or 'case committee', though such terms can be applied to quite differently formulated mechanisms. The object, however, is to explore the underlying logic informing such generic processes of redress as may develop within established administrative structures.

Redress in the form of an *appeal* is premised on a doctrinal conception of rights and a concern that the state should properly meet its obligations. The individual is constituted as a juridical subject, and the classic forum or mechanism is a tribunal, which may or may not be chaired by a lawyer but which performs a formal function that is quasi-judicial. Tribunals can also be introduced for the social regulation of private disputes (e.g. between employees and employers, or between tenants and landlords) and case-review committees (such as those that might deal, for example, with school admissions appeals) that do not necessarily operate under formal adjudicative procedures and may be mis-described as tribunals. But our particular concern is with tribunals that adjudicate on claims against the state. This can briefly be illustrated with reference to the development of social security tribunals in Britain, a process that began with the introduction of unemployment insurance in 1911. The concern at that time was that the ordinary courts had proved themselves to be ill-suited to the handling of industrial injury claims brought against employers by unrepresented workers and that a different sort of adjudicative forum was required. The government introduced a three-member 'Court of Referees' chaired by a lawyer but sitting with lay trades-unions and local business representatives. The sporting nomenclature symbolised the patronising assumption that this would be received by the working classes as a mechanism to ensure 'fair play' on terms they would understand (Wraith & Hutchinson, 1973). In the 1930s, another tribunal was introduced to adjudicate on social assistance benefits for unemployed people, though the government's motive for this was to provide a safety valve that might deflect public resentment against the increasingly unpopular household means-test associated with the benefit (Lynes, 1975). Tribunals for the adjudication of different benefits thereafter proliferated, but were then, by stages, consolidated and increasingly 'judicialised' as social security law became ever more complex (Leggatt, 2001; Thomas & Genn, 2013). What this story illustrates is an enduring tension between the need for accessible redress and a desire for technical rigour.

Redress in the form of a *petitionary complaint* is premised on a claims-based conception of rights but, once again, a concern that the state should properly meet its obligations. The individual is constituted as an aggrieved citizen, and the classic remedy is that of an ombudsperson. The mechanism is petitionary in the sense that it entails a process by which public attention may be drawn to a grievance, and it is possible for other forms of public or democratic community forum through which to channel disapproval or demands for a 'social response' (McCarthy et al., 1992; Mulcahy & Lloyd-Bostock, 1992). Such instances – though seemingly rare in practice – may at least approach something akin to a form of social reparation. The formal ombudsperson, however, had its origins in Scandinavian tradition, dating back more than two centuries (Stacey, 1978). It was a model based on the idea of a people's champion, specifically empowered to challenge state authority using investigatory powers, allowing them to 'dig where the courts and tribunals cannot trespass' (Lewis & Birkinshaw, 1993, p. 78). The substantive process, unlike that before a tribunal, is not adversarial but entirely inquisitorial. In the Nordic tradition, ombudspersons have been allowed to point up systemic weaknesses in policy and administration and propose improvements. The ombudsperson model – or at least the 'ombudsman' term or label – has been adopted in various forms by governments around the world (in Australia, Austria, Canada, France, New Zealand and the United Kingdom) and, incidentally, within different private business sectors as part of a variety of both voluntary and regulatory schemes. It can be applied in a social rights context as a mechanism for challenges to government departments and agencies in respect of social security, health and social care, education and housing. It is rare, however, for it to be implemented on terms that live up to the Nordic ideal. For example, in the case of the UK's Parliamentary Commissioner for Administration (a sort of ombudsperson), they can only be accessed through a citizen's MP, can only investigate restrictively defined instances of 'maladministration' (rather than substantive decisions), and have no power to enforce their public recommendations. The effectiveness of any ombudsperson scheme or public complaints forum depends largely on the willingness of governments to allow themselves to be subject to such scrutiny.

Redress in the form of a *personal complaint* is premised on a doctrinal conception of rights and a concern with satisfying or appeasing the demands of the individual. The individual is constituted as a 'heroic consumer' (Warde, 1994), and the classic remedy is a formal complaint procedure. The process is informed by managerialist doctrine that regards citizens as potentially vocal consumers of social services, the provision of which may be regarded as a business like any other (see Chapter 2, this volume). Customer grievances must be turned into complaints, and the information they generate must be regarded as a management tool by which to enhance the efficacy of the service (Pfeffer & Coote, 1991). Staff in health and social care, social security and educational institutions must share the mission of the institution and must be trained to deal proactively and expeditiously with complaints, to disarm aggrieved consumers and to ensure the institution's mission is achieved. The doctrinal fiction on which this depends assumes parity of power between welfare professionals and administrators on the one hand and their potentially vulnerable or disadvantaged patients, clients, claimants, parents or students on the other. And it assumes that the latter are 'consumers' through 'choice' rather than necessity. The object is more akin to the satisfaction of civil rights than the fulfilment of social rights. The trend towards the development of formal complaints procedures is characteristic of the managerial trend to which capitalist welfare states have lately been subject. Such procedures can be sophisticated in design and entail, for example, specialist staff and independently chaired complaints panels. In the British case, complaints procedures, particularly in relation to health and social care provision, have become increasingly complex and fragmented following reforms aimed at driving competitive local commissioning, such that at the time of writing one watchdog had declared the system to be 'utterly bewildering' (Healthwatch England, 2014). The effectiveness of individual complaint procedures in the social rights context is potentially limited if the focus is on the resolution or containment of the complaints rather than the satisfaction of complainants' needs (Brewer, 2007).

Redress in the form of a *review* is premised on a claims-based conception of rights and, once again, a concern with satisfying or appeasing the demands of the individual. The individual is constituted as a passive client or helpless supplicant, and the remedy might be a case committee or review panel, or failing that, some kind of administrative double check. The internal review represents the oldest means by which administrative review may be sought. In the days before the modern welfare state, the recipients of poor relief, like the eponymous hero of Charles Dickens novel, *Oliver Twist*, might dare to ask for more or to have their cases looked at again. Where elements of discretion persist in relation to the provision of social assistance or social care, it may still be common practice for case conferences, committees or panels to review the cases of clients who express dissatisfaction. Even where citizens have rights to social assistance, medical treatment, education, social care or re-housing, the form this takes may very well entail the exercise of discretion and deliberation, not with regard to a client's entitlement but the most appropriate form of help, treatment or placement. Where funds for particular forms of relief, facilities for particular kinds of treatment or care, or places in particular schools or types of housing are subject to budgetary limits or practical constraints, special panels may need to consider or perhaps re-consider to whom these should go. And even when rules of entitlement to a social benefit may be clear, if no right of appeal to an independent tribunal is provided, it is to be expected that some form of internal process of administrative or supervisory review of the facts of a case might be undertaken. The extension and development of social rights, even within the most developed welfare states, do not extinguish the use of such mechanisms, though of course the quality and consistency of the resultant decision-making will always be problematic and subject to challenge. In such circumstances, front-line welfare professionals and administrators, as decision-makers, become *ad hoc* policy-makers rather than rights adjudicators (Lipsky, 1980/2010).

CONCLUSION

This book has been concerned with the part played by social rights in promoting human welfare and has from the outset situated this concern in relation to an understanding of human **sociality**. Sociality represents a constitutive characteristic of the human species, albeit in the context of *Homo sapiens*' other defining characteristics. Human beings are possessed of a distinctive form of **consciousness** by which thinking is coterminous with being and entails a unique or particular sense of selfhood. And yet the individual self cannot be wholly autonomous, since human beings are of necessity socially interdependent; their welfare depends on their capacity not only to care for one another but also to **work** together. Work entails conscious and creative interaction with the natural environment and with other human beings, by which the species not only sustains itself but also socially evolves, and by which thereby human **history** is made.

Social rights have thus been presented as an expression of sociality – an expression that embraces, yet reaches beyond, the love expressed in intimate human relationships and the solidarity expressed in communal human activity. Social rights can articulate human needs at a wider institutional level. This book has introduced two rather different ways in which our understanding of social rights has come about. An explicit concept of social rights first crystallised with the development of capitalist welfare states in the global North and through an account of this process furnished – after the event – by T.H. Marshall. Marshall suggested that social rights had emerged as the culmination of the story by which modern citizenship had evolved. Social rights were a tangible product of capitalist development; we had *made* them. A related but differently inflected concept of social rights crystallised on the international stage as the world emerged from the second of the two world wars that had occurred during the first half of the twentieth century. Social rights, it was decided, were an essential component of our human rights, and they are necessary to peace and social order; we had *discovered* them.

The alternative argument in this book has been that social rights may be understood as articulations of human need. Human beings are and have always been both needy and social. By socially negotiating the ways in which together we satisfy our needs, we constitute customary expectations, practices and beliefs. Insofar as we can construct the claims we make upon one another through a discourse of rights and shared responsibilities, we might recognise that we have always had social rights. Their existence is neither the unique achievement of capitalist civilisation nor a revelatory insight of twentieth-century policymakers, jurists and ethicists. But having invented a discourse of rights, we have extended it to encompass the evolving processes by which human beings articulate and claim mutual recognition of each other's needs. It is a conflicted and elusive discourse on the one hand, but an evolving and powerful one on the other. Gathering together some of the unfinished threads from previous chapters, this chapter will consider the future of social rights as meaningful and effective social constructs.

The chapter will return to a critique of the Marshallian concept of social citizenship and argue for a more open understanding of the chaotic, multi-layered processes by which social rights may be constructed or negotiated. And it will return to a critique of the dominant human rights paradigm by which social rights are held to be progressively realisable and argue that as an approach to the recognition of human vulnerability, it is not sufficient. Advancing the case for a new humanist perspective which takes account of the existential challenges facing the human species. It will reconsider the significance of social rights as an expression of sociality and the part they may play in fashioning the welfare and history of the human species.

A post-Marshallian theory of social rights

Informing much of this book and other recent work by this author is what might be described as a post-Marshallian concept or account of social rights. It is post-Marshallian firstly, in the sense that it has a different story to tell than that told by Marshall; secondly, because it recognises social rights as contested outcomes of negotiation and struggle; thirdly, because we live increasingly in a post-national or global era to which the Marshallian account is no longer fully suited.

A different story: the rootedness of social rights in human sociality

It was argued in Chapter 1 of this volume that the character of human sociality not only marks human beings out from other species but also defines the conscious identity of every member of the species and the basis on which human beings recognise and communicate with each other. Sociality is a part of what defines being human. However, it will be evident that the form, depth and orientation of human sociality may vary over time and in different historical contexts. Human interdependency can be negotiated in different ways. Human individuals may be constrained or enabled to be more or less self-sufficient or more or less mutually supportive.

Social rights have been, and will most certainly remain, central to social policy. They are articulated through social policy and are framed legally through national constitutions and/or politically by social legislation. The 'Stone Age Economics' (Sahlins, 1974; and see Chapter 1, this volume) of pre-historic hunter-gathering societies determined how to align wants with means. But clearly such societies contrived customs and practices (implicit policies and immanent processes) by which they organised how resources should be shared, how their members should care for each other and who should look to whom for what. Douglas and Ney (1998) make the point that contemporary social scientific analysis can be paradoxically asocial: the whole person, as the locus of human transactions and the creator of meaning, goes missing! It is a charge that can be laid against Marshall, for whom social rights were primarily administrative rather than social constructs. The issue is expressed in similar terms by Isin et al. (2008) when they speak of 'recasting the social in citizenship'.

If we are now to think about social rights and social citizenship differently, we should accept that the origins of social rights lie deep in human history. Before they were ever constituted through the language of rights, they were immanently present, albeit masked, for example, by beliefs in magic or mediated by tradition and religious imperatives. They have been and are now negotiated or 'disputed' (see Clarke et al., 2014) in all sorts of different ways, at diverse sites and at a multiplicity of levels.

Negotiation and struggle

Negotiation is a fundamental component of everyday life and 'communicative action' (Habermas, 1987). However, the negotiation of rights can take place at a variety of levels and in the context of differing relations of power. It may occur in the context of intimate personal and familial relationships or at the level of high-powered international diplomacy. It may be informally governed through relations of trust or formally circumscribed by rules of procedure. It can be instigated by bottom-up demands, or by top-down imposition; by popular resistance, or by governmental intervention. Negotiation is the warp and weft of social existence. It is by no means confined to face-to-face dialogue, explicit argument or political debate but can take the form of subtly waged battles for hearts, minds or for popular approval;

of struggles for hegemonic ascendancy between dominant and subaltern discourses (Gramsci, 1971); of artful strategies of resistance (Scott, 1985). Negotiation is axiomatically a dialogic and dialectical process, though it may be more or less powerfully directed or shaped by hegemonic frames of reference.

The idea that social rights may be understood as 'sites of social struggle' or 'sites of dialogue' is prefigured, for example, by Nedelsky and Scott (1992, p. 62). In part, this is a reaffirmation of the argument that all rights are socially constructed (e.g. Scheingold, 1974/2004; Waters, 1996; Travers, 2010). Nedelsky and Scott, however, presciently affirmed the specific argument that is central to this book, namely that social rights are the means by which we structure relationships of interdependency: they are 'rights in relationship' (1992, p. 69). Such dialogue can take place at an infinite variety of sites, within and between households, communities, nations and global institutions. It can entail 'conversations' between combinations of individual actors and collective actors. At one level, a subsistence farmer (perhaps with the assistance of a community elder) may, through dialogue, establish customary rights for members of their household to access a water source on a neighbour's land. At another level, the rights of HIV/AIDS sufferers to antiretroviral drug treatment may be developed through a 'constructive constitutional conversation' between the judiciary and the government – as occurred in the celebrated case of *Cruz Bermudez v. Ministerio de Sanidad y Asistencia Social* (1999) before the Venezuelan Supreme Court (discussed, for example, in O'Mathúna et al., 2005). Such an approach is encapsulated in the case made by Roberto Gargarella (2015) as a quest for 'dialogic justice'. At a global level, complex multi-party negotiations may entail conversations across the boundaries of conflicting orthodoxies (between, for example, the characteristically utilitarian Washington Consensus perception of the World Bank and the more characteristically universalist perception of the ILO).

We might reflect upon different ways in which humans embrace, tolerate or resist the social arrangements around them. A classic account of the 'social bases of obedience and revolt' has been provided by Barrington Moore, who endeavoured through an insightful anthropological and social historical analysis to tease out recurring elements in the 'moral codes' (Moore, 1978, ch. 1) by which all human societies have sought – whether successfully or unsuccessfully – internally to co-ordinate the exercise of authority, the division of labour and the distribution of resources. His central observation is that hitherto every social order has both beneficiaries and victims, and for a social order to be sustainable, its victims must apparently submit to a form of 'social anaesthesia'. Moore's chosen task was that of determining 'how people awake from anaesthesia, how they overcome a sense of inevitability and how a sense of injustice may take its place' (1978, pp. 460–461). Along the way, however, he throws out a number of hints about how human beings accommodate different notions of justice. Table 11.1 is loosely informed by

TABLE 11.1 Popular notions of social justice and correlated perceptions of social rights

Notions of social justice	Correlated perceptions of social rights
People will accommodate an unequal distribution of resources in society, *provided* it is in the context of:	
Just reward People must be persuaded there is broad equality of reward in proportion to skill, effort and achievement.	*Utilitarian.* Social rights assure **my best interests.** The rights claimed are rights to equal chances and 'fair' rather than equal outcomes; to guaranteed opportunities and equal treatment; albeit with a reliable social safety net in case of misfortune.
Just restraint People must be persuaded that nobody is hoarding scarce resources or free loading.	*Survivalist.* Social rights assure that **I can get by**. This reflects what Moore (1978, p. 38) characterises as the 'dog in the manger taboo'. The rights it claims are ambiguously 'social', since their priority is to preserve the habits by which the individual survives and ensure that the individual should not be disadvantaged by the greed of others.
Just advantage People must be persuaded that those with power and privilege fulfil their proper obligations.	*Communitarian.* Social rights assure that, through ordered social cohesion, **we can get by**. Moore makes the point that in a hierarchical society, 'A secure but lowly status is much easier to bear than no position at all ... [because] ... the individual can trade obedience and loyalty for security if the relationship has some colour of justice and affection' (1978, p. 463). The advantage of those with wealth and high status is just or tolerable so long as they observe the principles of *noblesse oblige* and their responsibilities to the poor.
Just shares People must be persuaded that risks and responsibilities are equally shared.	*Universalist.* Social rights, by systematic means, assure **our collective wellbeing**, reflecting a more substantive understanding of equality and a concern for optimal human welfare. It is consistent with a rule of equality characterised by Moore (1978, p. 38) as 'a form of general social insurance against misfortune'. [**Note:** however, as explained in Chapters 7 and 8 of this volume, social insurance-based rights do not necessarily guarantee universal risk sharing, though their coverage can be extended in that direction, as has been achieved, for example, in Nordic welfare states.]

Moore's argument and suggests how popular notions of social justice might equate with or support the ideal-typical perceptions of social rights outlined in Figure 5.1 in this volume, each of which is imbued with a different logic and normative underpinning. As human societies became more complex and unequal, human sociality has come to be expressed in terms of very different aspirations and notions of social justice.

Marshall's theory of social rights was premised on a conception of citizenship within a democratic welfare capitalist state. A post-Marshallian conception of social rights should contend not only with the competing perceptions characterised in Table 11.1 and the reality that even within capitalist welfare states social rights are negotiated and realised in a multiplicity of ways, but it must also acknowledge the extent to which social rights are or should not necessarily be conditional on the citizenship of a nation-state. If it is accepted that social rights are the outcome of struggles to achieve recognition for human needs, it may be grasped firstly that this is a *continuous* struggle that occurs at a variety of sites and levels, and it is likely that it will sometimes give rise to rights that are objectively suboptimal or unsustainable; secondly, that it is a *dynamic* struggle, and it is unlikely that the form and substance of the rights that emerge will conform or even approximate to just one of the ideal-type perceptions outlined in Table 11.1. It might nevertheless be supposed that a 'just shares' notion of social justice and a 'universalist' perspective come closest to Marshall's own ideal of institutionalised social rights. And it has been seen (see Chapter 2, this volume) that the organised labour movement and social democratic political parties have played a role in demanding and shaping social rights in this mould.

Methodological premises

The Marshallian conception of social citizenship can be transcended in order to account for social rights as a global human phenomenon, and it has been noted in Chapter 4 of this volume that overlapping notions of 'cosmopolitan' or 'global' citizenship have already entered emerging debates about universalist forms of inclusive citizenship in a post-national context. The universalism favoured by advocates of more 'generous' or inclusive social-democratic welfare state regimes in the global North may be described as *cosmopolitan* in an overarching 'methodological sense' (Beck, 1992, 2003). Universality is equated with an acknowledgement of social diversity and the principle of equality of recognition of individuals, regardless of age, gender, family or occupational status. A cosmopolitan methodological perspective begins potentially to blur the boundaries between citizenship rights and human rights. Arguing from an explicitly cosmopolitan outlook, Robert Fine revisits critiques of the human rights agenda that draw a strict distinction between top-down rights as imperialistic instruments of social control and redemptive bottom-up rights as instruments of emancipation, arguing that in reality 'everything interesting occurs in the in-between' (Fine, 2007, p. 141). This would seem to chime with the contention that substantive social rights may be forged at the points where competing perspectives collide. This has already been illustrated in the discussion of refugee rights in Chapter 9 of this volume.

The reality, however, is that practical thinking around social rights – even from a cosmopolitan perspective – remains mired in 'methodological nationalism'. That term has been coined by Wimmer and Schiller (2002) and alludes to a tendency to assume that 'the nation-state is the natural social and political form of the modern world'. This tendency remains more or less implicit even, for example, among ardent advocates of universality such as those who focus on the potential for Universal Basic Income and/or Universal Basic Services schemes (Torry, 2018; Sloman et al., 2021; and see, e.g., https://basicincome.org; Social Prosperity Network, 2017; Gough, 2019). Some leading campaigners prefer explicitly to frame Basic Income as a 'Citizen's Income' on the premise that it is through the citizenship of a state that entitlement should unconditionally arise. Some purely experimental BI schemes in the global South have been implemented in smaller provincial or village localities (e.g. Haarman & Haarman, 2012), and some BI advocates have argued – albeit to no effect – for a pan-European EU Citizen's Income (see Dean, 2018). Nonetheless, the prevailing assumption is that basic income and public services are, or are most likely in practice to be, rights of citizenship. Implicitly, it is assumed that national citizenship takes a form that was established in the Westphalian era (i.e. following the Treaty of Westphalia of 1648, briefly mentioned in Chapter 2 of this volume, which established the principle of national sovereignty). That form of citizenship developed in the capitalist global North and was, in part at least, bequeathed to the global South during the colonial era and, thereafter, by way of international aid conditions (e.g. Mamdani, 1996; and see earlier discussion of the 'cultural critique' in Chapter 9, this volume).

Bridget Anderson (2020), citing the case of the Roma people as a racialised minority group across Europe, argues for what she calls 'methodological de-nationalism', a switch with relevance for other transnational ethnic minorities, wider diasporic communities, migrants and refugees. But what perhaps is warranted is a broader and deeper methodological humanism, by which social rights may be construed as an essential manifestation of human sociality. The narrative account of the 'unnatural' development of the human species with which this book began sketched out the part played by global processes of human migration and colonisation. That process led to the creation of social divisions and more or less arbitrary geographical boundaries, culminating in the invention of the sovereign nation-state as the basis of the form of citizenship upon which the nationalist methodological framework and the realisation of social rights currently depend. The process of globalisation that began towards the end of the twentieth century (e.g. Held & McGrew, 2007) and which supposedly portended a new post-Westphalian era (Fraser, 2008) may have changed the context in which nation-states function, but it has not eliminated the constraints their existence impose on human development and on the scope for universal social rights.

The humanist approaches to social development identified in Chapter 4 of this volume clearly embody an element of methodological humanism insofar as they identify poverty, whether in the global South or the global North, as a violation of human rights and therefore a global concern. And it is to social rights as human rights that we must now return.

Humanising the social rights agenda

To further an understanding of social rights as an essential element of human sociality, it is necessary firstly, to de-mystify the illusion of individual sovereignty that lies at the heart of the dominant human rights tradition; secondly, to adopt, as suggested, a form of methodological humanism; third, to consider the arguably limited steps by which it may (or may not) be possible to reform the international human rights framework; and finally, to bring a human scale to bear upon the realisation of social rights at the level of everyday human lives.

'Dignity' and the illusion of individual sovereignty

In Chapter 3 of this volume, a distinction was drawn between the dominant and (after Woodiwiss, 2005) the 'minor' traditions in prevailing human rights discourse: the former being essentially individualistic and the latter essentially solidaristic. Central to the dominant tradition is the totemic concept of dignity. The term appears in nearly all international instruments pertaining to human rights. The preamble to the UDHR calls at its outset for the recognition of the 'inherent dignity ... of all members of the human family'. Such recognition may be normatively interpreted as a claim to equal integrity and personal autonomy amidst a family of atomistic, self-seeking individuals, though, potentially, it might also be interpreted as a claim to inclusion and ontological security within a diverse and interdependent human family. It is the former interpretation that overwhelmingly dominates, and in Chapter 3 of this volume, we noted the excoriating critique of Hannah Arendt, for whom the claim to some kind of *inborn* human dignity – if indeed that is what 'inherent' dignity means – is hubris: an 'arrogant myth'.

Arendt's argument needs to be understood in context. Her scholarship revolved around a critical analysis of totalitarianism. The immense significance claimed for the post-second world war human rights agenda was that it could address the rights of stateless persons and those who had been denied citizenship; and, in a fundamental sense, the rights of those whose experiences of war and atrocity had stripped them of their very humanity. Reflecting on such horrors as the Nazi concentration camps, Arendt concluded:

> The assumption of human rights, based upon the assumed existence of a human being as such, broke down at the very moment when those who professed to believe in it were for the first time confronted with people who had indeed lost all other qualities and special relationships - except they were still human. The world saw nothing sacred in the abstract nakedness of being human.
>
> *(1951, p. 295)*

For Arendt, humanity is not an abstract quality; it arises through membership in a concrete political community. Her complaint was that 'Today we consider both history and nature alien to the essence of man' (1951, p. 435). An appeal to inherent or intrinsic human dignity was for her a negation of the reality of the human condition. Paradoxically, although Arendt was supremely critical of Marx, she shared with him the belief that humanity is defined not only by human biology but also essentially by human history and sociality. In different ways, Arendt and Marx each recognised the constitutive character of human interdependence. In both analyses, however, there was some ambiguity as to the place of social rights. Arendt drew a distinction between public rights and private interests (1977); a distinction that, confusingly and perhaps perversely, appears to correspond pretty much to the now familiar distinction between, on the one hand, civil and political rights (which she saw as 'public') and, on the other, social rights (which she saw as 'private') (Parekh, 2008, p. 93). For Arendt, our humanity is defined through participation in the public sphere, while the means by which human beings satisfy their biological needs are seen as a private, not a social, matter. Nevertheless, she conceded that the meeting of what she called private interests is a necessary foundation for the exercise of public freedom and 'public happiness'. Poverty, she argues, must be overcome for the sake of political life (Parekh, 2008, p. 27). There is a sense in which Arendt's conception of the private and public realms equates with the Aristotelian notions of hedonic wellbeing (private existence) and eudaimonic wellbeing (public existence) (see Chapters 2 and 3, this volume). The fullness of our humanity is realised through public participation in a political (and axiomatically, therefore, social) community.

This is, up to a point, consistent with an alternative definition of dignity: a dignity that is not inherent but achieved. Jones (2012) suggests three broad definitions of dignity: the 'intrinsic' dignity assumed by human rights discourse; the 'attributed' dignity associated with high social status and/or with dignitaries; and the kind of dignity that may be defined on the basis of a virtue ethics approach (see Chapter 5, this volume). Differently inflected versions of the latter view may be seen, for example, in the work of MacIntyre (1999) or Harris (1997). It is a view that looks for dignity in interdependence. Since humans are all vulnerable creatures, there can be as much dignity in receiving as in giving care and support, and a complementarity between awareness of one's human limitations (humility) and one's willingness to help others (compassion). Here we are concerned with everyday virtues, including and especially those associated with a public service ethos; with, for example, the vocational commitment of healthcare professionals and welfare administrators in their dealings with vulnerable individuals; and with the public spiritedness entailed when people take part in public deliberation and lend support to the collective provision of social services. However, this is, perhaps, too tenuous a defence of the use of the word dignity to define a foundational human right. If dignity is a virtue or a spiritual quality, it may be admirable or desirable, but it is not innate. Dignity 'in practice' (Wright et al., 2014, pp. 60–61) is socially constructed and realised or experienced through interdependence and solidarity with others.

Yet we have seen in Chapter 4 that one of the principal justifications for social rights and social development has been that poverty is held to be a violation of human dignity. Relative poverty is widely understood as something more than material deprivation, but in terms of its relational and symbolic aspects: the humiliation, the shame and the loss of dignity with which it is associated (Smith, 1776; Lister, 2004; Walker et al., 2013). Poverty is not an economic phenomenon but a human experience (Boltvinik, forthcoming). Poverty in this sense is a social construct, as are the social rights by which we might lay claim to counter poverty. The right not to be poor can be a right, but it may be argued that it is not best achieved by appeals to inherent dignity. People can be so anaesthetised to suffering that they accept their lot and suffer *with dignity*. As Moore has put it – 'The human capacity to withstand suffering and abuse is impressive, tragically so' (1978, p. 13). The international anti-poverty movement ATD Fourth World, which was mentioned in Chapter 4 of this volume, seeks to promote the dignity of poor people. The ATD acronym originally stood for '*Aide à Toute Détresse*' (help for all in distress), but it has lately been anglicised so as to stand for 'All Together in Dignity'. This was not simply a concession to the forces of linguistic imperialism but an acknowledgement of the movement's philosophy, which focuses on enabling people experiencing poverty to fight stigma and prejudice by establishing a sense of shared dignity. Just as Alcoholics Anonymous requires members publicly to confess their alcoholism, ATD Fourth World requires its members publicly to acknowledge their own poverty. The difference is that alcoholics must struggle throughout their lives to cope with their addiction, but people experiencing poverty should surely be enabled to escape from poverty rather than to find dignity in poverty.

Other social movements have sought to foster not dignity, but indignation. An example is the worldwide Occupy movement that sprang up in opposition to the austerity measures and associated curtailment of social rights following the global financial crisis that began in or about 2008 and whose ramifications rumbled on (Kerton, 2012; Pickerill & Krinsky, 2012). The Spanish wing of that movement was known as *Indignados* (Castañeda, 2012), which translated to English means 'outrage', a name directly influenced by the title of a manifesto entitled *Indignez-Vous* in the original French language edition, by the former resistance fighter, human rights campaigner and supporter of myriad radical causes, Stéphane Hessel (2011). As a loosely networked global movement, Occupy and/or *Indignados* was concerned with a range of discontents within which social rights did not always feature that explicitly, but its potential impact, it might be argued, stemmed from a refusal to suffer with what might conventionally be described as 'dignity'.

Attempts to connect abstract notions of human dignity with the practical business of realising social rights are rather scarce. A notable exception is a thoughtful account provided by Chan & Bowpitt (2005), which is very much concerned with welfare *systems*, rather than with social rights and discourses of rights. For Chan and Bowpitt, human dignity 'resides in our possession of intrinsic capacities which strive for autonomy and mutuality' (2005, p. 22). If human dignity can be said to equate with personal autonomy (Doyal & Gough, 1991), it may be argued that autonomy is not synonymous with sovereign independence and should amount to far more than mere self-sufficiency (Williams, 1999). As for mutuality, it is a slippery concept. It may refer to a narrow utilitarian calculus of reciprocity, rather than to inclusive social relations of interdependency. In Chan and Bowpitt's case, mutuality is addressed in a teleological manner by drawing on classic psychological literature (specifically, Bowlby, 1969) to demonstrate that social interaction is *necessary* for personal development and self-identity, whereas Tomasello (2021; and see discussion in Chapter 1 of this volume) suggests a more dynamic understanding of the association between ontogenetic *sociality* and individual *sociability*. The focus remains on what is allegedly intrinsic to the individual rather than what is intrinsic to the human species.

However, we need not accept, as some suggest (e.g. Macklin, 2003), that we should banish the term 'dignity' from public discourse. Bioethicists remind us that we live in era, when, as a result of new technologies, the definition of what it is in biological terms to be human is quite literally in question (Pellegrino, et al., 2009), and it behoves us in the wider context 'to understand and acknowledge the variations in [the] meanings [of human dignity]' (*ibid.* p. 535). However, just as we can now manipulate the genetics of the human organism, we have long had the capacity to eradicate poverty, which, though it may be a condition symbolically devoid of dignity, is the objective result of a failure of human solidarity and of social rights.

Asserting methodological humanism

Returning for a moment to Tom Campbell's plea for humanity before justice (2007; and see Chapter 4, this volume), poverty may be said to be a violation of human rights because it amounts to inhumanity, not injustice. This approach, by demanding a global response, is founded implicitly on a humanist methodology.

It may be argued that at the very least this requires a recalibration of our understanding of human rights in favour of what we have been referring to as the minor tradition. If the object of social rights is not so much to underwrite some abstract standard of human dignity as to respond to humanitarian indignation, the principle that social rights may be 'progressively realised' is to be questioned: it is not good enough. The assertion of this book is that social rights are constituted through the naming and claiming of needs at a multiplicity of sites and levels. The idea of what would be 'good-enough' is suggested by Fiona Williams' reflections on 'good-enough principles for welfare' (1999; and mentioned in Chapter 3, this volume). Drawing on Winnicott's (1953) notion of 'good-enough parenting', Williams suggests that 'good-enough' indicates 'a morality grounded in the relational conditions of everyday life sufficient for the recognition of moral worth' (1999, p. 675). Williams' principles of welfare cover issues of interdependence, care, intimacy, bodily integrity, identity, transnationality and voice. A full exposition warrants more space than is available in this chapter, but here lies the basis of a bid for the kind of social rights where human subjects' identities:

> are sustained through interdependence, through striving for the mutual recognition of worth and a tolerance of diversity, and whose capacity for self-interested action is mediated through bonds of belonging and meanings of identity and structured by local, national and international relations of power and inequality.
>
> *(1999, p. 685)*

Notions of dignity remain wholly relevant, but humanity is *socially* contextualised. Insofar as needs may be translated into rights, they are *social* rights. What they demand is more than dignity; they demand the recognition of needs and good-enough responses to need.

We have seen that when social rights are translated into rights of citizenship within a welfare state, the right to social security provides some degree of protection (or 'asylum' in its literal and non-pejorative sense) against the hazards of life, including the risks of an exploitative labour market and of poverty in old age; the right to housing provides some protection against the hazards of exclusive housing markets and the risks of homelessness; and the right to social care provides protection against the risks of social exclusion and socially produced disability. Whether as human rights or citizenship rights, social rights, as we might wish to define them, are concerned with social negotiation around human needs. Their full realisation requires more than a defence of human dignity (however defined); it requires a recognition of human sociality, both globally as a species characteristic and at the locus of interdependent human lives. 'Think globally - act locally' is the slogan adopted in 1971 by Friends of the Earth, though it is thought originally to have been coined early in the twentieth century by a pioneering town planner and social activist, Partick Geddes (see Boardman, 1978). It is an apposite slogan for a methodological humanist approach to social rights. Human beings are definitively characterised by their capacity to think on the one hand and purposefully act on the other. The realisation of human sociality has both global and local significance since it relates potentially to a shared consciousness of our global interdependency as a species and to the collaborative activities ('the work') by which we may shape our own and each other's lives. It is a slogan that bypasses the arbitrary boundaries and potential constraints of the nation-state and embraces humanity both as a global species and in the quotidian realities of being human.

The de-nationalisation of social rights?

This begs many questions. Since the UDHR is a declaration negotiated in another era by representatives of nation-states with a spectrum of competing interests, should we seek to re-write it? It is difficult, however, to see the circumstances in which the currently deeply conflicted international 'community' might in the foreseeable future convene a legitimate forum through which to approach such a task, nor how any other kind of legitimate forum might be convened.

Critics of the UN point to the democratic deficit that results not merely from its organisational structure but more fundamentally from the extent to which it exists to serve the diverse and conflicting interests of its member states, rather than humanity as a whole. They seek reforms that might subject the UN to greater influence from civil society organisations and individual citizens of the world. The organisation, *Democracy Without Borders*, advocates for a UN Parliamentary Assembly as a step towards a world parliament and a global constitution and for a World Citizenship Initiative by which to give every human being a voice (see www.peoplesassembly.global/en/). The organisation asserts that 'the UNDHR and the International Covenant on Civil and Political Rights constitute a right to democracy at all levels of public authority, from the local to the global', but conspicuously makes no mention of the ICESCR and offers no discussion of the role of social rights. The *Earth Federation Movement* advocates for a World Parliament: 'A democratic non-military government based on peace and solving environmental problems' (see http://worldparliament-gov.org/). It proposes an extensive and procedurally elaborate 'Earth Constitution', which promisingly foresees a new age 'when the earth's total resources shall be equitably used for human welfare'. And yet, while including a briefly drawn 'Bill or Rights for Earth Citizens', this entirely omits any mention of social rights.

The Spanish Society for International Human Rights Law has elaborated a Declaration on the Human Right to Peace, a final version of which was adopted in 2010 at an International Congress convened in Santiago de Compostela under the auspices of the World Social Forum on Education for Peace (SIIHRL, 2010). On the premise that poverty and social exclusion are regarded as a form of structural, as opposed to armed, violence, the authors contend they are incompatible with peace. The declaration accordingly makes express provision for social rights to combat poverty, albeit that these amount to little more than a restatement or reaffirmation of existing provisions in the UDHR. Though it has no legal standing, this alternative declaration is significant first as an attempt to situate social rights in a broader context, but also as a tactic through which to influence working groups reporting to the UN's HRC. In 2016, the HRC (RES/32/28) eventually agreed to a somewhat different version of a Declaration on the Right to Peace, which guardedly asserts that 'States should … guarantee freedom from fear and want as a means to build peace within and between societies' (Article 2). Read in context, the inclusion of 'and want' in this clause seems almost incidental and adds little by way of emphasis to the fundamental importance of social rights.

More radical reforms to the machinery of the UN would require changes to its basic architecture (see Chapter 9, this volume). The innovations necessary to establish institutions capable, for example, of administering global taxation mechanisms and redistribution through, for example, a global basic income (see www.globalincome.org) or an international social security system (Townsend, 2002) would require a significant strengthening of the powers of ECOSOC relative to those of other organs of the UN and probably, therefore, amendments to the UN Charter. This would in turn be dependent on the effective democratisation of the Security Council and General Assembly procedures (Patomäki & Teivainen, 2004). Nevertheless, enhanced co-ordination between and within existing UN agencies and further strengthening of regional supranational co-ordinating bodies clearly could have some part to play in the development and enforcement of social rights worldwide. Optimists have claimed there is scope for the promotion of some degree of 'global social reformist hegemony' in relation to social rights (Deacon, 2007, p. 189), and it might be acknowledged that provision under the SDGs (see Box 9.1, this volume) for a Global Partnership for Sustainable Development constitutes a 'baby-step' in that direction.

In particular, as discussed in Chapter 9 of this volume, international migration – fuelled by global poverty, geo-political conflicts and the consequences of climate change – is increasingly recognised as one of the most enduring challenges. The International Convention on the Protection of the Rights of All

Migrant Workers and Members of Their Families of 1990 (which came into force in 2003) provides to migrants rights to participate in contributory social security schemes (where these exist), to urgent medical care and to education for their children. But the Convention has been neither signed nor ratified by any of the economically advanced countries of the world (albeit that many of them do begrudgingly comply, more or less, with its main provisions). A form of global citizenship that would allow for migration without borders would seem to be a remote possibility, though it has been afforded serious consideration in a UNESCO report (Pecoud & de Guchteneire, 2005). The UNDHR provides for a right to emigration under Article 13 (that is, a right to leave a country, including one's own), but no corresponding right to immigration (that is, to enter any other country). To provide an open right of mobility – as broadly applies within the EU – would be logical, but open up the question of the extent to which social rights can indeed be universal. Entzinger (2007) has suggested that for established welfare states there are four possible solutions: speeding up the integration of immigrants into the labour market; limiting safety net entitlements for established citizens and immigrants alike; allowing restricted entitlement for immigrants; deterritorialising entitlements (i.e. allowing greater portability of entitlements 'earned' over the life course through working or residing in different countries). In practice, most developed welfare states employ a mixture of such solutions, but the underlying assumption is that there are limits to the human solidarity upon which the provision of social rights depends (Alesina & Glaeser, 2004; Goodhart, 2006). This assumption has been challenged on empirical grounds (Banting & Kymlicka, 2006), but from an ethical perspective, the point made, for example, by Honneth (1995; and see discussion in Chapter 1, this volume) is that the framing of rights transcends feelings of solidarity: they are concerned with the recognition of the claims of distant strangers, without regard for territorial boundaries.

For the foreseeable future, social rights – whether for established citizens or recent migrants – will for the most part be framed in a national context. To those who press the cause of social rights, the nation-state that currently governs most of our social rights may yet be regarded:

> ... as a link in a chain of historical development. Hence it by no means constitutes '[human beings'] natural environment' but merely a real fact whose actual power must be reckoned with but which has no inherent right to determine our actions. The state and the laws shall be seen as having no more than an empirical validity. In the same way as yachts[persons] must take exact note of the direction of the wind without letting the wind determine [their] course; on the contrary, [they] defy it and exploit it in order to hold fast to [their] original course.
>
> *(Lukács, 1971, p. 262) [non-gender-specific nouns and pronouns substituted]*

Questions of human scale

The sociality of the human species is necessary to the personality of its members in real-time and at their actual location. Human lives are lived locally and currently, therefore, within nation-states. The locality of human lives may be determined by accidents of birth or by circumstances (and sometimes choices) associated with processes of migration. The course of human lives is therefore affected in specific ways by 'the state and the laws' to which human beings may immediately be subject, but with or against which individually or collectively they may react. Though social rights may now be for the most part systematically and abstractly constructed, they nonetheless have meaningful consequences and institutional impacts in what Habermas (1987) refers to as the 'life world' and Lefebvre (1991, 2014) as the 'social space'. Within the life world or social space, the incursions of the state and the law can be 'steered' in whole or in part by various means: by strategic legal intervention; by grassroots movements; and/or by policy-driven community engagement initiatives.

- Strategic legal intervention. Within nation-states, there will be – as discussed in Chapter 10 of this volume – more or less immediate proactive and reactive legal remedies available in relation to the functioning of welfare policies and institutions. In spite of the limitations faced by community-based activists and welfare lawyers working at local levels, it is often through their ingenuity that pressure for observance, reform and further development of social rights is maintained. It is important to acknowledge the contribution that legal activism can play as a tactic within wider strategies (Scheingold, 1974/2004). The contention of the legal realist movement within socio-legal studies has been that although legally framed rights are top-down constructions, they provide a discursive resource that can be deployed in bottom-up political tactics. Scheingold has suggested that a new politics of rights might 'decentre' law in a quite radical sense. He presents 'a vision of the interpenetration of multiple levels of legality' (2004, p. xxii) and of a role for law and 'cause lawyering' (see also Sarat & Schiengold, 2001) within a context where rights can be accorded not fixed meanings but a plurality of everyday meanings. When it comes to social rights, legal meanings are only one kind of meaning within that plurality, albeit a strategically important kind of meaning.

  Street-level welfare activists can engage locally with people not necessarily as sovereign individual citizens but as vulnerable and essentially interdependent human beings. Such work may proceed out of moral conviction, but the quotidian reality is that social policies and national legislation are but a means, not the end of social rights. Social legislation may provide, for example, for the administration of a particular social welfare scheme and do nothing either more or less than assign or regulate the responsibilities and conduct of officials or professionals appointed to fulfil specified tasks (Hirst, 1980). When help is withheld under any such scheme, a welfare rights worker or lawyer who assists a legal challenge or appeal is not so much upholding a right to social support as, in many instances, challenging the propriety of a particular administrative ruling or regulation. As a Social Security Commissioner, rejecting a social assistance appeal in the United Kingdom once said: 'At the end of the day, the [prevailing social assistance provision] is not something to which there is a divine right: it is nothing more than an arbitrary compromise, sanctioned by Parliament, between the demand for benefits on the one hand and the availability of public funds to finance it' (case R(SB)55/83 – reported in *Welfare Rights Bulletin*, 60, July 1984). Substantive social rights do indeed arise from more or less arbitrary compromises between competing interests. But they can also be the outcome of campaigns for less conditionality and for more generous provision – in short, for better compromises – campaigns in which welfare rights casework and cause lawyering can play a supporting role.

- Grassroots movements. While the constitutional and legal context matters, of equal or, in some respects, greater importance is the everyday context of the life world, which is the role of grassroots struggles and informal demands. That world is never wholly disconnected from the systemic legal and formal constitutional sphere, since it exists in continual communication with it: reacting to, resisting and informing it. Political activity of various kinds spans the divide between these contexts. The post-Marshallian conception of social citizenship enables us to understand that the social negotiation of social rights permeates every level of human existence, from the global to the most local. At the level of everyday relations of interdependency, we can see that the realisation of social rights might entail the 'publicising' of 'privately' experienced needs. This is the essence of the 'politics of needs interpretation' espoused by Nancy Fraser (1989, ch. 8, and Dean, 2020, ch. 9). Fraser's original argument was that needs discourse is generated in three spheres: the political, the economic and the domestic. Fraser's particular idea of a politics of needs interpretation is of a struggle to project the needs associated with everyday livelihoods and household survival from the domestic to the political sphere and to prevent the subordination of such needs to the demands of the economic sphere. This entails a notion of 'private' and 'public' realms quite similar to that of Hannah Arendt (see above), albeit that Fraser is seeking to erode the barriers between them so as to achieve a fundamental 're-balancing' of democracy.

This opens further the possibility for negotiating social rights; for translating hidden or neglected needs – especially those experienced by women and marginalised social groups – into rights-based claims-making; for expanding our understanding of social rights, not least as rights that can be 'enjoyed' without necessarily being formally implemented through legislation (Davy & Pellissery, 2013). Practical instances of something like this may be seen, for example, in the resistance practices of the Malaysian peasants studied by Scott (1985); practices Scott refers to as a form of 'infra-politics'. It can be seen that the practices adopted within informal settlements can amount, according to Holston (2009), to a form of 'insurgent citizenship'. Active struggles for gender equality, for sustainable living standards and social justice may be initiated and fomented at grassroots sites. The resultant social practices may well be far from perfect in terms of the levels of equality and inclusion that they achieve, and they may or may not lead to the realisation of more formal forms of social citizenship, but nonetheless, they matter. At the local scale – beneath that of a city, the nation, a continent, the world – an individual can cease to be a mere inhabitant or denizen but can be recognised as a member of an active, collaborating, caring social unit.

Grassroots sites can now, of course, be global as well as local. Infra-politics can be virtually as well as physically located. The power and penetration of social media based on new information technologies dissolves the significance of territorial boundaries and facilitates communication within virtual communities with shared needs and interdependencies (Williams, 2007). It is this that has made possible the resistances of the Occupy and *Indignados* movements mentioned above. The potential of movements such as these for the promotion of social rights has still, perhaps, to be realised. At one stage the emergence of the *World Social Forum* had been regarded as the foundation though which global resistance to global capitalist hegemony might be articulated (Callinicos, 2003; Kaldor, 2003), though it has since been criticised, for example, by Bob Deacon for resolving 'not to fashion a manifesto, preferring instead a thousand voices to bloom' (2007, p. 190). One example of a popular manifesto that could perhaps be globally promoted through such channels would be Guy Standing's proposed *Precariat Charter* (2014). This is an informal charter that gives expression to Standing's call for a form of global occupational citizenship (mentioned in Chapter 9, this volume). The demands made in the Charter include a redefinition of work, the removal of systemic poverty and precarity traps, the decommodification of education and a move towards universal basic income. The Charter also has its critics (e.g. Harris, 2014), but it exemplifies a campaigning tool that draws on the language of rights and an alternative to more formal attempts to develop or amend human rights treaties and conventions.

- Policy-driven community engagement. Community engagement in the development and implementation of social policy and social rights will not necessarily be insurgent in origin. It can, after a fashion, be manufactured, though its effectiveness may be limited. In Britain, for example, there were experiments in the 1970s with non-statutory urban Neighbourhood Councils, with local Community Relations Councils, and locally elected Community Health Councils. Such bodies could be effective, if only marginally or occasionally, in mobilising local rights-based demands (Cockburn, 1977; Loney, 1983), but none have survived. In Brazil, the 1988 Constitution made specific provision for social rights and sought to embed principles of citizen participation. This has led to the creation of an extensive federal and local network of public policy management councils, with responsibility for formulating and managing policy in areas such as education, health and welfare, with parity of representation from community representatives on the one hand and representatives of government and service providers on the other (Coelho, 2004). Admittedly, the ability of such councils at the local level effectively to mobilise people proved to be extremely variable. However, a much-hailed example of such a process has been the participatory budget-making process in Porto Allegre (Wainwright, 2003). Elsewhere in Latin America, in Venezuela in 2005, the Chavez regime sought to create a 'new geometry of power' (Massey, 2008) through the promotion of Communal Councils, autonomous from existing local government structures and governed by Citizens Assemblies. These self-organising Councils could be locally instigated and established by groups of families in urban, rural and indigenous areas (Marcano, 2009). It was intended that they would incorporate local grassroots committees concerned, inter alia, with health, education, water and energy provision and that they should establish a Communal Bank and bid for government funds for infrastructural and housing projects. Their impact, it would seem, was, in practice, modest and their functioning compromised by the persistence of social inequalities, as well as by resistance from career bureaucrats and the Venezuelan right wing, but as a model for bottom-up engagement having the potential for the framing of social rights, such initiatives set interesting precedents (Azzellini, 2013).

Among the proposals contained in a Draft Social Charter proposed by the Canadian Anti-Poverty Organisation in 1992 (Nedelsky & Scott, 1992; Hunt, 1996, pp. 185–190) was provision for a national Social Rights Council that would evaluate compliance with the Charter, conduct investigations and make representations for reform or improvements in social rights provision. The Council would function explicitly according to 'dialogic' principles; that is to say, it would embrace the idea that social rights are constituted through negotiation. The Social Charter was never adopted, but the idea of a Social Rights Council remains attractive, not only at a national level but at more *local* levels. Local social rights councils might in principle provide a site for debate relating specifically and immediately to the needs of local people, where not only would grievances be aired, but vernacular discourses of need could be promoted, and rights-based demands could be framed. They could perhaps constitute a bottom-up forum through which to conduct a politics of needs interpretation. There is inevitably a danger that local fora of this nature will co-opt as much as empower local people and that, however constituted, they would be insufficiently socially inclusive. Such bodies are unlikely to be entrusted with direct executive powers, but they could be accorded some measure of influence over local human service providers and a voice in national policy-making processes.

Shifts in perception: being human and doing good

The range of ideas just presented are not blueprints or even suggestions; they are merely examples of ways in which human sociality could unfold and in which new approaches to social rights and human welfare may develop. More important, perhaps, is the need to reframe the terms of debate through which we consider social rights and human welfare. It has already been implied that we might inflect the approach to social rights as human rights from what has been defined as the hegemonic/dominant to the subaltern/minor tradition. This requires a shift in perception.

Consciousness of sociality

We have noted how Moore speaks of the 'social anaesthesia' by which human populations can be numbed against suffering. Medically speaking, a general anaesthetic entails a complete loss of consciousness (Seth, 2021); the curtailment of an essential human characteristic upon which all other characteristics depend. The argument that is developed in this book is that consciousness of our sociality can be suppressed. Anaesthetics can, of course, be partial or local rather than general, and, in any event, Moore was using the term metaphorically to refer to distortions of perception that can also be captured through concepts of fetishism, as already discussed both in Chapter 1 and elsewhere in this volume with particular reference to currently prevailing fetishised perceptions of individual sovereignty – perceptions which impair the understanding of human interdependency and the essential sociality upon which human welfare depends. It is important to stress that such a fetish, like the commodity fetish identified by Marx, is neither a psychological aberration nor a conspiratorially conjured illusion; it is an immanent phenomenon attributable to a dominant logic. In a similar way, it is a dominant logic that sustains the conventions of methodological nationalism and so obscures a wider awareness of the global character of the human species and its shared existence.

BOX 11.1 LINGUISTIC FOIBLES: A REFLECTION ON THE MEANING OF BEING OR DOING GOOD

A relatively recent fashion in common English language parlance when responding to the ritual greeting, 'Hello, how are you?', is not necessarily to say 'I'm well, thank you', but 'I'm good, thanks'. The response is meant succinctly to convey (whether truthfully or not) that the respondent is feeling well or that they feel their life is going well; it is *not* meant to assert that they are a good or a caring person! In this instance, the *adjective* 'good' has been ungrammatically substituted for the *adverb* 'well'. English is an adaptable language, however, and the unnoticed use of 'good' as an adverb and, in this instance, as a synonym for 'well' has already, it would seem, lapsed into acceptability. The pedantic objections of grammarians are all but forgotten. But the ambiguity entailed remains significant. The linguistic shift cuts across recent controversies around:

- on the one hand, the competing definitions and uses of the terms *well*being and *wel*fare and their relationship between being and doing;
- and on the other, the fact that – as a noun *and* an adjective – 'good' has potentially, if not necessarily, moral connotations.

To say 'I'm well' is simply to reflect (subjectively or objectively) on one's current state of well-being, but to say 'I'm good', when *meaning* 'I'm well', elides the potential moral implications of being or doing good. Claiming explicitly to be virtuous might open one to accusations of hubris or immodesty. Claiming to be a 'do-gooder' might – in unsympathetic company – open one to ridicule. However, the meaning and the significance of 'being good' or 'doing good' in this instance have been obscured or compromised.

Even at the level of trends in everyday language, latent or inadvertent contradictions can go unnoticed (for a minor example, see Box 11.1). Perceptions and meanings can be changed or switched.

Human well-being depends on human beings doing good for one another. The premise of the concept of sociality is that human beings 'do good' for other human beings not only because they may be (in part at least) genetically hardwired to do so, not necessarily because they calculate that it will be good for themselves, not because they may be commanded to do so (whether by God or the Law), but because they are human. These other factors may all play a part in motivating human beings to do good, and together, they can contribute to making us not natural beings but social beings. Human beings uniquely learn, work and make their lives with each other. To that end, the 'goals' (cf. Bulmer et al., 1989) of institutionalised social policy and social rights self-evidently extend beyond the minimalist ethical imperative that policymakers and human service providers should merely 'do no harm'. Though seldom expressed in such terms, such goals have an implied aim that, so far as possible, social welfare policies should 'do good' by and for the human species. The question of what exactly is good for our species may be contested, and the intentions of individual 'do-gooders' and the effectiveness of collective 'do-gooding' may sometimes be questioned. The argument of this book, however, is that it is through an extended sociality – as a constitutive species characteristic – that the good of the species is realised and that social rights, as an expression of that sociality, are means by which the species may succeed or fail to provide for the good of all its members. This, however, is not a picture that is generally recognised.

Switching to a humanistic perspective

It has been argued that what is required is 'a conceptual gestalt switch by which to transcend fetishised or illusory perceptions as to the basis on which everyday individual wellbeing is attained' (Dean, 2023, p. 266). In psychology, gestalt refers to a perception that makes sense of something as a whole rather than as an assembly of constituent parts. It is the way we generally interpret our experiences of the world, save that things that are complex and/or ambiguous may be capable of perception in more than one way. Figure 11.1

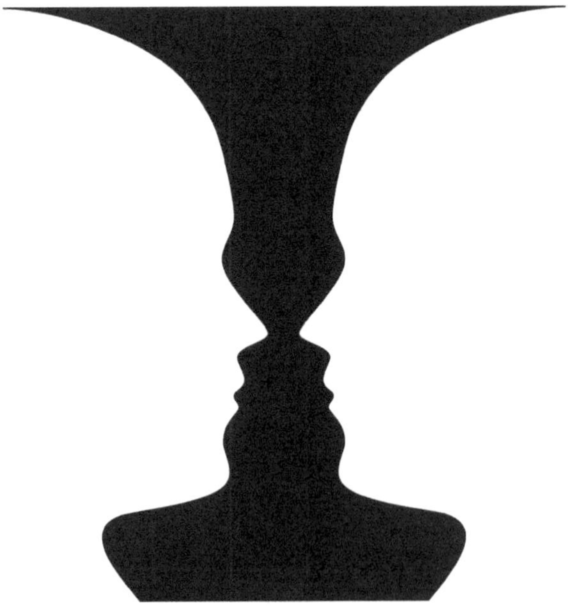

FIGURE 11.1 An inanimate vase or two human beings facing one another? A classic ambiguous image to illustrate perceptual gestalt switching.

is a classic (and no doubt familiar) example of an image that may be perceived in two ways. Anyone observing the image for the first time may perceive it only one way, depending perhaps on contextual cues or their frame of mind at that moment. But once they are aware of the ambiguity of the image, they can switch at will between the different perceptions.

Big pictures can be differently interpreted, and their component elements may be differently perceived. When we consider the forms of creative co-operation that are required both locally and globally to sustain human life and the mechanisms by which care, goods and services are exchanged between intimates, neighbours and strangers, our perceptions can be led, directed, or shaped in a multiplicity of ways. The switch in perception advocated in this book prioritises a form of species awareness. This may be variously described as the adoption of a life-first principle (Dean, 2020) or a needs-first ethic (Dean, 2015). But it is humanistic not necessarily in a moralising sense but more pertinently in a material or methodological sense. By embracing the encompassing concept of sociality as a substantive species characteristic, the perspective captures an overarching view of human welfare or well-being, and of social citizenship as an open process of social negotiation. Social rights are conceived as a requirement for human welfare and a 'good life'; that is to say, a fully human life. A humanistic perspective entails an acceptance of 'doing good' as a collective responsibility for the attainment of fully human lives. Doing good, therefore, entails no more and no less than realising our human sociality.

It is, inevitably, a perception that can be inflected in a variety of ways. Within the realms of conventional political or ideological discourse, a humanistic perspective is a challenge to narrow utilitarian and managerial thinking, since it recognises that life's meaning precedes the things that people might choose, or be made, to do. From within the spectrum of liberal thinking, social liberals and 'reluctant collectivists' (George & Wilding, 1985, ch. 3) are likely – implicitly or explicitly – to subscribe to some brand of Kantian deontological ethics (see Chapter 5, this volume) that can accommodate elements of collective responsibility and which may be attracted, for example, to a Rawlsian conception of social justice, on the one hand, or to Sen's capability approach, on the other. Similarly, inheritors of the civic republican tradition, radical democrats and left-communitarians, might rally in various ways around a humanistic perspective that emphasises the significance of life guarantees through risk sharing and social insurance. There is scope for discussion of a humanistic perspective within contemporary liberal and communitarian discourses.

However, the humanistic perspective and its understanding of sociality are informed by and resonate most strongly with a Marxian theory of human need and of the material human essence. Marx's particular vision was of a society that might succeed from capitalism – a society in which the measure of things would flow from inclusive understandings of *need* (premised on fully human lives) rather than from fetishised conceptions of *value* (premised on the commodity form). We might envisage how a humanistic emphasis upon the development of social rights and democratic social planning might constitute the beginnings of what Soper (1981) has alluded to as a politics of human need. Essentially the same insight is captured by de Sousa Santos' conceptualisation (mentioned in Chapter 9) of an 'axiology of care': a theory that values care, not economic progress or commodities. De Sousa Santos was suggesting that as a means to challenge the orthodoxies of global capitalism, we might explore alternative ways of thinking that emanate from the global South. In Chapter 7, we touched on the ideas of Ivan Illich and Paulo Friere, who have each radically challenged the professionalised premises on which human service provision imported by the global South from the global North is founded, arguing instead for rights to health and educational provision to be premised on 'conviviality' and shared consciousness raising. There is also an important connection that can be made with the feminist ethic of care that was discussed in Chapter 5 of this volume – an ethic which, once again, puts care centre stage, emphasising the extent to which human wellbeing depends on the social negotiation of responsibilities and relationships. The point about the humanistic perspective is that it construes the human individual's need for autonomy not in terms of self-sufficiency but in the context of social interdependency; it prioritises the integrity of the human being as a living social actor rather than as a competitive utility-maximising individual and agent of economic production.

Marx is best known for his writings in the fields of sociology and political economy and, for example, the architectonic or structural metaphor by which he posited the primary importance of the relations of economic production as the 'base' upon which human society's political, cultural and legal 'superstructure' is constructed (1859). The base/superstructure metaphor has been variously interpreted, reinterpreted and 'strained' (Thompson, 1978, p. 303), but its premise can be both reframed and critiqued by applying the analysis distilled from Marx's own philosophical writings. Is it the case that the existential necessity of 'work' (human beings' productive metabolism with Nature) determines the development of human consciousness, sociality and historical development? Taken as a whole, Marx's writings would seem by implication to acknowledge that 'work', consciousness, sociality and human development are interdependent; any one of these species-characteristics may be said to be foundational for the other. Without suggesting an alternative architectonic metaphor, we might reflect on the ways in which sociality is 'foundational' for the other three species' characteristics: for creative consciousness, productive activity, human development and the social rights that may promote them.

In conclusion

The often deeply troubled yet hitherto resilient human species is currently exposed to a range of existential threats against which its members must *together* struggle: a climate emergency; intransigent global poverty and inequalities; frightening geo-political instabilities; heightened risks from pandemics and degenerative diseases. In this context we might reflect upon sociality and its relationship to other constitutive characteristics of the human species and, thereby, upon the spectrum of social rights discussed in this book and their underpinning relevance to human welfare. Let us again – through both a local and a global lens – consider:

- ***Sociality and care-fullness.*** Advocating for a 'care full' social policy agenda Marian Barnes (2012, p. 18) captures something of what may be entailed by the humanistic perspective suggested above. Sociality entails an essential – if often unrealised – human capacity to care for and about other members of the species. At one level, this may be expressed through rights of people when they are vulnerable to be cared for and of those who provide such care to be fully recognised. At other levels, it may entail universal rights to the means of subsistence, to collectively financed and compassionately delivered healthcare services, and to collectively guaranteed housing provision. Beyond this, it is through sociality that extensions of social rights may sustain other essential characteristics of the species.
- ***Consciousness and thought-fullness.*** A case can similarly be made for a 'thought full' social policy agenda: an agenda that promotes not individual self-sufficiency but 'critical autonomy' (Doyal & Gough 1991, p. 67), ethical reasoning and reflective thinking. This requires a universal right to education that extends beyond basic institutional instruction in literacy, numeracy and practical skills but which more effectively fosters the development of human personality and social awareness. The right to education therefore intersects with a right to developmental care during childhood and to cultural and political participation during adulthood.
- ***'Work' and creative-ness.*** The social policy agenda has conventionally been connected, if not subservient, to labour-market policy, but a perspective driven by an understanding of human sociality must embrace an understanding that 'work' means more than labour-market participation: it is about human beings' creative 'metabolism with Nature' (Marx, 1887, pp. 83–40). Social rights relating to the protection of livelihoods and to economic production, as discussed in Chapter 8 of this volume, can be extended to embrace the enablement and protection of the full spectrum of purposeful human activity, including unpaid care work and cultural and political engagement.

- ***Human development and human-ness.*** The humanistic perspective discussed above is concerned with the 'right to have rights' (Arendt, 1951) including and especially social rights. The unique sociality of the human species implies not only negative rights – to be protected from the dehumanising effects of war, authoritarianism, exploitation, poverty, discrimination and the consequences of past and present abuses of the natural environment – but positive rights that make possible the social participation, inclusion and involvement necessary to human life and human development.

REFERENCES

Alcock, P. (2006). *Understanding Poverty* (3rd edn.). Basingstoke: Palgrave.
Alesina, A., & Glaeser, E. (2004). *Fighting Poverty in the US and Europe*. Oxford: OUP.
Alinsky, S. (1969). *Reveille for Radicals*. New York: Random House.
Allen, G. (2011). *Early Intervention*. London: Cabinet Office.
The Alliance for Legal Aid. (2014). *Legal Aid Today - LAPSO reform*. At www.save-legalaid.co.uk/legalaidunderlaspo.html
Alstadsaeter, A., Godar, S., Nicolaides, P., & Zucman, G. (2023). *Global Tax Evasion Report 2004*. Paris: EU Tax Observatory.
Alston, P. (1990). US ratification of the covenant on economic, social and cultural rights. *American Journal of International Law*, *84*(2).
Alston, P., & Quinn, G. (1987). The nature and scope of states parties' obligations under the international covenant on economic, social and cultural rights. *Human Rights Quarterly*, *9*(1).
Amin, S. (1997). *Capitalism in the Age of Globalization*. London: Zed Books.
Anderson, B. (2020). Justice, Citizenship and Methodological De-Nationalism. In T. Knijn & D. Lepianka (Eds.), *Justice and Vulnerability in Europe*. Cheltenham: Elgar.
Andreassen, B., & Marks, S. (Eds.). (2010). *Development as a Human Right* (2nd edn.). Antwerp: Intersentia.
Annetts, J., Law, A., McNeish, W., & Mooney, G. (Eds.). (2009). *Understanding Social Movements and Social Welfare*. Bristol: Policy Press.
Apel, K. (1980). *Towards the Transformation of Philosophy*. London: Routledge.
Apel, K. (1991). A Planetary Macro-Ethics for Humankind. In E. Deutsch (Ed.), *Culture and Modernity*. Honolulu: University of Hawaii Press.
Arendt, H. (1951). *The Burden of Our Time*. London: Secker & Warburg.
Arendt, H. (1977). Public Rights and Private Interests. In M. Mooney & F. Stuber (Eds.), *Small Comforts for Hard Times*. New York: Columbia University.
Aristotle. (c. 350 BCE). *Eudemian Ethics - Books I. II and VIII (1982 edn. translated by M. Woods)*. Oxford: Clarendon Press.
Aristotle. (1981). *The Politics*. Harmondsworth: Penguin.
Ashton, E. (2011). The Alleged Dichotomy between Positive and Negative Rights and Duties. In C. Beits & R. Goodin (Eds.), *Global Basic Rights*. Oxford: OUP.

ATD Fourth World. (2014). *Challenge 2015*. Paris: ATD Fourth World.
Atkin, L., Shalom, H., & West, R. (2014). *The Behavioural Change Wheel*. Bream, Gloucestershire: Silverback.
Atkinson, A. (Ed.) (2004). *New Sources of Development Finance*. Oxford: OUP.
Azzellini, D. (2013). The communal state: Communal councils, communes and workplace democracy. *NACLA Report on the Americas*, *46*(2).
Bagilhole, B. (2009). *Understanding Equal Opportunities and Diversity*. Bristol: Policy Press.
Baker, J., Lynch, K., Cantillon, S., & Walsh, J. (2004). *Equality: From Theory to Action*. Basingstoke: Macmillan.
Ball, S. (2008). *The Education Debate*. Bristol: Policy Press.
Balloch, S., & Hill, M. (Eds.). (2007). *Care, Community and Citizenship*. Bristol: Policy Press.
Bankowski, Z., & Mungham, G. (1976). *Images of Law*. London: Routledge & Kegan Paul.
Banting, K., & Kymlicka, W. (2006). *Multiculturalism and the Welfare State*. Oxford: OUP.
Baptiste, W., & Bricker-Jenkins, M. (2002). A View from the Bottom. In R. Albelda & A. Withorn (Eds.), *Lost Ground*. Cambridge, MA: South End Press.
Barnes, M. (2012). *Care in Everyday Life*. Bristol: Policy Press.
Barnes, C., & Mercer, G. (2010). *Exploring Disability* (2nd edn.). Cambridge: Polity.
Barr, N. (2010). Long-term care. *Social Policy & Administration*, *44*(4).
Barrientos, A. (2001). Welfare regimes in Latin America. Paper presented at the *Social Policy in Developing Contexts* workshop, 1–2 March, University of Bath.
Barrientos, A. (2004). Latin America. In I. Gough, G. Wood, A. Barrientos, P. Bevan, P. Davis & G. Room (Eds.), *Insecurity and Welfare Regimes in Asia, Africa and Latin America*. Cambridge: CUP.
Barry, A., Osborne, T., & Rose, N. (Eds.). (1996). *Foucault and Political Reason*. London: UCL Press.
Bastagli, F. (2009). *From Social Safety Net to Social Policy? The Role of Conditional Cash Transfers in Welfare State Development in Latin America*. Brasilia: International Policy Centre for Inclusive Growth.
Batchelet, M. (2011). *Social Protection Floor for a Fair and Inclusive Globalization*. Geneva: ILO.
Bauman, Z. (1987). *Legislators and Interpreters*. Cambridge: Polity.
Bauman, Z. (1998). *Work, Consumerism and the New Poor*. Buckingham: Open University Press.
Beck, U. (1992). *Risk Society*. London: Sage.
Beck, U. (2003). Toward a new critical theory with a cosmopolitan intent. *Constellations*, *10*(4).
Beck, U., & Beck-Gernsheim, E. (1995). *The Normal Chaos of Love*. Cambridge: CUP.
Beck, W., Van der Maesen, L., & Walker, A. (Eds.). (1997). *The Social Quality of Europe*. Bristol: Policy Press.
Bell, D. (1973). *The Coming of Post-Industrial Society*. London: Heinemann.
Belyaev, D. (1979). Destabilizing selection as a factor in domestication. *Journal of Heredity*, *70*(5).
Bentham, J. (1789). An Introduction to the Principles and Morals of Legislation. In M. Warnock (Ed.), *Utilitarianism* (1962 ed.). Glasgow: Collins.
Berlin, I. (1967). Two Concepts of Liberty. In A. Quinton (Ed.), *Political Philosophy*. Oxford: OUP.
Bevan, P. (2004). The Dynamics of Africa's in/security Regimes. In I. Gough & G. Wood (Eds.), *Insecurity and Welfare Regimes in Asia, Africa and Latin America*. Cambridge: CUP.

Beveridge, W. (1942). *Social Insurance and Allied Services*. London: HMSO.

Billis, D., & Glennerster, H. (1998). Human services and the voluntary sector. *Journal of Social Policy*, *27*(1).

Blyth, M. (2013). *Austerity*. Oxford: OUP.

Boardman, P. (1978). *The Worlds of Pastrick Geddes*. London: Routledge & Kegan Paul.

Bochel, H. (2005). Ethics, Risk and Social Policy. In C. Bochel, H. Bochel, R. Page & R. Sykes (Eds.), *Social Policy*. Harlow: Pearson.

Boehm, C. (1993). Egalitarian behaviour and reverse dominance hierarchy. *Current Anthropology*, *34*, 227–254.

Boltvinik, J. (forthcoming). *From Poverty to Well-Being and Human Flourishing*. (Vol. 2. A Marxian Approach to Human Poverty). Bristol: Policy Press.

Boratav, K., & Özuğurlu, M. (2006). Social Policies and Distributional Dynamics in Turkey. In M. Karshenas & V. Moghadam (Eds.), *Social Policy in the Middle East*. Basingstoke: Palgrave.

Bornat, A., Pereira, C., Pilgrim, D., & Williams, F. (Eds.). (1993). *Community Care*. Basingstoke: Macmillan.

Bottomore, T. (1992). Citizenship and Social Class, Forty Years on. In T. Marshall & T. Bottomore (Eds.), *Citizenship and Social Class*. London: Pluto.

Bowlby, J. (1969). *Attachment and Loss* (Vol. Attachment). New York: Basic Books.

Boyle, A. (2007). *Human Rights or Environmental Rights? A Reassessment*. Edinburgh: School of Law.

Braathen, E. (2000). New Social Corporatism. In Comparative Research on Poverty (Ed.), *A Critical Review of the World Development Report 2000/200*. Bergen: CROP.

Braathen, E. (2005). Social Funds in Africa: A Technocratic-Clientalistic Response to Poverty? In A. Cimadamore, H. Dean & J. Siqueira (Eds.), *The Poverty of the State*. Buenos Aires: CLACSO/CROP.

Bradshaw, J. (1972). The Concept of Social Need. *New Society*, 30 March.

Bradshaw, J. (2017). Why the two-child policy is the worst social security policy ever. *Social Policy Association 50th Anniversary Blog Series*. https://social-policy.org.uk/category/50-for-50/page/5/

Bregman, R. (2020). *Humankind*. London: Bloomsbury.

Brewer, B. (2007). Citizen or customer? *International Review of Administrative Sciences*, *73*(4).

Brixton Advice Centre. (1976). *Tenth Annual Report*. London: Brixton Advice Centre.

Brundtland, G. (1987). *Our Common Future*. Oxford: OUP.

Bulmer, M., Piachaud, D., & Lewis, J. (Eds.). (1989). *The Goals of Social Policy*. London: Unwin Hyman.

Burchardt, T. (1997). *Boundaries between Public and Private Welfare*. CASE Paper 2. London: LSE.

Burchardt, T. (2013). *Re-Visiting the Conceptual Framework for public/private Boundaries in Welfare*. Social Policy in a Cold Climate Research Note 2. London: LSE.

Burrows, R., Pleace, N., & Quilgars, D. (Eds.). (1997). *Homelessness and Social Policy*. London: Routledge.

Bynum, W. (2008). *The History of Medicine*. Oxford: OUP.

Cahill, M. (2002). *The Environment and Social Policy*. London: Routledge.

Callender, C. (2010). Bursaries and institutional aid in higher education in England. *Oxford Review of Education*, *36*(1).

Callinicos, A. (2003). *An Anti-Capitalist Manifesto*. Cambridge: Polity.

Callinicos, A. (2007). *Social Theory: A Historical Introduction* (2nd edn.). Cambridge: Polity.

Callinicos, A. (2010). *Bonfire of Illusions*. Cambridge: Polity.

Campbell, T. (1983). *The Left and Rights*. London: Routledge & Kegan Paul.
Campbell, T. (1988). *Justice*. Basingstoke: Macmillan.
Campbell, T. (2006). *Rights*. London: Routledge.
Campbell, T. (2007). Poverty as a Violation of Human Rights. In T. Pogge (Ed.), *Freedom from Poverty as a Human Right: Who Owes What to the Very Poor*. Oxford: OUP.
Carlin, J., Howard, J., & Messinger, S. (1967). *Civil Justice and the Poor*. New York: Russell Sage.
Carter, M. (2003). *T.H. Green and the Development of Ethical Socialism*. Exeter: Imprint Academic.
Castañeda, E. (2012). The indignados of Spain. *Social Movement Studies*, *11*(3–4).
Castells, M. (1983). *The City and the Grassroots*. London: Arnold.
Castles, F. (1982). *The Impact of Parties*. London: Sage.
Cerami, A. (2013). *Permanent Emergency Regimes in Sub-Saharan Africa*. Basingstoke: Palgrave.
Cerami, A., & Vanhuysse, P. (2009). *Post-Communist Welfare Pathways*. Basingstoke: Palgrave.
Chambers, R., & Conway, G. (1992). Sustainable Rural Livelihoods. Discussion Paper 296. Brighton: Institute of Development Studies.
Chan, J. (1999). A Confucian Perspective on Human Rights for Contemporary China. In J. Bauer & D. Bell (Eds.), *The East Asian Challenge for Human Rights*. Cambridge: CUP.
Chan, C.-K., & Bowpitt, G. (2005). *Human Dignity and Welfare Systems*. Bristol: Policy Press.
Chan, C.-K., Ngok, K.-L., & Phillips, D. (2008). *Social Policy in China*. Bristol: Policy Press.
Chant, S. (2008). The feminization of poverty and the feminisation of ant-poverty programmes. *Journal of Development Studies*, *44*(2), 165–197.
Chattoo, S., Atkin, K., Craig, G., & Flynn, R. (Eds.). (2019). *Understanding 'Race' and Ethnicity* (2nd edn.). Bristol: Policy Press.
Chenwi, L. (2020). The African System. In M. Langford, B. Porter, R. Brown & J. Rossi (Eds.), *Research Handbook on Economic, Social and Cultural Rights*. Cheltenham: Elgar.
Children's Rights Alliance for England. (2013). *State of Children's Rights in England: Review of Government Action on UN Recommendations for Strengthening children's Rights in the UK*. London: CRAE.
Chitty, C. (2009). *Education Policy in Britain* (2nd ed.). Basingstoke: Palgrave.
Clarke, B. (1996). *Deep Citizenship*. London: Pluto.
Clarke, J. (1999). Coming to Terms With Culture. In H. Dean & R. Woods (Eds.), *Social Policy Review 11*. Luton: Social Policy Association.
Clarke, J., Coll, K., Dagnino, E., & Neveu, C. (2014). *Disputing Citizenship*. Bristol: Policy Press.
Clarke, J., & Newman, J. (1997). *The Managerial State*. London: Sage.
Coates, D. (2007). *The National Minimum Wage*. London: Work Foundation.
Cockburn, C. (1977). *The Local State*. London: Pluto Press.
Coelho, V. (2004). Brazil's health councils. *IDS Bulletin*, *35*(2).
Coles, B. (1995). *Youth and Social Policy*. London: UCL Press.
Comola, M., & de Mello, L. (2010). Enhancing the Effectiveness of Social Policies in Indonesia. *OECD Economics Department Working Papers*, *810*.
Comte, A. (1851). *System of Positive Polity* (1973 edn.). New York: Burt Franklin.
Comte, A. (1896). *Positive Philosophy* (Vol. 1–4). London: Bell and Sons.
Conant, L. (2010). Regional Legal Frameworks for Human Rights and Social Policy in Europe. In A. Nevile (Ed.), *Human Rights and Social Policy*. Cheltenham: Elgar.

Craig, G. (2008). The Limits of Compromise? In G. Craig, T. Burchardt & D. Gordon (Eds.), *Social Justice and Public Policy*. Bristol: Policy Press.
Cranston, M. (1976). Human Rights, Real and Supposed. In N. Timms & D. Watson (Eds.), *Talking about Welfare*. London: Routledge & Kegan Paul.
Cranston, R. (1985). *Legal Foundations of the Welfare State*. London: Weidenfeld & Nicholson.
Craven, M. (1995). *The International Covenant on Economic, Social and Cultural Rights*. Oxford: Clarendon Press.
Crompton, R. (2008). *Class and Stratification* (3rd edn.). Cambridge: Polity.
Crosland, C. A. R. (1956). *The Future of Socialism*. London: Jonathan Cape.
da Silva, J.-G., Belik, W., & Takagi, M. (2005). The Challenges of a Policy of Food Security in Brazil. In A. Cimadamore, H. Dean & J. Siqueira (Eds.), *The Poverty of the State*. Buenos Aires: CLACSO/CROP.
Daly, M. (2002). Care as a good for social policy. *Journal of Social Policy*, *31*(2).
Daly, M. (2011). *Welfare*. Cambridge: Polity.
Daniel, P., & Ivatts, J. (1998). *Children and Social Policy*. Basingstoke: Macmillan.
Darwin, C. (1871). *The Descent of Man* (2013 edn.). Hertfordshire: Wordworth Editions.
Davidova, N., & Manning, N. (2009). Russia. In P. Alcock & G. Craig (Eds.), *International Social Policy: Welfare Regimes in the Developed World* (2nd edn.). Basingstoke: Palgrave.
Davies, M. (2008). Stigma, Shame and Sense of Worth. In J. Strelitz & R. Lister (Eds.), *Why Money Matters*. London: Save the Children.
Davis, P. (2004). Rethinking the Welfare Regime Approach in the Context of Bangladesh. In I. Gough & G. Wood (Eds.), *Insecurity and Welfare Regimes in Asia, Africa and Latin America*. Cambridge: CUP.
Davis, K., & Moore, W. (1945). Some principles of stratification. *American Sociological Review*, *10*(2).
Davy, B. (2012). *Land Policy*. Farnham: Ashgate.
Davy, U. (2013). Social citizenship going international: Changes in the reading of UN-sponsored economic and social rights. *International Journal of Social Welfare*, *22*(Supplement 1).
Davy, B., & Pellissery, S. (2013). The citizenship promise (un)fulfilled. *International Journal of Social Welfare*, *22*(Supplement 1).
Dawkins, R. (1976). *The Selfish Gene* (1978 edn.). St Albans: Granada Publishing.
de Brosses, C. (1765). On the Worship of Fetish Gods. In R. Morris & D. Leonard (2017) (Eds.), *The Returns of Fetishism*. Chicago: UoC Press.
de Haas, H., Castles, S., & Miller, M. (2019). *The Age of Migration* (6th edn.). London: Bloomsbury.
de Schweinitz, K. (1961). *England's Road to Social Security*. Pennsylvania: Perpetua.
de Sousa Santos, B. (2001). *Toward a New Legal Common Sense* (2nd edn.). London: Butterworths.
de Sousa Santos, B. (2006). *The Rise of the Global Left*. London: Zed Books.
Deacon, B. (1993). Developments in East European Social Policy. In C. Jones (Ed.), *New Perspectives on the Welfare State in Europe*. London: Routledge.
Deacon, B. (2007). *Global Social Policy and Governance*. London: Sage.
Deacon, B., Hulse, M., & Stubbs, P. (1997). *Global Social Policy*. London: Sage.
Dean, H. (1991). *Social Security and Social Control*. London: Routledge.
Dean, H. (1992). Poverty discourse and the disempowerment of the poor. *Critical Social Policy* (35).
Dean, H. (1998). Popular paradigms and welfare values. *Critical Social Policy*, *18*(2).
Dean, H. (2000). Towards an Embodied Account of Welfare. In K. Ellis & H. Dean (Eds.), *Social Policy and the Body*. Basingstoke: Macmillan.

Dean, H. (Ed.) (2004). *The Ethics of Welfare*. Bristol: Policy Press.

Dean, H. (2007). The ethics of welfare-to-work. *Policy and Politics*, *35*(4).

Dean, H. (2009). Critiquing capabilities. *Critical Social Policy*, *29*(2).

Dean, H. (2011). The ethics of migrant welfare. *Ethics and Social Welfare*, *5*(1).

Dean, H. (2012a). The Experience of Welfare. In J. Baldock, L. Mitton, & S. Vickerstaff (Eds.), *Social Policy* (4th ed.). Oxford: OUP.

Dean, H. (2012b). Welcome relief or indecent subsidy? *Policy and Politics*, *40*(3).

Dean, H. (2013). The translation of needs into rights. *International Journal of Social Welfare*, *22*(Supplement 1), S32–S49.

Dean, H. (2015). *Social Rights and Human Welfare*. Abingdon: Routledge.

Dean, H. (2016). Eudaimonia and Species Being. In J. Vittersø (Ed.), *Handbook of Eudaimonic Well-Being*. Cham, Switzerland: Springer International.

Dean, H. (2018). EU Citizenship and 'Work' Tensions between Formal and Substantive Equality. In S. Seubert, O. Eberl & F. van Waarden (Eds.), *Reconsidering EU Citizenship: Contradictions and Constraints*. Cheltenham: Elgar.

Dean, H. (2020). *Understanding Human Need* (2nd edn.). Bristol: Policy Press.

Dean, H. (2023). From altruism to sociality. *Journal of International Social Welfare*, *32*(2).

Dean, H., & Khan, Z. (1997). Muslim perspectives on welfare. *Journal of Social Policy*, *26*(2).

Dean, H., & Platt, L. (Eds.). (2016). *Social Advantage and Disadvantage*. Oxford: OUP.

Dean, H., & Rodgers, R. (2004). Popular Discourses of Dependency, Responsibility and Rights. In H. Dean (Ed.), *The Ethics of Welfare*. Bristol: Policy Press.

Dean, H., & Taylor-Gooby, P. (1992). *Dependency Culture*. Hemel Hempstead: Harvester Wheatsheaf.

Dean, H. with Melrose, M. (1999). *Poverty, Riches and Social Citizenship*. Basingstoke: Macmillan.

Delanty, G. (2000). *Citizenship in a Global Age*. Buckingham: Open University Press.

Deneulin, S. (2006). *The Capability Approach and the Praxis of Development*. Basingstoke: Palgrave.

Destremau, B. (2000). Poverty, Exclusion and the Changing Role of the State in the Middle East. In H. Dean, R. Sykes & R. Woods (Eds.), *Social Policy Review 12*. Newcastle: Social Policy Association.

Dicey, A. (1885). *Introduction to the Law of the Constitution* (1939 edn.). London: Macmillan.

Donnelly, J. (2013). *Universal Human Rights in Theory and Practice* (3rd edn.). Ithaca: NY: Cornell UP.

Donzelot, J. (1979). *The Policing of Families*. London: Hutchinson.

Doogan, K. (2009). *New Capitalism? The Transformation of Work*. Cambridge: Polity.

Douglas, M. (1977). *Natural Symbols*. Harmonsworth: Penguin.

Douglas, M., & Ney, S. (1998). *Missing Persons*. Berkeley: University of California Press.

Doyal, L. (1979). *The Political Economy of Health*. London: Pluto.

Doyal, L., & Gough, I. (1991). *A Theory of Human Need*. Basingstoke: Macmillan.

Drakeford, M. (2000). *Privatisation and Social Policy*. Harlow: Longman.

Drescher, S. (2009). *Abolition*. Cambridge: CUP.

Dunbar, R., & Shultz, S. (2007). Evolution in the social brain. *Science*, *317*(5843).

Durbach, A. (2008). The Right to Legal Aid in Social Rights Litigation. In M. Langford (Ed.), *Social Rights Jurisprudence*. Cambridge: CUP.

Dutta, P., Murgai, R., Ravallion, M., & van de Walle, D. (2012). Does India's employment guarantee scheme guarantee employment? *Economic & Political Weekly*, *XLVII*(16).

Dworkin, R. (1977). *Taking Rights Seriously*. London: Duckworth.
Dwyer, P. (2000). *Welfare Rights and Responsibilities*. Bristol: Policy Press.
Dwyer, P. (2004). Creeping conditionality in the UK. *Canadian Journal of Sociology, 25*(2).
Dwyer, P. (2010). Understanding Social Citizenship - 2nd Edn. Bristol: Policy Press.
Easterlin, R. (2005). Building a Better Theory of Well-Being. In L. Bruni & P. Porta (Eds.), *Economics and Happiness*. Oxford: OUP.
The Economist. (2012). Special Report: 'State Capitalism'. 21–27 January. See https://www.economist.com/leaders/2012/01/21/the-rise-of-state-capitalism.
Edmonds, E., & Pavcnik, N. (2005). Child labor in the global economy. *Journal of Economic Perspectives, 19*(1).
Eide, A. (2001). Cultural Rights as Individual Human Rights. In A. Eide, C. Krause & A. Rosas (Eds.), *Economic, Social and Cultural Rights*. Dordrecht: Martinus Nijhoff.
Eide, A., Krause, C., & Rosas, A. (Eds.). (2001). *Economic Social and Cultural Rights*. (2nd edn.). Dordrecht: Martinus Nijhoff.
Elliott, B., & McCrone, D. (1987). Class, culture and morality. *Sociological Review, 35*(3).
Ellis, E. (2018). *Anthropocene*. Oxford: OUP.
Elsinger, P. (1998). *Toward an End to Hunger in America*. Washington, DC: Brookings.
Engels, F. (1884). *Origin of the Family, Private Property, and the State* (2010 edn.). London: Penguin.
Entzinger, H. (2007). Open Borders and the Welfare State. In A. Pecoud (Ed.), *Migration Without Borders*. Paris: Berghahn Books.
Equalities Review (2007). *Fairness and Freedom*. London: Cabinet Office.
Escobar, A. (2012). *Encountering Development* (2nd ed.). Princeton, NJ: PUP.
Esping-Andersen, G. (1990). *Three Worlds of Welfare Capitalism*. Cambridge: Polity.
Esping-Andersen, G. (1999). *The Social Foundations of Post-Industrial Economies*. Oxford: OUP.
Esping-Andersen, G. (2002). *Why We Need a New Welfare State*. Oxford: OUP.
Etzioni, A. (1995). *The Spirit of Community*. London: Fontana.
Fairbairns, Z. (1985). The Cohabitation Rule. In C. Ungerson (Ed.), *Women and Social Policy*. Basingstoke: Macmillan.
Falk, R. (1994). The Making of a Global Citizenship. In B. van Steenbergen (Ed.), *The Condition of Citizenship*. London: Sage.
Falkingham, J., & Hills, J. (1995). *The Dynamic of Welfare*. Hemel Hempstead: Harvester Wheatsheaf.
Fanon, F. (1967). *The Wretched of the Earth*. Harmondsworth: Penguin.
Farnsworth, K., & Irving, Z. (Eds.). (2015). *Social Policy in Times of Austerity*. Bristol: Policy Press.
Fenger, H. (2007). Welfare regimes in Central and Eastern Europe. *Contemporary Issues and Ideas in Social Science, 3*(2).
Ferguson, C. (1999). *Global Social Policy*. London: Department for International Development.
Finch, J. (1989). *Family Obligations and Social Change*. Cambridge: Polity.
Finch, J., & Mason, J. (1993). *Negotiating Family Responsibilities*. London: Routledge.
Fine, B. (1984). *Democracy and the Rule of Law: Liberal Ideals and Marxist Critiques*. London: Pluto.
Fine, B. (2002). Marxism and the Social Theory of Law. In R. Banakar & M. Travers (Eds.), *An Introduction to Law and Social Theory*. Oregon: Hart Publishing.
Fine, R. (2007). *Cosmopolitansim*. London: Routledge.
Fitzpatrick, P. (1992). Law as Resistance. In I. Grigg-Spall & P. Ireland (Eds.), *The Critical Lawyers' Handbook*. London: Pluto.

Fitzpatrick, T. (1999). *Freedom and Security*. Basingstoke: Macmillan.
Fitzpatrick, T. (2008). *Applied Ethics and Social Problems*. Bristol: Policy Press.
Fitzpatrick, T. (2018). *How to Live Well*. Cheltenham: Elgar.
Fitzpatrick, S., & Stephens, M. (2007). *An International Review of Homlessness and Social Housing Policy*. London: Department for Communities and Local Government.
Forder, A. (1974). *Concepts in Social Administration*. London: Routledge & Kegan Paul.
Forster, W. (1870). Speech Introducing Elementary Education Bill, House of Commons. In S. Maclure (Ed.), *Education Documents* (1996 edn.). London: Methuen.
Foster, J. (1999). Marx's theory of metabolic rift. *American Journal of Sociology, 105*(2).
Foucault, M. (1977). *Discipline and Punish*. Harmondsworth: Penguin.
Foucault, M. (1980). Power/Knowledge. In C. Gordon (Ed.). Hemel Hempstead: Harvester Wheatsheaf.
Foucault, M. (1991). Govermentality. In G. Burchell, C. Gordon & P. Miller (Eds.), *The Foucault Effect*. Chicago: UoC Press.
Foweraker, J., & Landman, T. (1997). *Citizenship Rights and Social Movements*. Oxford: OUP.
France, A. (1894). *Le Lys Rouge* (14th edn. – 2018). Vanves: Hatchette Livre.
Frank, A. (1971). *Capitalism and Underdevelopment in Latin America*. Harmondsworth: Penguin.
Fraser, D. (2017). *The Evolution of the British Welfare State* (5th edn.). London: Red Globe Press.
Fraser, I. (2011). Fidelity is confident its MINTs won't suck. *Bloomsbury Information QFINANCE* (10 May).
Fraser, N. (1989). *Unruly Practices*. Minneapolis: UoM Press.
Fraser, N. (2008). *Scales of Justice*. Cambridge: Polity.
Fraser, N. (2010). Scales of Justice: Reimagining Political Space in a Globalizing World. New York: Columbia UP.
Freeman, M. (2000). The future of children's rights. *Children & Society*, *14*(4).
Freeman, M. (2011). *Human Rights* (2nd edn.). Cambridge: Polity.
Freud, S. (1905). *Three Essays on Sexuality* (2017 edn.). London: Verso.
Friere, P. (1972). *Pedagogy of the Oppressed*. Harmondsworth: Penguin.
Fromm, E. (1961). *Marx's Concept of Man*. New York: Frederick Unger Publishing.
Fromm, E. (Ed.) (1965). *Socialist Humanism*. London: Allen Lane.
Fukuyama, F. (1992). *The End of History and the Last Man*. New York: Basic Books.
Gaia, E., Hujo, K., & Bennett, F. (2011). The use of conditions in social welfare programmes. *The Journal of Poverty and Social Justice*, *19*(1).
Galanter, M. (1976). Delivering legality: Some proposals for the direction of research. *Law and Society Review*, *11*(2).
Galbraith, K. (1992). *The Culture of Contentment*. Harmondsworth: Penguin.
Garfinkel, I., Miller, C., McLanahan, S., & Hanson, T. (1998). Deadbeat dads or inept states? *Evaluation Review*, *22*(6).
Gargarella, R. (2015). Deliberative Democracy, Dialogic Justice and the Promise of Social and Economic Rights. In H. Garcia, K. Klare & L. Williams (Eds.), *Social and Economic Rights in Theory and Practice*. Abingdon: Routledge.
Gargarella, R., Domingo, P., & Roux, T. (Eds.). (2006). *Courts and Social Transformation in New Democracies*. Burlington, VT: Ashgate.
Garland, D. (1981). The birth of the welfare sanction. *British Journal of Law and Society*, *8*(1).
Garnham, A., & Knights, E. (1994). *Putting the Treasury First*. London: CPAG.
Gauri, V., & Brinks, D. (Eds.). (2008). *Courting Social Justice*. Cambridge: CUP.

Gauthier, S., Rosa-Neto, P., Morais, J., & Webster, C. (2021). *World Alzheimer Report 2021*. London: Alzheimer's Disease International.
Gearty, C. (2011). Against Judicial Enforcement. In C. Gearty & V. Mantouvalou (Eds.), *Debating Social Rights*. Oxford: Hart Publishing.
Gearty, C., & Mantouvalou, V. (2011). *Debating Social Rights*. Oxford: Hart Publishing.
George, V. (1988). *Wealth, Poverty and Starvation*. Hemel Hempstead: Harvester Wheatsheaf.
George, V. (1993). Poverty in Russia. In R. Page & J. Baldock (Eds.), *Social Policy Review 5*. Canterbury: Social Policy Association.
George, V. (2010). *Major Thinkers in Welfare*. Bristol: Policy Press.
George, V., & Howards, I. (1991). *Poverty Amidst Affluence*. Aldershot: Edward Elgar.
George, V., & Page, R. (Eds.). (1995). *Modern Thinkers on Welfare*. Hemel Hempstead: Harvester Wheatsheaf.
George, V., & Wilding, P. (1985). *Ideology and Social Welfare*. London: Routledge & Kegan Paul.
George, V., & Wilding, P. (1994). *Welfare and Ideology*. Hemel Hempstead: Harvester Wheatsheaf.
Giddens, A. (1998). *The Third Way*. Cambridge: Polity.
Gilbert, A. (1992). Marx's Moral Realism. In G. McCarthy (Ed.), *Marx and Aristotle: Nineteenth Century German Social Theory and Classical Antiquity*. Maryland: Rowman & Littlefield.
Gilbert, B. (1966). *The Evolution of National Insurance in Great Britain*. London: Michael Joseph.
Gilbert, N. (2004). *Transformation of the Welfare State*. Oxford: OUP.
Gittens, D. (1993). *The Family in Question* (2nd ed.). Basingstoke: Macmillan.
Glasby, J. (2022). Social Care. In P. Alcock, T. Haux, V. McCall, & M. May (Eds.), *The Student's Companion to Social Policy* (6th edn.). Chichester: Wiley-Blackwell.
Goldthorpe, J., Llewellyn, C., & Payne, C. (1982). *Social Mobility and Class Structure in Modern Britain* (2nd ed.). Oxford: Clarendon Press.
Goodhart, D. (2006). *Progressive Nationalism*. London: Demos.
Goodman, R., & Peng, I. (1996). The East Asian Welfare States. In G. Esping-Andersen (Ed.), *Welfare States in Transition*. London: Sage.
Gorz, A. (1999). Reclaiming Work: Beyond the Wage-Based Society. Cambridge: Polity.
Gorz, A. (2010). The Immaterial: Knowledge, Value and Capital. Kolkata: Seagull Books.
Gough, I. (1979). *The Political Economy of the Welfare State*. Basingstoke: Macmillan.
Gough, I. (1997). Social Aspects of the European Model and Its Economic Consequences. In W. Beck, L. van der Maesen & A. Walker (Eds.), *The Social Quality of Europe*. Bristol: Policy Press.
Gough, I. (2019). Universal basic services. *Political Quarterly*, *90*(3).
Gough, I., & McGregor, J. (Eds.). (2007). *Wellbeing in Developing Countries*. Cambridge: CUP.
Gough, I., Wood, G., Barrientos, A., Bevan, P., Davis, P., & Room, G. (2004). Insecurity and Welfare Regimes in Asia, Africa and Latin America: Social Policy in Development Contexts. Cambridge: CUP.
Graeber, D., & Wengrow, D. (2022). *The Dawn of Everything*. London: Penguin.
Gramsci, A. (1971). *Prison Notebooks*. London: Lawrence & Wishart.
Gregory, L., & Matthews, P. (2022). Social policy and queer lives? *Journal of Social Policy*, *51*(3).

Griffin, J. (2008). *On Human Rights*. Oxford: OUP.
Griffiths, J. (1997). *The Politics of the Judiciary* (5th edn.). London: Fontana.
Grover, A. (2011). Thematic Study on the Realization of the Right to Health of Older Persons. Geneva: UNHRC.
Guterres, A. (2023). *Global Sustainable Development Report 2023*. New York: UN.
Haarman, C., & Haarman, D. (2012). Namibia. In *Basic Income Worldwide*. London: Palgrave.
Haarmann, C., Haarmann, D., Shindonola-Mote, H., Nattrass, N., van BNiekerk, I., & Samson, M. (2009). *Making the Difference!* Windhoek, Namibia: Basic Income Group Coalition.
Habermas, J. (1987). *The Theory of Communicative Action: Vol 2*. Cambridge: Polity.
Habermas, J. (1996). *Between Facts and Norms*. Cambridge: Polity.
Hadley, R., & Hatch, S. (1981). *Social Welfare and the Failure of the State*. London: Allen and Unwin.
Hall, S., & Held, D. (1989). Citizens and Citizenship. In S. Hall & M. Jacques (Eds.), *New Times*. London: Lawrence and Wishart.
Halmos, P. (1973). *The Faith of the Counsellors*. London: Constable.
Harden, I., & Lewis, N. (1986). *The Noble Lie*. London: Hutchinson.
Hardoy, J., & Satterthwaite, D. (1989). *Squatter Citizen*. London: Earthscan.
Hardt, M., & Negri, A. (2000). *Empire*. Cambridge, MA: Harvard UP.
Harari, Y. (2011). *Sapiens: A Brief History of Humankind*. London: Vintage.
Harris, D. (2009). Collective Complaints Under the European Social Charter. In K. Kaikobad & M. Bohlander (Eds.), *International Law and Power*. The Netherlands: Koninklijke Brill.
Harris, G. (1997). *Dignity and Vulnerability*. Oakland, CA: University of California Press.
Harris, J. (2014). A Precariat Charter - review. *The Guardian* (9 April).
Hayek, F. (1976). *Law, Legislation and Liberty: Vol.2*. London: Routledge & Kegan Paul.
Hayter, T. (1971). *Aid as Imperialism*. Harmondsworth: Penguin.
Healthwatch England. (2014). Health and care complaints system is 'utterly bewildering' for people. At www.healthwatch.co.uk/news/health-and-care-complaints-system-is-utterly-bewildering-people
Hegel, G. (1807). *The Phenomenology of Spirit* (1977 edn.). Oxford: Clarendeon Press.
Hegel, G. (1821). *Elements of the Philosophy of Rights* (1991 edn.). Cambridge: CUP.
Held, D. (1987). *Models of Democracy*. Cambridge: Polity.
Held, D. (2004). *Global Covenant*. Cambridge: Polity.
Held, D. (2010). *Cosmopolitanism*. Cambridge: Polity.
Held, D., & McGrew, A. (2007). *Globalization/Anti-Globalization* (2nd edn.). Cambridge: Polity.
Heller, A. (1974). *The Theory of Need in Marx* (2018 edn.). London: Verso.
Helliwell, J., Layard, R., Sachs, J., De Neve, J., & Wang, S. (Eds.). (2024). *World Happiness Report*. Oxford: University of Oxford Wellbeing Research Centre.
Henman, P., & Fenger, M. (Eds.). (2006). *Administering Welfare Reform*. Bristol: Policy Press.
Hessel, S. (2011). *Time for Outrage! (Indignez-Vous!)*. London: Quartet Books.
Hewitt, M. (1993). Social movements and social need. *Critical Social Policy*, *13*(37), 52–74.
Hickel, J. (2022). *More is Less*. London: Penguin.
Hill, M. (2006). *Social Policy in the Modern World*. Oxford: Blackwell.
Himmelfarb, G. (1995). *The De-Moralisation of Society*. London: Institute of Economic Affairs.

Hindess, B. (1987). *Freedom, Equality and the Market*. London: Tavistock.
Hirsch, F. (1977). *The Social Limits to Growth*. London: Routledge & Kegan Paul.
Hirst, P. (1980). Law, Socialism and Rights. In P. Carlen & M. Collison (Eds.), *Radical Issues in Criminology*. Oxford: Martin Robertson.
Hirst, P., & Thompson, G. (1996). *Globalization in Question*. Cambridge: Polity.
Hobbes, T. (1651). *Leviathan* (1991 edn.). Cambridge: CUP.
Hobsbawm, E. (1962). *The Age of Revolution: 1789-1848*. New York: Mentor.
Hohfeld, W. (1946). *Fundamental Legal Conceptions as Applied in Judicial Reasoning*. New Haven, CT: Yale University Press.
Holden, C. (2022). International Trade, Global Economic Governance and Welfare. In N. Yeates & C. Holden (Eds.), *Understanding Global Social Policy*. Bristol: Policy Press.
Holliday, I. (2000). Productivist welfare capitalism. *Political Studies*, *48*(4).
Hollifeld, J. (1992). *Immigrants, Markets and States*. Cambridge, Mass: Harvard UP.
Holloway, J., & Picciotto, S. (Eds.). (1978). *State and Capital*. London: Arnold.
Holston, J. (2009). Insurgent citizenship in an era of global urban peripheries. *City and Society*, *21*(2).
Holzmann, R., & Hinz, R. (2005). *Old-Age Income Support in the 21st Century*. Washington, DC: World Bank.
Honneth, A. (1995). *The Struggle for Recognition*. Cambridge: Polity.
Honneth, A. (2017). *The Idea of Socialism*. Cambridge: Polity.
Hood, C. (1991). A public management for all seasons? *Public Administration*, *69*(1).
Howe, D. (2009). *A Brief Introduction to Social Work Theory*. Basingstoke: Palgrave.
Huizinga, J. (1949). *Homo Ludens* (2016 edn.). Kettering OH: Angelico Press.
Hulme, R., & Hulme, M. (2008). The Global Transfer of Social Policy. In N. Yeates (Ed.), *Understanding Global Social Policy*. Bristol: The Policy Press.
Humpage, L. (2010). Revisioning comparative welfare state studies. *Policy Studies*, *31*(5).
Hunt, A. (1978). *The Sociological Movement in Law*. Basingstoke: Macmillan.
Hunt, A. (1990). Rights and social movements. *Journal of Law and Society*, *17*(3).
Hunt, P. (1996). *Reclaiming Social Rights*. Aldershot: Dartmouth/Ashgate.
Hunt, P. (2006). Report of the Special Rapporteur on the Right of Everyone to the Enjoyment of the Highest Attainable Standard of Physical and Mental Health to the UN Economic and Social Council. Geneva: UN.
Hunt, P., Nowak, M., & Osmani, S. (2004). *Human Rights and Poverty Reduction*. Geneva: OHCHR.
Ignatieff, M. (1984). *The Needs of Strangers*. London: Chatto & Windus.
Ikawan, D. (2020). The International Covenant on Economic, Social and Cultural Rights and the Optional Protocol. In J. Dugard, B. Porter, D. Ikawan & L. Chenwi (Eds.), *Research Handbook on Economic, Social and Cultural Rights*. Cheltenham: Elgar.
Illich, I. (1971). *Deschooling Society*. London: Calder & Boyers.
Illich, I., McKnight, J., Zola, I., Caplan, J., & Shaiken, H. (1977). *Disabling Professions*. London: Marion Boyars.
Inglehart, R. (1990). *Culture Shift in Advanced Industrial Society*. Princeton NJ: Princeton UP.
Inglehart, R., & Welzel, C. (2005). *Modernization, Cultural Change and Democracy*. New York: Cambridge University Press.
International Labour Organization. (1919). *ILO Constitution* (with amendments up to 2015). At: www.ilo.org/publications/ilo-constitution-0
International Labour Organization. (1944). *Declaration Concerning the Aims and Purposes of the International Labour Organization*. Adopted, Philadelphia, ILO, 10 May.

International Labour Organization. (1995). *Protection Against Unjustified Dismissal*. Geneva: ILO.
International Labour Organization. (1999). *Decent Work*. Director General's Report. Geneva: ILO.
International Labour Organization. (2009). General Survey Concerning the Occupational Safety and Health Convention. Geneva: ILO.
International Labour Organization. (2011). *Equality at Work*. Geneva: ILO.
International Labour Organization. (2012). *Social Protection Floors Recommendation*. Geneva: ILO.
International Labour Organization. (2022). *Global Wage Report 2022/23*. Geneva: ILO.
Ishkanian, A., & Szrerter, S. (Eds.). (2012). *The Big Society Debate: A New Research Agenda for Social Policy*. Cheltenham: Edward Elgar.
Isin, E., Brodie, J., Juteau, D., & Stasiulis, D. (2008). Recasting the Social in Citizenship. In E. Isin (Ed.), *Recasting the Social in Citizenship*. Toronto: UoT Press.
Jackson, T. (2009). Prosperity Without Growth. London: Sustainable Development Commission.
Jacobs, H. (2013). Private property and human rights. *International Journal of Social Welfare*, *22*(Supplement 1).
James, S. (2008). *A Forgotten Right? The right to clothing in international law*. Paper presented at the Sixteenth Annual Australian and New Zealand Society of International Law (ANZIL) Conference, Canberra.
Jawad, R. (2022a). Social Policy in the Middle East and North Africa Region. In P. Alcock, T. Haux, V. McCall, & M. May (Eds.), *The Student's Companion to Social Policy* (6th edn.). Oxford: Wiley/Blackwell.
Jawad, R. (2022b). The Role of Religion. In P. Alcock, T. Haux, V. McCall, & M. May (Eds.), *The Student's Companion to Social Policy* (6th edn.). Oxford: Wiley/Blackwell.
Jessop, B. (2002). *The Future of the Capitalist State*. Cambridge: Polity.
Jo, Y., & Walker, R. (2014). Self-Sufficiency, Social Assistance and the Shaming of Poverty. In E. Gubrium, S. Pellissery & I. Lodemel (Eds.), *The Shame of It*. Bristol: Policy Press.
Johnson, N. (1987). *The Welfare State in Transition*. Brighton: Wheatsheaf.
Jones, C. (1993). The Pacific Challenge. In C. Jones (Ed.), *New Perspectives on the Welfare State in Europe*. London: Routledge.
Jones, D. (2012). Human Dignity in Healthcare. Paper presented at the Anscombe Bioethics Centre conference on *Human Dignity*, 18 June, Blackfriars Hall, Oxford.
Jones, P. (1994). *Rights*. Basingstoke: Macmillan.
Jordan, B. (1973). *Paupers*. London: Routledge & Kegan Paul.
Jordan, B. (1996). *A Theory of Poverty and Social Exclusion*. Cambridge: Polity.
Jordan, B. (1998). *The New Politics of Welfare*. London: Sage.
Jordan, B. (2008). *Welfare and Well-Being*. Bristol: Policy Press.
Jowell, J. (1975). *Law and Bureaucracy*. New York: Dunellan.
Jung, C., Hirschl, R., & Rosevar, E. (2013). *Economic and Social Rights in National Constitutions*. Social Science Research Network. At http://dx.doi.org/10.2139/ssrn.2349680
Kabeer, N. (2004). Globalization, labor standards, and women's rights. *Feminist Economics*, *10*(1), 3–35.
Kaldor, M. (2003). *Global Civil Society*. Cambridge: Polity.
Kamenka, E., & Tay, A. (1975). Beyond Bourgeois Individualism. In E. Kamenka & R. Neale (Eds.), *Feudalism, Capitalism and Beyond*. London: Edward Arnold.
Kananen, J. (2014). *The Nordic Welfare States in Three Eras*. Farnham: Ashgate.
Kant, I. (1785). *Groundwork of the Metaphysics of Morals* (1991 edn.). London: Routledge

Karshenas, M., & Moghadam, V. (2006). *Social Policy in the Middle East*. Basingstoke: Palgrave.

Kelly, A. (1994). *The National Curriculum*. London: Chapman.

Kendall, J., & Knapp, M. (1995). A Loose and Baggy Monster. In J. Davis Smith, C. Rochester & R. Hedley (Eds.), *An Introduction to the Voluntary Sector*. London: Routledge.

Kennet, P., & Retief, A. (2022). Social Policy in Low-Income Countries. In P. Alcock, T. Haux, V. McCall, & M. May (Eds.), *Student's Companion to Social Policy* (6th edn.). Oxford: Wiley.

Kerton, S. (2012). Tahrir, here? *Social Movement Studies*, *11*(3–4).

Kim, S.-Y. (2011). *The Politics of Struggle in a State-Civil Society Partnership*, PhD Thesis. London School of Economics and Political Science,

King, D. (1999). *In the Name of Liberalism*. Oxford: Oxford University Press.

Klein, R. (2011). *Sociality as the Human Condition*. Leiden: Brill.

Klein, R., & Edgars, B. (2002). *The Dawn of Human Culture*. New York: Wiley.

Klug, F. (2000). *Values for a Godless Age*. London: Penguin.

Knijn, T., Martin, C., & Millar, J. (2007). Activation as a common framework for social policies towards lone parents. *Social Policy & Administration*, *41*(6).

Köhler, G., & Pogge, T. (2014). Big holes in the SDG draft. *CROP Poverty Brief* (August 2014 - www.crop.org).

Korpi, W. (1983). *The Democratic Class Struggle*. London: Routledge & Kegan Paul.

Kuznets, S. (1955). Economic growth and income inequality. *American Economic Review*, *45*(1).

Kymlicka, W. (1995). *Multicultural Citizenship*. Oxford: Clarendon Press.

Landau, D., & Dixon, R. (2019). Constitutional Non-Transformation? In J. Dugard, B. Porter, D. Ikawan & I. Chenwi (Eds.), *The Future of Social and Economic Rights*. Cambridge: CUP.

Langan, M., & Ostner, I. (1991). Gender and Welfare. In G. Room (Ed.), *Towards a European Welfare State?* Bristol: SAUS.

Langford, M. (2008). The Justiciability of Social Rights. In *Social Rights Jurisprudence*. Cambridge: CUP.

Langford, M., & King, J. (2008). Committee on Social, Economic and Cultural Rights. In M. Langford (Ed.), *Social Rights Jurisprudence*. Cambridge: CUP.

Langford, M., Porter, B., Brown, R., & Rossi, J. (Eds.). (2016). *The Optional Protocol to the International Covenant on Economic, Social and Cultural Rights*. Pretoria: University Law Press.

Langford, M., Rodriguez-Garavito, C., & Rossi, J. (Eds.). (2017). *Social Rights Judgements and the Politics of Compliance*. Cambridge: CUP.

Law Society. (2023). A decade of cuts At www.lawsociety.org.uk/contact-or-visit-us/press-office/press-releases/a-decade-of-cuts-legal-aid-in-tatters

Lederer, K. (1980). *Human Needs*. Cambridge, MA: Oelgeschlager, Gunn & Hain.

Lee, S., McCann, D., & Messenger, J. (2007). *Working Time Around the World*. London: Routledge.

Lefebvre, H. (1991). *The Production of Space*. Oxford: Blackwell.

Lefebvre, H. (2014). *Critique of Everyday Life* (One Volume Edn.). London: Verso.

Le Grand, J. (1982). *The Strategy of Equality*. London: Allen and Unwin.

Leggatt, A. (2001). Tribunals for Users. London: Lord Chanceller's Office.

Leisering, L. (2022). Global Social Security Policy. In Y. N & C. Holding (Eds.), *Understanding Global Social Policy*. Bristol: Policy Press.

Leisering, L., & Barrientos, A. (2013). Social citizenship for the global poor? *International Journal of Social Welfare*, *22*(Supplement1).

Lenaghan, J. (1997). Citizens' Rights to Health Care in the UK. In J. Lenaghan (Ed.), *Hard Choices in Health Care*. London: BMJ.

Leung, J. (1994). Dismantling the "Iron rice bowl. *Journal of Social Policy*, *23*(3).
Levinas, E. (1'969). *Totality and Infinity*. Pittsburgh, PA: Duquesne University Press.
Levitas, R. (Ed.) (1986). *The Ideology of the New Right*. Cambridge: Polity.
Lewis, J. (2000). Work and Care. In H. Dean, R. Sykes, & R. Woods (Eds.), *Social Policy Review 12*. Newcastle: Social Policy Association.
Lewis, J. (2001). Family Change and Lone Parents as a Social Problem. In M. May, R. Page & E. Brunsdon (Eds.), *Understanding Social Problems*. Oxford: Blackwell.
Lewis, J. (2006). Work/family reconciliation, equal opportunities and social policies. *Journal of European Public Policy*, *13*(3).
Lewis, J. (2009). *Work-Family Balance, Gender and Policy*. Cheltenham: Edward Elgar.
Lewis, N., & Birkinshaw, P. (1993). *When Citizens Complain*. Buckingham: Open University Press.
Lewis, G., Gewirtz, S., & Clarke, J. (Eds.). (2000). *Rethinking Social Policy*. London: Sage.
Lewis, J., & Surender, R. (Eds.). (2004). *Welfare State Change*. Oxford: OUP.
Liebenberg, S. (2008). South Africa. In M. Langford (Ed.), *Social Rights Jurisprudence*. Cambridge: CUP.
Lipset, M. (1963). *Political Man*. London: Mercury Books.
Lipsky, M. (1980/2010). Street-Level Bureaucracy. New York: Russell Sage Foundation.
Lister, R. (1990). *The Exclusive Society: Citizenship and the Poor*. London: CPAG.
Lister, R. (1998). Citizenship, sexual identity and social exclusion. *International Journal of Sociology and Social Policy*, *28*(9–10).
Lister, R. (2003). *Citizenship: Feminist Perspectives*, (2nd edn.). Basingstoke: Macmillan.
Lister, R. (2004). *Poverty*. Cambridge: Policy.
Lister, R. (2010). *Understanding Theories and Concepts in Social Policy*. Bristol: Policy Press.
Lock, F. (1999). *Edmund Burke* (Vol. 1). Oxford: Clarendon Press.
Locke, J. (1690). *Two Treatises on Civil Government* (1960 edn.). New York: Mentor.
Lockwood, D. (1996). Civic integration and class formation. *British Journal of Sociology*, *47*(3).
Lødemel, I., & Trickey, H. (Eds.). (2000). *'An Offer You Can't Refuse*. Bristol: Policy Press.
Loney, M. (1983). *Community Against Government*. London: Heinemann.
Lukács, G. (1971). *History and Class Consciousness*. London: Merlin Press.
Lund, F. (2008). *Changing Social Policy*. Cape Town: HSRC Press.
Lynes, T. (1975). Unemployment Assistance Tribunals in the 1930s. In M. Adler & A. Bradley (Eds.), *Justice, Discretion and Poverty*. Abingdon: Professional Books.
Lyotard, J. (1984). *The Postmodern Condition*. Manchester: Manchester UP.
M'Baye, K. (1972). Le droit au développement comme un droit de l'Homme. *Revue Des Droits De l'Homme*, *5*, 503–505.
MacIntyre, A. (1999). *Dependent Rational Animals*. Peru, IL: Carus Publishing.
MacIntyre, A. (2007). *After Virtue* (3rd ed.). Notre Dame, Indiana: Notre Dame Press.
Macklin, R. (2003). Dignity is a useless concept. *British Medical Journal*, *327*, 1419–1420.
Malik, K. (2001). *Man, Beast, Zombie*. London: Phoenix.
Mamdani, M. (1996). *Citizen and Subject*. Princeton, NJ: Princeton UP.
Mameli, A. (1997). Poverty and Group Consciousness. In A. Kjønstad & J. Veit-Wilson (Eds.), *Law, Power and Poverty*. Bergen: CROP.
Mann, M. (1987). Ruling class strategies and citizenship', *Sociology*. *21*(3).

Manning, N. (2007). Turkey, The EU and social policy. *Social Policy & Society*, *6*(4).

Mantouvalou, V. (2011). In Support of Legalisation. In C. Gearty & V. Mantouvalou (Eds.), *Debating Social Rights*. Oxford: Hart Publishing.

Marcano, C. (2009). From the neo-liberal barrio to the socialist commune. *Human Geography*, *2*(3).

Marcuse, H. (1964). *One Dimensional Man*. Boston, Mass: Beacon Press.

Marks, N. (2006). *The Unhappy Planet Index*. London: New Economics Foundation.

Marks, S. (2004). The human right to development. *Harvard Human Rights Journal*, *17*, 137–168.

Marks, S. (2013). The Emergence and Scope of the Human Right to Health. In M. Zuniga, S. Marks & L. Gostin (Eds.), *Advancing the Human Right to Health*. Oxford: OUP.

Márkus, G. (1978). *Marxism & Anthropology: The Concept of 'human essence' in the Philosophy of Marx* (2014 edn.). NSW, Australia: modem-Verlag.

Marmot, M. (2010). *Fair Society, Healthy Lives*. London: The Marmot Review.

Marshall, G. (1997). *Repositioning Class*. London: Sage.

Marshall, T. (1950). Citizenship and Social Class. In T. Marshall & T. Bottomore (Eds.), *Citizenship and Social Class* (1992 ed.). London: Pluto.

Marx, K. (1843). *Critique of Hegel's Philosophy of Right* (1970 edn.). Cambridge: CUP.

Marx, K. (1844). Economic and Philosophical Manuscripts. In L. Colletti (Ed.), *Early Writings (1975 edn.)*. Harmondsworth: Penguin.

Marx, K. (1845). *Theses on Feuerbach*. In T. Bottomore & M. Rubel (Eds.), Karl Marx Harmondsworth: Penguin.

Marx, K. (1857). *Grundrisse* (1973 edn.). London: Penguin.

Marx, K. (1859). Preface to a Contribution to the Critique of Political Economy. In *Marx and Engels Selected Works* (1969 edn, Vol. 1). Moscow: Progress.

Marx, K. (1887). *Capital* (1970 edn. Vol. I). London: Lawrence & Wishart.

Marx, K. (1893). *Capital* (1956 edn. Vol. 2). London: Lawrence & Wishart.

Marx, K. (1894). *Capital* (1959 edn. Vol. 3). London: Lawrence & Wishart.

Marx, K., & Engels, F. (1848). *The Communist Manifesto*. (1970 Merit Pamphlet). New York: Pathfinder Press.

Maslow, A. (1943). A theory of human motivation. *Psychological Review*, *50*, 370–396.

Massey, D. (2008). Notas sobre la geometria del poder. *Dio-critica*, *5*, 56–59.

Mauss, M. (1925). *The Gift* (2002 edn.). Abingdon: Routledge.

Maxwell, S. (2005). The Washington Consensus is Dead! Working Paper 243. London: Overseas Development Institute.

McArthur, J., & Rasmussen, K. (2017). *Change of Pace*. Washington DC: Brookings.

McCarthy, P., Simpson, B., Hill, M., Walker, J., & Corlyon, J. (1992). *Grievances, Complaints and Local Government*. Aldershot: Avebury.

McGregor, J. (2007). Researching Wellbeing. In I. Gough & J. McGregor (Eds.), *Wellbeing in Developing Countries*. Cambridge: CUP.

McLaughlin, E. (1999). Social Security and Poverty. In J. Ditch (Ed.), *Introduction to Social Security*. London: Routledge.

McQueen, J. (2022). *Guide to Landlord and Tenant Law* (revised edn.). London: Emerald Publishing.

Mead, G. (1934). *Mind, Self and Society from the Standpoint of a Social Behaviorist*. Chicago: Chicago UP.

Mead, L. (1997). *From Welfare to Work*. London: IEA Health & Welfare Unit.

Meadows, D., Randers, J., & Behrens, W. III (1972). *The Limits to Growth*. London: Pan.

Mehedi, M. (1999). *The content of the right to education*. Working paper presented to the Sub-Commission on Prevention of Discrimination and Protection of Minorities. New York: ECOSOC.
Meiksins-Wood, E. (1995). *Democracy Against Capitalism*. Cambridge: CUP.
Menger, C. (1871). *Principles of Economics* (1950 edn.). Glencoe, Ill: Free Press.
Meyer, J. (2007). Globalization: Theory and trends. *International Journal of Comparative Sociology*, *48*(4).
Meyer, J. (2009). The Nation State. In G. Krucken & G. Drori (Eds.), *World Society*. Oxford: OUP.
Meyer, J., Boli, J., Thomas, G., & Ramirez, F. (1997). World society and the nation state. *American Journal of Sociology*, *103*(1).
Midgley, J. (1995). *Social Development*. London: Sage.
Midgley, J. (2013). Social Development and Social Welfare. In P. Kennett (Ed.), *Comparative Social Policy* (2nd edn.). Cheltenham: Elgar.
Milanovic, B. (2007). Globalization and Inequality. In D. Held & A. Kaya (Eds.), *Global Inequality*. Cambridge: Polity.
Miles, R. (1989). *Racism*. London: Routledge.
Mill, J. S. (1859). *On Liberty*. [1972 edn.]. London: JM Dent.
Miller, J. (2021). Hugo Grotius. In E. Zalta (Ed.), *The Stanford Encyclopedia of Philosophy*. Stanford University Press. At https://plato.stanford.edu/archives/spr2021/entries/grotius/
Mishra, R. (1984). *The Welfare State in Crisis*. Hemel Hempstead: Harvester Wheatsheaf.
Mishra, R. (1990). *The Welfare State in Capitalist Society*. Hemel Hempstead: Harvester Wheatsheaf.
Mishra, R. (1999). *Globalisation and the Welfare State*. Hemel Hempstead: Harvester Wheatsheaf.
Modood, T. (2013). *Multiculturalism* (2nd edn.). Cambridge: Polity.
Moore, B. J. (1978). *Injustice*. New York: Macmillan.
Morabito, C., Vandenbroek, M., & Roose, R. (2013). 'The greatest of Equalisers'. *Journal of Social Policy*, *42*(3).
Morgan, L. (1887). *Ancient Society* (1907 edn.). New York: Henry Holt & Co.
Morris, J. (1991). Pride against Prejudice. London: Women's Press.
Morris, J. (2003). Community Care or Independent Living? In N. Ellison & C. Pierson (Eds.), *Developments in British Social Policy 2*. Basingstoke: Palgrave.
Morris, L. (2002). *Managing Migration*. London: Routledge.
Morris, L. (2006). Social Rights, Trans-National Rights and Civic Stratification. In L. Morris (Ed.), *Rights*. London: Routledge.
Morris, R. (2017). After De Brosses. In R. Morris & D. Leonard (Eds.), *The Returns of Fetishism*. Chicago: University of Chicago Press.
Moss, P. (2005). Learning With Other Countries. In Daycare Trust (Ed.), *Learning with Other Countries*. London: Daycare Trust.
Mulcahy, L., & Lloyd-Bostock, S. (1992). Complaining. In R. Dingwall & P. Fenn (Eds.), *Quality and Regulation in Health Care*. London: Routledge.
Munck, R. (2005). *Globalization and Social Exclusion*. Bloomfield, CT: Kumarian Press.
Muralidhar, S. (2008). India. In M. Langford (Ed.), *Social Rights Jurisprudence*. Cambridge: CUP.
Musgrave, R. (1959). *The Theory of Public Finance*. New York: McGraw Hill.
Naandi Foundation. (2018). *HUNGaMA Survey Report*. Hyderabad: Naandi Foundation.
National Consumer Council. (1977). *The Fourth Right of Citizenship*. London: NCC.

Nedelsky, J., & Scott, C. (1992). Constitutional Dialogue. In J. Bakan & D. Schneiderman (Eds.), *Social Justice and the Constitution*. Ottawa: Carleton UP.

Neuberger, J. (2010). *The Report of the Advisory Panel on Judicial Diversity*. London: Ministry of Justice.

New Economics Foundation. (2012). Happy Planet Index: 2012 Report. London: NEF.

Newby, H. (1996). Citizenship in a Green World. In M. Bulmer & A. Rees (Eds.), *Citizenship Today*. London: UCL Press.

Newman, B., & Thompson, R. (1989). Economic growth and social development. *World Development*, *17*(4).

Nissanke, M. (2003). *The Revenue Potential of the Currency Transfer Tax for Development Finance*. (WIDER discussion paper no. 2003/81). Helsinki: UN.

Novak, T. (1988). *Poverty and the State*. Milton Keynes: Open University Press.

Nowak, M. (2001). The Right to Education. In A. Eide, C. Krause, & A. Rosas (Eds.), *Economic, Social and Cultural Rights* (2nd edn.). Dordrecht: Martinus Nijhoff.

Nowak, M. (2011). Informal oral presentation to The Road to Global Social Citizenship Co-operation Group, convened at Center for Interdisciplinary Studies (ZiF) (Bielefeld, Germany, 19 May).

Nozick, R. (1974). *Anarchy, State and Utopia*. Oxford: Blackwell.

Nussbaum, M. (1999). Virtue ethics. *Journal of Ethics*, *3*(3).

Nussbaum, M. (2011). *Creating Capabilities*. Cambridge, MA: Belknap Press.

Nyers, P. (Ed.) (2009). *Securitizations of Citizenship*. Abingdon: Routledge.

O'Connor, J. (1973). *Fiscal Crisis of the State*. New York: St. Martin's Press.

O'Mathúna, D., Scott, A., McAuley, A., Walsh-Daneshmandi, A., & Daly, B. (2005). *Health Care Rights and Responsibilities*. Dublin: Irish Patients' Association.

O'Neill, J. (2001). Building Better Global Economic BRICs. *Global Economic Paper*, 66. New York: Goldman Sachs.

O'Neill, O. (1986). *Faces of Hunger*. London: Allen & Unwin.

O'Neill, O. (2005). The dark side of human rights. *International Affairs*, *81*, 427–439.

Offe, C. (1972). Advanced capitalism and the welfare state. *Politics and Society*, *2*(4).

Offe, C. (1984). *Contradictions of the Welfare State*. Cambridge, Mass: MIT Press.

Office of the High Commissioner for Human Rights. (2006). *Principles and Guidelines for a Human Rights Approach to Poverty Reduction Strategies*. Geneva: OHCHR.

Office of the High Commissioner for Human Rights. (2013). *Directory of Special Procedures Mandate Holders*. Geneva: OHCHR.

Oliver, M. (1990). *The Politics of Disablement*. Basingstoke: Macmillan.

Organisation for Economic Co-operation and Development. (2019). *Society at a Glance 2019*. Paris: OECD.

Organisation for Economic Co-operation and Development. (2023). *PISA 2022 Results* (Volume I). Paris: OECD.

Padley, M., Stone, J., & Robinson, E. (2024). *Households Living Below a Minimum Income Standard 2008-2022*. York: Joseph Rowntree Foundation.

Paine, T. (1791). *The Rights of Man* (1984 edn.). Harmondsworth: Penguin.

Palmer, E. (2007). *Judicial Review, Socio-Economic Rights and the Human Rights Act*. Oxford: Hart Publishing.

Papadakis, E., & Taylor-Gooby, P. (1987). The Private Provision of Public Welfare: State, Market and Community. Brighton: Wheatsheaf.

Parekh, S. (2008). *Hannah Arendt and the Challenge of Modernity*. Abingdon: Routledge.

Pascal, B. (1670). *Pensèes* (1958 ed.). Louisville, KY: GLH Publishing.

Pascall, G. (1986/1997). *Social Policy*. London: Tavistock.

Pascall, G. (2012). *Gender Equality in the Welfare State*. Bristol: Policy Press.

Pashukanis, E. (1978). *General Theory of Law and Marxism*. London: Ink Links.
Patomäki, H., & Teivainen, T. (2004). *A Possible World*. London: Zed Books.
Peck, J. (2001). *Workfare States*. New York: Guildford Press.
Peck, J., & Tickell, A. (2012). Neoliberalism resurgent? *South Atlantic Quarterly*, *111*(2).
Pecoud, A., & de Guchteneire, P. (2005). Migration Without Borders. Global Migration Perspectives Research Paper No. 27. Paris: UNESCO Global Commission on International Migration.
Pellegrino, E., Schulman, A., & Merrill, T. (Eds.). (2009). *Human Dignity and Bioethics*. Notre Dame, IN: Notre Dame UP.
Peng, I. (2002). Social care in crisis. *Social Politics*, *9*(3).
Perry, R. (Ed.). (1964). *Sources of Our Liberties*. New York: McGraw-Hill.
Pfeffer, N., & Coote, A. (1991). Is Quality Good for You? London: IPPR.
Phillips, A. (1999). Which Equalities Matter? Cambridge: Policy Press.
Phillips, A. (2007). Multiculturalism Without Culture. Princeton, NJ: PUP.
Piachaud, D. (1981, 10 September). Peter Townsend and the Holy Grail. *New Society*.
Pickerill, J., & Krinsky, J. (2012). Why does occupy matter? *Social Movement Studies*, *11*(3–4).
Picketty, T. (2014). *Capital in the Twenty-First Century*. Cambridge, MA: Belknap Press.
Pierson, C. (1998). *Beyond the Welfare State*. Cambridge: Polity.
Pierson, C. (2001). *Hard Choices*. Cambridge: Polity.
Piovesan, F. (2008). Brazil. In M. Langford (Ed.), *Social Rights Jurisprudence*. Cambridge: CUP.
Piven, F., & Cloward, R. (1977). *Poor People's Movements*. New York: Pantheon Books.
Plant, R. (1992). Citizenship, Rights and Welfare. In A. Coote (Ed.), *The Welfare of Citizens*. London: IPPR/Rivers Oram Press.
Plant, R., Lesser, H., & Taylor-Gooby, P. (1980). *Political Philosophy and Social Welfare*. London: Routledge & Kegan Paul.
Pogge, T. (2002). *World Poverty and Human Rights*. Cambridge: Polity.
Pogge, T. (Ed.) (2007). *Freedom from Poverty as a Human Right*. Oxford: OUP.
Pointer, F. (1896). *A History of Education* (2006 Replica ed.). Boston, MA: Elibron Claasics.
Polanyi, K. (1944). *The Great Transformation*. New York: Rinehart.
Polis, A., & Schwab, P. (1979). Human Rights. In A. Polis & P. Schwab (Eds.), *Human Rights*. New York: Praeger.
Pollock, A., & Price, D. (2013). *Duty to Care*. London: Centre for Labour and Social Studies.
Porter, D., & Craig, D. (2004). The third way and the third world. *Review of International Political Economy*, *11*(2).
Powell, E. (1972). *Still to Decide*. London: Elliot Right Way Books.
Powell, F. (2007). *The Politics of Civil Society*. Bristol: Policy Press.
Powell, M. (Ed.) (2007). *Understanding the Mixed Economy of Welfare*. Bristol: Policy Press.
Prendergast, R. (2005). The concept of freedom and its relation to economic development. *Cambridge Journal of Economics*, *29*, 1145–1170.
Prime Minister's Office. (1991). *The Citizen's Charter*. Cm.1599. London: HMSO.
Prosser, T. (1983). *Test Cases for the Poor*. London: CPAG.
Putnam, R. (1993). *Making Democracy Work*. Princeton, NJ: Princeton UP.
Ramani, S. (2021). Russia And China in Africa, *Policy Insights*, 120. At www.jstor.org/stable/resrep38659

Ramose, M. (2003). The Philosophy of Ubuntu and Ubuntu as a Philosophy. In P. Coetee & A. Roux (Eds.), *The African Philosophy Reader* (2nd ed.). London: Routledge.
Rand, A. (1964). *The Virtue of Selfishness*. New York: New American Library.
Raphael, D. (1989). Enlightenment and Revolution. In N. MacCormick & Z. Bankowski (Eds.), *Enlightenment, Rights and Revolution*. Aberdeen: Aberdeen UP.
Rawls, J. (1972). *A Theory of Justice*. Oxford: OUP.
Reader, S. (2006). Does a basic needs approach need capabilities? *The Journal of Political Philosophy*, *14*(3).
Reich, C. (1964). The new property. *Yale Law Journal*, *73*.
Richardson, D. (1998). Sexuality and citizenship. *Sociology*, *32*(1).
Richardson, K., Steffeb, W., & Lucht, W., et al. (2023). Earth beyond six of nine planetary boundaries. *Science Advances*, *9*(37).
Ridge, T. (2002). *Childhood Poverty and Social Exclusion*. Bristol: Policy Press.
Rieger, E., & Leibfried, S. (2003). *Limits to Globalization*. Cambridge: Polity.
Roche, M. (1992). *Re-Thinking Citizenship*. Cambridge: Polity.
Rodgers, G., Gore, C., & Figueiredo, J. (Eds.). (1995). *Social Exclusion*. Geneva: ILO.
Rolnik, R. (2013). Report of the Special Rapporteur on Adequate Housing as a Component of the Right to an Adequate Standard of Living, and on the Right to non-Discrimination in This Context on her Mission to the United Kingdom of Great Britain and Northern Ireland (29 August–11 September 2013). Geneva: UN.
Roosevelt, F. (1941). *State of the Union address to Congress 6 January*: http://www.ourdocuments.gov/doc.php?flash=false&doc=70&page=transcript.
Roosevelt, F. (1944). State of the Union Address to Congress 11 January. In S. Rosenman (Ed.), *The Public Papers and Addresses of Franklin D. Roosevelt* (1950 edn., Vol. XIII). New York: Harper.
Rorty, R. (1982). *Consequences of Pragmatism*. Minnesota: University of Minnesota.
Rosanvallon, P. (2021). *The Populist Century*. Cambridge: Polity.
Rosas, A. (2001). The Right to Development. In A. Eide, C. Krause, & A. Rosas (Eds.), *Economic, Social and Cultural Rights* (2nd ed.). Dordrecht: Nijhoff.
Rose, N. (1996a). Governing "advanced" Liberal Democracies. In A. Barry, T. Osborne & N. Rose (Eds.), *Foucault and Political Reason*. London: UCL Press.
Rose, N. (1996b). The death of the social? *Economy and Society*, *25*(3).
Rose, R. (1988). *Ordinary People in Public Policy*. London: Sage.
Rostow, W. (1971). *The Stages of Economic Growth*. Cambridge: CUP.
Roulstone, A., & Barnes, C. (Eds.). (2005). *Working Futures?* Bristol: Policy Press.
Roulstone, A., & Prideaux, S. (2012). *Understanding Disability Policy*. Bristol: Policy Press.
Rousseau, J.-J. (1762). Of the Social Contract or Principles of Political Right. In V. Gourevitch (Ed.), *Rousseau* (1997 ed.). Cambridge: CUP.
Rys, V. (2010). *Reinventing Social Security Worldwide*. Bristol: Policy Press.
Sachs, A. (2009). *The Strange Alchemy of Life and Law*. Oxford: OUP.
Sachs, W. (Ed.) (2010). *The Development Dictionary*. (2nd ed.). London: Zed Books.
Sahlins, M. (1974). *Stone Age Economics*. London: Tavistock.
Salomon, M. (Ed.) (2005). *Economic, Social and Cultural Rights*. London: Minority Rights Group International.
Salomon, M. (2007). *Global Responsibility for Human Rights*. Oxford: OUP.
Salomon, M. (2010). International Human Rights Obligations in Context. In B. Andreassen & S. Marks (Eds.), *Development as a Human Right*. Antwerp: Intersentia.
Sandel, M. (1982). *Liberalism and the Limits of Justice*. Cambridge: CUP.

Sarat, A., & Schiengold, S. (Eds.). (2001). *Cause Lawyering and the State in a Global Era*. Oxford: OUP.
Saunders, P. (1984). Beyond housing classes. *International Journal of Urban and Regional Research*, *8*(2).
Saville, J. (1958). The welfare state. *New Reasoner*, *1*(3).
Sawyer, M. (2003). Employer of last resort. *Journal of Economic Issues*, *37*(4), 881–907.
Scaff, L. (1998). Max Weber. In R. Stones (Ed.), *Key Sociological Thinkers*. Basingstoke: Palgrave.
Scheingold, S. (1974/2004). *The Politics of Rights*. Ann Arbor, MI: University of Michigan Press.
Schmidt, J., & Matthews, N. (2018). From state to system. *Geoforum*, *92*, 151–159.
Schwartz, S. (1992). Universals in the content and structure of values. *Advances in Experimental Social Psychology*, *25*(1).
Schwartz, S., Cieciuch, J., & Michele et al. (2012). Refining the theory of basic individual values. *Journal of Personality and Social Psychology*, *103*(4).
Scott, J. (1985). *Weapons of the Weak*. New Haven: Yale University Press.
Scott, J. (1990). *Domination and the Arts of Resistance*. New Haven: Yale University Press.
Scruton, R. (Ed.) (1991). *Conservative Texts*. Basingstoke: Macmillan.
Sen, A. (1981). *Poverty and Famines*. Oxford: Clarendon Press.
Sen, A. (1982a). Equality of What? In A. Sen (Ed.), *Choice, Welfare and Measurement*. Oxford: Blackwell.
Sen, A. (1982b). Rights and agency. *Philosophy and Public Affairs*, *11*(1).
Sen, A. (1985). *Commodities and Capabilities*. Amsterdam: Elsevier.
Sen, A. (1999). *Development as Freedom*. Oxford: OUP.
Sen, A. (2004). Elements of a theory of human rights. *Philosophy & Public Affairs*, *32*(4), 315–356.
Sengupta, A. (2000). Realizing the right to development. *Development and Change*, *31*, 553–578.
Sengupta, A. (2010). The Human Right to Development. In B. Andreassen & S. Marks (Eds.), *Development as a Human Right* (2nd edn.). Antwerp: Intersentia.
Seth, A. (2021). *Being You*. London: Faber & Faber.
Sevenhuijsen, S. (1998). *Citizenship and the Ethics of Care*. London: Routledge.
Sevenhuijsen, S. (2000). Caring in the third way. *Critical Social Policy*, *20*(1).
Shakespeare, T. (2006). *Disability Rights and Wrongs*. London: Routledge.
Shi, S.-J. (2012). Towards inclusive citizenship? *Journal of Social Policy*, *41*(4).
Shue, H. (1980). *Basic Rights*. Princeton: PUP.
Shutes, I. (2016). Citizenship and Migration. In H. Dean & L. Platt (Eds.), *Social Advantage and Disadvantage*. Oxford: OUP.
Sivanandan, A. (1990). *Communities of Resistance*. London: Verso.
Slimak, L. (2023). *The Naked Neanderthal*. London: Allen Lane.
Sloman, P., Varga, D., & Pinto, P. (Eds.). (2021). *Universal Basic Income in Historical Perspective*. London: Palgrave.
Slorach, R. (2016). *A Very Capitalist Condition*. London: Bookmarks Publications.
Slote, L. (2001). *Morals from Motives*. Oxford: OUP.
Smith, A. (1759). *The Theory of Moral Sentiments* (1976 edition ed.). Indianapolis: Liberty Fund.
Smith, A. (1776). *An Inquiry into the Nature and Causes of the Wealth of Nations* (1900 edn.). London: Routledge.
Smith, T., & Noble, M. (1995). *Education Divides*. London: CPAG.
Social Prosperity Network. (2017). *Social Prosperity for the Future*. London: Institute for Global Prosperity.

Soper, K. (1981). *On Human Needs*. Brighton: Harvester.
Soper, K. (1993). The Thick and Thin of Human Needing. In G. Drover & P. Kerans (Eds.), *New Approaches to Welfare Theory*. Aldershot: Elgar.
Soysal, Y. (1994). *Limits of Citizenship*. Chicago: Chicago UP.
Spanish Society for International Human Rights Law. (2010). *Santiago Declaration on the Human Right to Peace*. At http://mail.aedidh.org/?q=node/1853
Squires, P. (1990). *Anti-Social Policy*. Hemel Hempstead: Harvester Wheatsheaf.
Stacey, F. (1978). *Ombudsmen Compared*. Oxford: OUP.
Standing, G. (1996). Social Protection in Central and Eastern Europe. In G. Esping-Andersen (Ed.), *Welfare States in Transition*. London: Sage.
Standing, G. (2009). *Work after Globalization*. Cheltenham: Edward Elgar.
Standing, G. (2011). *The Precariat*. London: Bloomsbury.
Standing, G. (2013). India's experiment in basic income grants. *Global Dialogue*, *3*(5).
Standing, G. (2014). *A Precariat Charter*. London: Bloomsbury.
Starr, P. (1988) The meaning of privatisation. *Yale Law and Policy Review*, *6*(1).
Steinberg, J. (2011). *Bismark*. Oxford: OUP.
Stephens, M. (1982). Law Centres and Citizenship. In P. Thomas (Ed.), *Law in the Balance*. Oxford: Martin Robertson.
Stephenson, S. (2000). Civil Society and its Agents in the Post-Communist World. In H. Dean, R. Sykes & R. Woods (Eds.), *Social Policy Review 12*. Newcastle: Social Policy Association.
Stewart, J., & Lynch, Z. (2018). *Environmental Health and Housing*. (2nd ed.). Abingdon: Routledge.
Stiglitz, J. (2003). Globalizarion and Its Discontents. London: Penguin.
Stiglitz, J., Sen, A., & Fitoussi, J. (2009). *Report by the Commission on the Measurement of Economic Performance and Social Progress*: see https://ec.europa.eu/eurostat/documents/8131721/8131772/Stiglitz-Sen-Fitoussi-Commission-report.pdf
Streeten, P., Burki, S., Ul Haq, M., Hicks, N., & Stewart, F. (1981). *First Things First*. Oxford: OUP.
Sumner, W. (1906). *Folkways*. (1940 ed.). Boston, MA: Ginn.
Sunstein, C. (2005). Why Does the American Constitution Lack Social and Economic Guarantees? In M. Ignatieff (Ed.), *American Exceptionalism and Human Rights*. Princeton, NJ: PUP.
Task Force on Justice. (2019). *Justice for All*. New York: Centre on International Co-operation.
Tawney, R. (1913). Poverty as an Industrial Problem. In R. Tawney (Ed.), *Memoranda on the Problems of Poverty* (Vol. 2). London: William Morris Press.
Taylor, C. (1992). The Politics of Recognition. In A. Gutmann (Ed.), *Multiculturalism*. Princeton: PUP.
Taylor, D. (1998). Social identity and social policy. *Journal of Social Policy*, *27*(3).
Taylor-Gooby, P. (1994). Postmodernism and social policy.? *Journal of Social Policy*, *23*(3).
Taylor-Gooby, P. (2013). *The Double Crisis of the Welfare State*. Basingstoke: Palgrave.
Teubner, G. (Ed.) (1987). *Dilemmas of Law in the Welfare State*. Berlin: Walter de Gruyter.
Thomas, C., & Genn, H. (2013). Understanding Tribunal Decision-Making. London: Nuffield Foundation.
Thompson, E. (1968). *The Making of the English Working Class*. Harmondsworth: Penguin.
Thompson, E. (1975). *Whigs and Hunters*. New York: Parthenon.
Thompson, E. (1978). *The Poverty of Theory and Other Essays*. London: Merlin.
Thompson, E. (1993). *Customs in Common*. New York: New Press.
Thomson, G. (1987). *Needs*. London: Routledge & Kegan Paul.

Thompson, C., & Brook, Y. (2011). *Neoconservatism*. Boulder, CO: Paradigm.
Titmuss, R. (1955). Lecture at the University of Birmingham in Honour of Eleanor Rathbone. In P. Alcock, H. Glennerster, A. Oakley, & A. Sinfield (Eds.), *Welfare and Wellbeing: Richard Titmuss' Contribution to Social Policy* (2001 edn.). Bristol: Policy Press.
Titmuss, R. (1958). *Essays on the Welfare State*. London: Allen & Unwin.
Titmuss, R. (1968). *Commitment to Welfare*. London: Allen and Unwin.
Titmuss, R. (1970). *The Gift Relationship* (1997 edn.). New York: New Press.
Titmuss, R. (1971). Welfare rights, law and discretion. *Political Quarterly*, *42*(2).
Toebs, B. (2001). The Right to Health. In A. Eide, C. Krause & A. Rosas (Eds.), *Economic, Social and Cultural Rights*. Dordrecht: Martinus Nijhoff.
Tomasello, M. (2021). *Becoming Human*. Cambridge, MA: Harvard UP.
Torry, M. (2016). Religious Advantage and Disadvantage. In H. Dean & L. Platt (Eds.), *Social Advantage and Disadvantage*. Oxford: OUP.
Torry, M. (2018). *Why We Need a Citizen's Basic Income*. Bristol: Policy Press.
Townsend, P. (1979). *Poverty in the UK*. Harmondsworth: Penguin.
Townsend, P. (1991). The structured dependency of the elderly. *Ageing and Society*, *1*(1).
Townsend, P. (1993). *The International Analysis of Poverty*. Hemel Hempstead: Harvester Wheatsheaf.
Townsend, P. (2002). Poverty, Social Exclusion and Social Polarisation. In P. Townsend & D. Gordon (Eds.), *World Poverty*. Bristol: Policy Press.
Townsend, P. (2007). *The Right to Social Security and National Development*. Discussion Paper 18. Geneva: ILO.
Townsend, P. (Ed.) (2009). *Building Decent Societies*. Basingstoke: Palgrave.
Townsend, P., & Donkor, K. (1996). *Global Restructuring and Social Policy*. Bristol: Policy Press.
Townsend, P., & Gordon, D. (Eds.). (2002). *World Poverty*. Bristol: Policy Press.
Townsend, P., & Walker, A. (1981). *Disability in Britain*. Oxford: Martin Robertson.
Tranter, K., Sleep, L., & Stannard, J. (2008). The cohabitation rule. *Melbourne University Law Review*, *32*(2), 698–738.
Travers, M. (2010). A Sociological Critique of Rights. In R. Banakar (Ed.), *Rights in Context*. Farnham: Ashgate.
Tronto, J. (1994). *Moral Boundaries*. New York: Routledge.
Tronto, J. (2013). *Caring Democracy*. New York: New York UP.
Tudor-Hart, J. (1971). The inverse care law. *Lancet* (27 February), 405–412.
Turner, B. (1990). Outline of a theory of citizenship. *Sociology*, *24*(2).
Turner, B. (1991,). *Prolegomena to a general theory of social order*. Paper presented 23 February at ESRC workshop: Citizenship, Civil Society and Social Cohesion, London.
Turner, B. (1993). Outline of a theory of human rights. *Sociology*, *27*(3).
Turner, B. (2006). *Vulnerability and Human Rights*. Pennsylvania: Pennsylvania State University.
Tweedie, J., & Hunt, A. (1994). The future of the welfare state and social rights. *Journal of Law and Society*, *21*(3).
Twine, F. (1994). *Citizenship and Social Rights*. London: Sage.
United Nations. (1993). *Vienna Declaration and Programme of Action*. Adopted by the World Conference on Human Rights on 25 June. Vienna: UN.
United Nations. (1995). *The Copenhagen Declaration and Programme of Action*. World Summit for Social Development. New York: UN.
United Nations. (2000). *United Nations Millennium Declaration*. Res 2/55. New York: UN.
United Nations. (2012). Human Rights and Extreme Poverty (Resolution Adopted 20 December on Report of Third Committee). New York: UN.

United Nations. (2015). Transforming Our World. Res. 70/1. New York: UN.
United Nations Committee on Economic Social and Cultural Rights. (2001). *Poverty and the International Covenant on Economic, Social and Cultural Rights*. Geneva: UN.
United Nations Development Programme. (1993). *Human Development Report 1993*. New York: UNDP.
United Nations Development Programme. (2000). *Human Development Report 2000*. New York: Oxford University Press.
United Nations Development Programme. (2003). *Human Development Report 2003 - Millennium Development Goals*. New York: Oxford University Press.
United Nations Development Programme. (2010). *Human Development Report 2010*. Basingstoke: Palgrave Macmillan.
United Nations Development Programme. (2022). *Human Development Report 2021/2022*. New York: UNDP.
United Nations Educational Scientific and Cultural Organization. (1994). *Salamanca Statement and Framework for Action on Special Needs Education*. Paris: UNESCO.
United Nations Educational Scientific and Cultural Organization. (2007). *EFA Global Monitoring Report*. Paris: UNESCO.
United Nations Educational Scientific and Cultural Organization. (2011). *Global Education Digest 2011*. Montreal: UNESCO_UIS.
United Nations Educational Scientific and Cultural Organization. (2013). *Education for All Global Monitoring Report Fact Sheet*. Paris: UNESCO.
United Nations Educational Scientific and Cultural Organization. (2024). *#HerEducationOurFuture*. Global Education Monitoring Research Team paper. At https://doi.org/10.54676/WTPE4528
United Nations Human Settlements Programme. (2003). *The Challenge of Slums*. London: Earthscan.
United Nations Human Settlements Programme. (2023). *Rescuing SDG 11 for a Resilient Urban Panet*. Nairobi: UN-Habitat.
United Nations Office on Drugs and Crime and United Nations Development Programme. (2016). *Global Study on Legal Aid: Global Report*. New York: UN.
Vail, J. (1999). Insecure Times. In J. Vail, J. Wheelock & M. Hill (Eds.), *Insecure Times*. London: Routledge.
Van Steenbergen, B. (1994). Towards a Global Ecological Citizen. In B. Van Steenbergen (Ed.), *The Condition of Citizenship*. London: Sage.
Vandermoortele, J. (2015). A serene look at the SDGs. *CROP Poverty Brief*. At www.crop.org/viewfile.aspx?id=809
Visser, J. (2006). Union membership statistics in 24 countries. *Monthly Labour Review*, *129*(1).
Vizard, P., & Burchardt, T. (2007). *Developing a Capability List*. CASEpaper 121. London: CASE/STICERD.
Vygotsky, L. (1978). Mind and Society: The Development of Higher Mental Processes. Cambridge, MA: Harvard UP.
Wainwright, H. (2003). *Reclaim the State*. London: Verso.
Walker, G. (2015). The right to energy. *European Institute*, *374*(4). doi:10.3917/eufor.378.0026.
Walker, R. (2005). *Social Security and Welfare*. Maidenhead: Open University Press.
Walker, R., Kyomuhendo, G., Chase, E., Choudry, S., Gubrium, E., Nicola, J., & Ming, Y. (2013). Poverty in global perspective. *Journal of Social Policy*, *42*(2).
Walker, P., & Walker, A. (2018). The golden rule revisited. *Philosophy Now*, *125*. At https://philosophynow.org/issues/125/The_Golden_Rule_Revisited
Walker, A., & Wong, C. (Eds.). (2005). *East Asian Welfare Regimes in Transition*. Bristol: Policy Press.

Walzer, M. (1983). *Spheres of Justice*. Oxford: Blackwell.
Walzer, M. (1994). *Thick and Thin*. Notre Dame, Indiana: UND Press.
Warde, A. (1994). Consumers, Consumption and Post-Fordism. In R. Burrows & B. Loader (Eds.), Towards a Post-Fordist Welfare State? London: Routledge.
Warnock, M. (1978). *Special Educational Needs*. London: HMSO.
Waterman, P. (2001). *Globalization, Social Movements and the New Internationalisms*. London: Continuum.
Waters, M. (1996). Human rights and the universalisation of interests. *Sociology*, *30*(3).
Watson, A. (1990). Roman law and English law. *Loyola Law Review*, *36*(2).
Watson, D. (1980). *Caring for Strangers*. London: Routledge & Kegan Paul.
Watson, P. (Ed.) (2013). *Health Care Reform and Globalisation*. London: Routledge.
Watson, T. (1995). *Sociology, Work and Industry* (3rd edn.). London: Routledge.
Weaite, M. (2013). The United Kingdom. In M. Zuniga, S. Marks & L. Gostin (Eds.), *Advancing the Human Right to Health*. Oxford: OUP.
Webb, B., & Webb, S. (1935). *Soviet Communism*. London: Longman.
Weeks, J. (1990). *Sex, Politics and Society* (2nd edn.). London: Longman.
White, S. (2003). *The Civic Minimum*. Oxford: OUP.
Whitworth, A., & Wilkinson, K. (2013). Tackling child poverty in South Africa. *Development South Africa*, *30*(1).
Wikeley, N. (2006). *Child Support*. Portland, OR: Hart Publishing.
Wilensky, H. (1975). *The Welfare State and Equality*. Berkeley: University of California Press.
Wilkinson, R. (2005). *The Impact of Inequality*. New York: New Press.
Wilkinson, R., & Pickett, K. (2009). *The Spirit Level*. London: Allen Lane.
Williams, F. (1989). *Social Policy*. Cambridge: Polity.
Williams, F. (1999). Good-enough principles of welfare. *Journal of Social Policy*, *28*(4).
Williams, M. (2007). Non-Territorial Boundaries of Citizenship. In S. Benhabib, I. Shapiro & D. Petrovic (Eds.), *Identities, Affiliations and Allegiances*. Cambridge: CUP.
Williamson, J. (1990). What Washington Means by Policy Reform. In J. Williamson (Ed.), *Latin American Adjustment*. Washington: Institute for International Economics.
Wimmer, A., & Schiller, N. (2002). Methodological nationalism and beyond. *Global Networks*, *2*(4), 301–334.
Winnicott, D. (1953). Transitional objects and transitional phenomena. *International Journal of Psychoanalysis*, *34*, 89–87.
Wolfensberger, W. (1972). *The Principle of Normalisation in Human Services*. Toronto: National Institute on Mental Retardation.
Women's Budget Group. (2023). *Gender Gaps in Access to Civil Legal Justice*. At https://wbg.org.uk/wp-content/uploads/2023/07/Gender-gaps-in-access-to-civil-legal-justice-WBG.pdf
Woodiwiss, A. (2005). *Human Rights*. London: Routledge.
World Bank. (1991). *Assistance Strategies to Reduce Poverty*. Washington, DC: World Bank.
World Bank. (1994). *Averting the Old Age Crisis*. Washington, DC: World Bank.
World Bank. (2001). *World Development Report 2000/2001*. Oxford: World Bank.
World Food Programme. (2022). *WFP Strategic Plan (2022-2025)*. Rome: WFP.
World Health Organization. (2008). *Commission on Social Determinants of Health*. Geneva: WHO.
World Health Organization. (2023). *Mental Health, Human Rights and Legislation*. Geneva: WHO/OHCHR.

World Values Survey. (2023). *WVS World Cultural Map 2023 Version*. At www.worldvaluessurvey.org/WVSNewsShow.jsp?ID=467
Worrel, M., & Krier, D. (2018). Totems, fetishes and enchanted modernity. *Logos*, *17*(1).
Wraith, R., & Hutchinson, P. (1973). *Administrative Tribunals*. London: Allen and Unwin.
Wright, G., Noble, M., Ntshongwana, P., Neves, D., & Barnes, H. (2014). *The Role of Social Security in Respecting and Protecting the Dignity of Lone Mothers in South Africa*. Oxford: Centre for the Analysis of South African Social Policy.
Yan, M. (2014). China's Dibao System. In E. Gubrium, S. Pellissery & I. Lodemel (Eds.), *The Shame of It*. Bristol: Policy Press.
Yeates, N. (2001). *Globalization and Social Policy*. London: Sage.
Yeates, N. (Ed.) (2008). *Understanding Global Social Policy*. Bristol: The Policy Press.
Yeates, N., & Piper, N. (2022). Global Migrations and Global Social Policy. In N. Yeates & C. Holden (Eds.), *Understanding Global Social Policy* (3rd ed.). Bristol: Policy Press.
Young, K. (Ed.) (2019). *The Future of Economic and Social Rights*. Cambridge: CUP.
Younghusband, E. (1964). *Social Work and Social Change*. London: Allen & Unwin.
Zander, M. (1978). *Legal Services for the Community*. London: Temple-Smith.
Zedillo, E. (2001). *Report of the High-Level Panel on Financing for Development*. New York: UN.
Žižek, S. (2005). Against human rights. *New Left Review*, *34*, 115–131.

INDEX

Note: *Italicized* page references refer to figures and **bold** references refer to tables.

FSC
www.fsc.org
MIX
Papier | Fördert gute Waldnutzung
FSC® C083411

Kolibri 360 GmbH
Ferdinand-Jühlke-Straße 7
99095 Erfurt, Deutschland
produktsicherheit@kolibri360.de